Molecular Pathology: An Update

Editor

MARTIN H. BLUTH

CLINICS IN LABORATORY MEDICINE

www.labmed.theclinics.com

Editor-in-Chief
MILENKO JOVAN TANASIJEVIC

June 2018 • Volume 38 • Number 2

ELSEVIER

1600 John F. Kennedy Boulevard • Suite 1800 • Philadelphia, Pennsylvania, 19103-2899

http://www.theclinics.com

CLINICS IN LABORATORY MEDICINE Volume 38, Number 2
June 2018 ISSN 0272-2712, ISBN-13: 978-0-323-61072-8

Editor: Stacy Eastman
Developmental Editor: Laura Fisher

Reprints. For copies of 100 or more, of articles in this publication, please contact the Commercial Reprints Department, Elsevier Inc., 360 Park Avenue South, New York, New York 10010-1710. Tel. 212-633-3874, Fax: 212-633-3820, E-mail: reprints@elsevier.com.

Clinics in Laboratory Medicine (ISSN 0272-2712) is published quarterly by Elsevier Inc., 360 Park Avenue South, New York, NY 10010-1710. Months of issue are March, June, September, and December. Business and Editorial offices: 1600 John F. Kennedy Blvd., Suite 1800, Philadelphia, PA 19103-2899. Periodicals postage paid at NewYork, NY and additional mailing offices. Subscription prices are $263.00 per year (US individuals), $507.00 per year (US institutions), $100.00 per year (US students), $347.00 per year (Canadian individuals), $617.00 per year (Canadian institutions), $185.00 per year (Canadian students), $402.00 per year (international individuals), $617.00 per year (international institutions), $185.00 (international students). Foreign air speed delivery is included in all Clinics subscription prices. All prices are subject to change without notice. POSTMASTER: Send address changes to *Clinics in Laboratory Medicine*, Elsevier Health Sciences Division, Subscription Customer Service, 3251 Riverport Lane, Maryland Heights, MO 63043. **Customer Service: 1-800-654-2452 (US). From outside of the US and Canada, call 1-314-447-8871. Fax: 1-314-447-8029. E-mail: journalscustomerservice-usa@elsevier.com (for print support) or journalsonlinesupport-usa@elsevier.com (for online support).**

Clinics in Laboratory Medicine is covered in *EMBASE/Exerpta Medica, MEDLINE/PubMed (Index Medicus), Cinahl, Current Contents/Clinical Medicine, BIOSIS* and *ISI/BIOMED*.

Contributors

EDITOR-IN-CHIEF

MILENKO JOVAN TANASIJEVIC, MD, MBA
Vice Chair for Clinical Pathology and Quality, Department of Pathology, Director of Clinical Laboratories, Brigham and Women's Hospital, Dana-Farber Cancer Institute, Associate Professor of Pathology, Harvard Medical School, Boston, Massachusetts

EDITOR

MARTIN H. BLUTH, MD, PhD
Founder, Bluth Bio Industries, Southfield, Michigan; Professor of Pathology, Wayne State University School of Medicine, Detroit, Michigan; Director of Pathology Laboratories, Michigan Surgical Hospital, Warren, Michigan; Medical Director, Kids Kicking Cancer, Southfield, Michigan

AUTHORS

EMAN ABDULFATAH, MD
PGY4, Department of Pathology, Detroit Medical Center Harper University Hospital, Wayne State University, Detroit, Michigan

QURATULAIN AHMED, MD
Staff Pathologist, Michigan Diagnostic Pathologists, Providence Hospital, Southfield, Michigan

ROUBA ALI-FEHMI, MD
Professor, Department of Pathology, Detroit Medical Center Harper University Hospital, Wayne State University, Detroit, Michigan

BARAA ALOSH, MD
PGY4, Department of Pathology, Detroit Medical Center Harper University Hospital, Wayne State University, Detroit, Michigan

SUDESHNA BANDYOPADHYAY, MD
Assistant Professor, Department of Pathology, Detroit Medical Center Harper University Hospital, Wayne State University, Detroit, Michigan

RAFIC BEYDOUN, MD
Associate Professor, Department of Pathology, Detroit Medical Center Harper University Hospital, Detroit, Michigan

AMARPREET BHALLA, MBBS, MD
Clinical Assistant Professor, Department of Pathology and Anatomical Sciences, Jacobs School of Medicine and Biomedical Sciences, University at Buffalo, The State University of New York, Buffalo General Hospital, Buffalo, New York

MARK J. BLUTH, PhD
Bluth Bio Industries, Southfield, Michigan

MARTIN H. BLUTH, MD, PhD
Founder, Bluth Bio Industries, Southfield, Michigan; Professor of Pathology, Wayne State University School of Medicine, Detroit, Michigan; Director of Pathology Laboratories, Michigan Surgical Hospital, Warren, Michigan; Medical Director, Kids Kicking Cancer, Southfield, Michigan

ROBERTSON D. DAVENPORT, MD
Department of Pathology, University of Michigan, Ann Arbor, Michigan

MATTHEW B. ELKINS, MD, PhD
Department of Pathology, SUNY Upstate Medical University, Syracuse, New York

MARILYNN RANSOM FAIRFAX, MD, PhD
Department of Pathology, Wayne State University School of Medicine, Medical Director, Clinical Microbiology Laboratories, DMC University Laboratories, Detroit, Michigan

ALI M. GABALI, MD, PhD
Associate Professor, Wayne State University School of Medicine, Head of Hematopathology Division, Director of Hematopathology Fellowship Program, Co-Director of Hematology Unit, Director of Core Hematology and Coagulation, Karmanos Cancer Center, Detroit Medical Center, Detroit, Michigan

TAREK JAZAERLY, MD
Assistant Professor, Wayne State University School of Medicine, Karmanos Cancer Center, Detroit Medical Center, Detroit, Michigan

KATRIN KIAVASH, MD
Department of Pathology, Wayne State University, DMC University Laboratories, Detroit, Michigan

RADHAKRISHNAN RAMCHANDREN, MD
Associate Professor, Wayne State University School of Medicine, Karmanos Cancer Center, Detroit Medical Center, Detroit, Michigan

HOSSEIN SALIMNIA, PhD, D(ABMM)
Department of Pathology, Wayne State University School of Medicine, Technical Chief, Clinical Microbiology Laboratories, DMC University Laboratories, Detroit, Michigan

SAJIV SETHI, MD
Department of Gastroenterology, University of South Florida, Tampa, Florida

SEEMA SETHI, MD
Assistant Professor, Department of Pathology, University of Michigan, Staff Pathologist, Department of Pathology and Laboratory Medicine, VA Ann Arbor Medical Center Healthcare System, Ann Arbor, Michigan

ANDREW DAVID THOMPSON, MD, PhD
Department of Pathology, Wayne State University, DMC University Laboratories, Karmanos Cancer Center, Detroit, Michigan

LEI ZHANG, MD, PhD
PGY-4, Department of Pathology and Anatomical Sciences, Jacobs School of Medicine and Biomedical Sciences, University at Buffalo, Buffalo General Hospital, Buffalo, New York

YINGTAO ZHANG, MD, PhD
PGY-3, Department of Pathology and Anatomical Sciences, Jacobs School of Medicine and Biomedical Sciences, University at Buffalo, Buffalo General Hospital, Buffalo, New York

MUHAMMAD ZULFIQAR, MD
Consultant Pathologist, Southeastern Pathology Associates (SEPA Labs), Brunswick, Georgia; Department of Pathology, Detroit Medical Center Harper University Hospital, Detroit, Michigan

Contents

The unprecedented expansion of molecular pathology continues to affect and influence the clinical laboratory. Technologic advances in high-throughput automation, cost containment, and refined methodology have improved the understanding of pathobiology through application of molecular pathology to multiple disease spaces. Incorporation of this field to emerging omics platforms, pharmacovigilance and biomarker discovery, and accessibility by lay consumers demonstrates the widespread reach of molecular pathology in the clinical marketplace. Pathologists should remain the stewards of this powerful and adaptable technology to provide guidance and appropriate laboratory application toward effective patient monitoring with respect to disease diagnosis and management.

Molecular pathology techniques continue to evolve. Although polymerase chain reaction (PCR) remains the cornerstone methodology for nucleic acid amplification, improvements in nucleic acid detection methodologies have increased the detection sensitivity by using fluorescent and bead-based array technologies. Single base pair lesions can be detected via sequencing and related techniques to discern point mutations in disease pathogenesis. Novel technologies, such as high-resolution melting analysis, provide fast high-throughput post-PCR analysis of genetic mutations or variance in nucleic acid sequences. These and other technologies such as hybrid capture, fluorophore, and chemiluminescence detection assays allow for rapid diagnosis and prognosis for expeditious and personalized patient management.

MicroRNAs (miRNAs) are poised to provide diagnostic, prognostic, and therapeutic targets for several diseases, including malignancies for precision medicine applications. The miRNAs have immense potential in the clinical arena because they can be detected in the blood, serum, tissues (fresh and formalin-fixed paraffin-embedded), and fine-needle aspirate specimens. The most attractive feature of miRNA-based therapy is that a single miRNA could be useful for targeting multiple genes that are deregulated in cancers, which can be further investigated through systems biology and network analysis that may provide cancer-specific personalized therapy.

Molecular biological techniques have evolved expeditiously and in turn have been applied to the detection of infectious disease. Maturation of these technologies and their coupling with related technologic advancement in fluorescence, electronics, digitization, nanodynamics, and sensors among others have afforded clinical medicine additional tools toward expedient identification of infectious organisms at concentrations and sensitivities previously unattainable. These advancements have been adapted in select settings toward addressing clinical demands for more timely and effective patient management.

Virtually all the red blood cell and platelet antigen systems have been characterized at the molecular level. Highly reliable methods for red blood cell and platelet antigen genotyping are now available. Genotyping is a useful adjunct to traditional serology and can help resolve complex serologic problems. Although red blood cell and platelet phenotypes can be inferred from genotype, knowledge of the molecular basis is essential for accurate assignment. Genotyping of blood donors is an effective method of identifying antigen-negative and/or particularly rare donors. Cell-free DNA analysis provides a promising noninvasive method of assessing fetal genotypes of blood group alloantigens.

Diagnosis of hematologic malignancies has matured to encompass molecular as well as phenotypic characteristics. Cytogenetic abnormalities are considered common events in this regard. These abnormalities generally consist of structural chromosomal abnormalities or gene mutations, which often are integral to the pathogenesis and subsequent evolution of an individual malignancy. Improvements made in identifying and interpreting these molecular alterations have resulted in advances in the diagnosis, prognosis, monitoring, and therapy for cancer. As a consequence of the increasingly important role of molecular testing in hematologic malignancy management, this article presents an update on the importance and use of molecular tests, detailing the advantages and disadvantages of each test when applicable.

The molecular pathogenesis and classification of colorectal carcinoma are based on the traditional adenoma-carcinoma sequence, serrated polyp pathway, and microsatellite instability (MSI). The genetic basis for hereditary nonpolyposis colorectal cancer is the detection of mutations in the MLH1, MSH2, MSH6, PMS2, and EPCAM genes. Genetic testing for Lynch syndrome includes MSI testing, methylator phenotype testing, BRAF mutation testing, and molecular testing for germline mutations in MMR genes. Molecular markers with predictive and prognostic implications include quantitative multigene reverse transcriptase polymerase chain reaction assay and KRAS and BRAF mutation analysis. Mismatch repair–deficient tumors have higher rates of programmed death-ligand 1 expression. Cell-free DNA analyses in fluids are proving beneficial for diagnosis and prognosis in these disease states toward effective patient management.

Neoplasms of the small intestine are rare in comparison with colorectal tumors. The most common tumor types arising in the small intestine are adenocarcinomas, well-differentiated neuroendocrine tumors, gastrointestinal stromal tumors, and lymphoma. Primary appendiceal neoplasms are rare and found in less than 2% of appendectomy specimens with an incidence of approximately 1.2 cases per 100,000 people per year in the United States. This article explores molecular diagnostics in the neoplasms of small intestine and appendix.

Esophageal cancer (EC) is rapidly increasing in incidence in the United States. Genetic changes associated with the development of EC involve the p16, p53, and APC genes. Human epidermal growth factor 2 (HER-2) overexpression is seen in gastroesophageal junction carcinoma and a subset gastric carcinoma (GC). Up to 50% cases of GC are related to *Helicobacter pylori* infection, and up to 16% are related to Epstein-Barr virus infection. Microsatellite instability is observed in up to 39% of GC, and cell-free nucleic acid analysis provides additional opportunities for diagnosis and prognosis of disease.

Pancreatic neoplasms, including ductal adenocarcinoma, solid pseudopapillary neoplasm, pancreatic endocrine neoplasms, acinar cell carcinoma, and pancreatoblastoma, are associated with different genetic abnormalities. Hepatic adenomas with beta-catenin exon 3 mutation are associated with a high risk of malignancy. Hepatic adenoma with arginosuccinate synthetase 1 expression or sonic hedgehog mutations are associated with a risk of bleeding. Hepatocellular carcinoma and cholangiocarcinoma display heterogeneity at both morphologic and molecular levels. Cholangiocellular carcinoma is most commonly associated with IDH 1/2 mutations.

Molecular genetic technologies are used to aid in the diagnosis and treatment of borderline melanocytic tumors as an adjuvant to the gold standard
histopathologic evaluation. A specific set of fluorescence in situ hybridization probes is widely used to aid in diagnosing challenging melanocytic
lesions. New melanoma probe cocktails have revealed increased sensitivity and specificity in ambiguous melanocytic cases. Array comparative
genomic hybridization is a more complex technology used for the workup
of diagnostically problematic Spitzoid melanocytic proliferations. Cutting-
edge technologies, including next-generation sequencing and cell-free
nucleic acid analysis, are promising biomarker applications for mutation
detection toward personalized patient management.

The most significant contribution of molecular subtyping of breast carcinomas has been the identification of estrogen-positive and estrogen-
negative tumor subtypes. Knowledge of genetic alterations in these tumors will help clinicians identify novel therapeutic targets. Understanding
the progression pathways involved in the transition of in situ carcinoma to
invasive carcinoma might lead to efficient risk stratification in these patients. The Cancer Genome Analysis Network has collected genomic
and epigenomic data to provide comprehensive information regarding
carcinogenesis and pathway interactions. Such information improves the
understanding of the disease process and also provides more accurate
information toward identifying targetable mutations for treatment.

Ovarian carcinoma continues to be a concern for women and maintains
significant morbidity and mortality. Emerging molecular markers are
providing additional opportunities for effective diagnosis and prognosis
of disease. An integrated clinicopathologic and molecular classification
of gynecologic malignancies has the potential to refine the clinical risk prediction of patients with cancer and to provide more tailored treatment
recommendations.

CLINICS IN LABORATORY MEDICINE

THE CLINICS ARE NOW AVAILABLE ONLINE!
Access your subscription at:
www.theclinics.com

Preface

Looking Good in Your Genes: Maximizing One's Personalized Molecular Fingerprint for Optimal Health

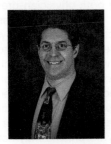

Martin H. Bluth, MD, PhD
Editor

The explosion in gene testing to determine one's risk of disease has created a tempest in the health care milieu. To find a piece of driftwood to cling to, various sources have sprung up to provide clarity, education, and guidance,[1] whereas others have offered a cloud of chaos, panic, and impetuousness.[2] Indeed, one can be overwhelmed by the onslaught of relative risk, odds ratios, and prognostication associated with a given gene mutation, polymorphism, and the like to a dizzying endpoint of frustration or despair. Lay press disseminations, which distill research studies into a bite-sized morsel, can overgeneralize published findings. Conversely, attention to a select aspect of a given study can underscore certain findings while obviating other key elements. For example, certain synopses may not highlight geography, sample size, methodology, or other limitations, thereby misrepresenting the uniqueness of a given study to a specific cohort, dose, technique, and so forth.

In addition, the aura of mystery and awe that shrouds gene testing has, in certain respects, mushroomed its significance way beyond its actual clinical application. Dr Sharon Moalem, in his book, *Survival of the sickest*, opens with a poignant statement: "genes are your history not your destiny."[3] This is not only comforting but is also true. Although there is no doubt that genes influence an individual's biology, it is equally evident that one is not exclusively and invariably defined by them in a static manner. During the early stages of genetic engineering, the sensationalism was overwhelming. The 1980s introduced Genentech's recombinant insulin, molecular technology matured at a rapid rate, restriction enzymes, *Taq* polymerase, and conjugated fluorophores gave rise to methodologies such as PCR, FISH, and microarray over time. The "one-gene-one-protein" idea predominated; biotechnology started to boom, and genes became big business. The turn of the century heralded an episode of genes gone wild, where genetic polymorphisms were identified for

Clin Lab Med 38 (2018) xiii–xvi
https://doi.org/10.1016/j.cll.2018.04.001
0272-2712/18/© 2018 Published by Elsevier Inc.

various disease states; the results of the Human Genome Project manifested human application, and population genetics interfaced with epidemiology. In certain circles marriages were considered only when predicated on one's genetic profile; insurance companies set their sails on assessing whether one's genes can affect disease probability and alter insurance premiums,[4] and forensic science began incorporating genetic interrogation for elucidating paternity as well as murder cases. For some choice to have children rested on the results of genetic testing and *designer genes*, modification of genes by genetic engineering, became a tantalizing topic of discussion to craft the child of your dreams like a genetic version of a Build a Bear Workshop.

The symphony of genes continued to crescendo by availing both physician-prescribed and direct-to-consumer gene testing opportunities. Various companies offered comprehensive gene testing, a forerunner of the "omics" panoply to "know thyself" as a means of identifying everything from one's ancestry, what foods to eat, forecasting disease, to the probability of which enzymes will catabolize which drugs, and so forth. Such noise can also transform into a cacophony if not taken with a grain of salt. While knowledge of certain genetic predispositions have proven clinically relevant, such as polymorphisms in single-carbon pathway metabolism where supplementation of methylated folate in those with select MTHFR polymorphisms polymorphism can be ideal,[5,6] other mutations or polymorphisms may not be clear and require additional interrogation.[7]

Furthermore, the influence of epigenetics, interfering RNAs (eg, siRNA), and enhancer effects among others has introduced additional variables that may affect the penetrance and expression of a gene.[8] Thus, the mere presence of a gene no longer mandates the expression and related clinical relevance with the same absolutism as before. One gene affecting many physiologic pathways has become the norm and has created an avenue for drug "repurposing" to treat various disease states where common pathways or mechanisms of action have been identified. Diet, polypharmacy, and environmental contexts among others can further influence the clinical effects of a gene as well as its disease relevance.

Although the variability and layered effects of such a multifactorial miasma may seem daunting, it can be considered a good thing. It in effect validates that we are fluid, ever-changing, adaptive, trending organisms that can, in certain respects, positively influence ourselves in the face of a seemingly deleterious polymorphism by changing our immediate or extended bio-focused environment. The term "biohacking" has a few connotations, including the idea of changing one's lifestyle to "hack" the biological status of the body toward optimum health.[9] Patients will explore various approaches to improve their health, including interrogating their genes, in cases where conventional medicine has failed them. This is not to say that physicians cannot provide diagnosis and management; rather, the ever-changing health care climate, cost containment, liability/privacy, insurance coverage networks, and the like can affect the time, diagnostic as well as management choices, and longevity that the physician has with the patient.

For example, those with joint disorders, GI disturbances, fatigue, and so forth, who have been to a multitude of physicians and received a plethora of prescription medications to no avail have sought other modalities, including diet alteration, polymorphism assessment, and/or environmental exposure interrogation, to discover that they were allergic to a food, deficient in an enzyme, or exposed to mold toxins, respectively. Those with select polymorphisms can further change their lifestyle, in addition to diet and environment, to include exercise and meditation to reduce or obviate pain, fatigue, and stressors to live optimal lives.[10,11] This personalization or precision medicine, which often incorporates analysis and interpretation of genes and polymorphisms, can highlight the uniqueness among individuals rather than the commonalities of the "one-size-fits-all" approach. This gestalt can further empower the individual by celebrating one's uniqueness and identify opportunities for health maintenance and growth.

Thus, the complicated variability of the ever-expanding domain of molecular pathology and personalized medicine can provide unprecedented opportunities for patient diagnosis and management by laboratory methods while appreciating the limitations inherent in this domain. It allows one to pause at the mention of disease and posit how these polymorphisms can be interpreted to improve the prognosis and quality of life. The idea that patients can "look good in their genes" provides a fresh perspective on patient management and health in general.

Martin H. Bluth, MD, PhD
Bluth Bio Industries
Southfield, MI 48034, USA

Wayne State University School of Medicine
Detroit, MI 48201, USA

Pathology Laboratories
Michigan Surgical Hospital
Warren, MI 48091, USA

Kids Kicking Cancer
Southfield, MI 48034, USA

E-mail addresses:
mbluth@med.wayne.edu; toxdocs@gmail.com

REFERENCES

1. Available at: https://www.ashg.org/education/Health_Professionals.shtml. Accessed April 13, 2018.
2. Available at: https://www.forbes.com/sites/elaineschattner/2017/10/29/3-lessons-from-an-alarming-case-of-mistaken-cancer-genetic-test-results/#553bfad16305. Accessed April 13, 2018.
3. Moalem S. Survival of the sickest: a medical maverick discovers why we need disease. New York: Harper Collins Publishers; 2012.
4. Andrews LB, Fullarton JE, Holtzman NA, et al, editors. Assessing genetic risks: implications for health and social policy. Institute of Medicine (US) Committee on Assessing Genetic Risks. Washington, DC: National Academies Press (US); 1994.
5. Nazki FH, Sameer AS, Ganaie BA. Folate: metabolism, genes, polymorphisms and the associated diseases. Gene 2014;533:11–20.
6. Jha S, Kumar P, Das A, et al. illness with MTHFR C677 T genetic polymorphism. Asian J Psychiatr 2016;22:74–5.
7. Dong SS, Zhang YJ, Chen YX, et al. Comprehensive review and annotation of susceptibility SNPs associated with obesity-related traits. Obes Rev 2018. https://doi.org/10.1111/obr.12677.
8. Available at: https://www.ncbi.nlm.nih.gov/probe/docs/techrnai/. Accessed April 13, 2018.
9. Available at: https://draxe.com/what-is-biohacking/. Accessed April 13, 2018.
10. Rosso AL, Metti AL, Glynn NW, et al, LIFE Study Group. Dopamine-related genotypes and physical activity change during an intervention: the lifestyle interventions

and independence for elders study. J Am Geriatr Soc 2018. https://doi.org/10.1111/jgs.15369.

11. Fenwick PH, Jeejeebhoy K, Dhaliwal R, et al. Lifestyle genomics and the metabolic syndrome: a review of genetic variants that influence response to diet and exercise interventions. Crit Rev Food Sci Nutr 2018;1–12. https://doi.org/10.1080/10408398.2018.1437022.

Introduction: Molecular Medicine in the Common Era
Applications and Impact of Molecular Pathology in Health and Disease

Martin H. Bluth, MD, PhD[a,b]

KEYWORDS

- Molecular pathology • Methods • Genomics • Omics • High throughput • Quality
- Polymorphisms

KEY POINTS

- Molecular pathology has profoundly influenced general pathology practice and the understanding of pathobiology and its techniques have provided medicine with accurate, sensitive, and rapid opportunities to diagnose and prognosticate disease in an unprecedented manner.
- Detection of abnormal genes and differences in patterns of gene expression can influence disease diagnosis and guide specific therapy in many disease settings.
- In addition to the clinical setting, molecular pathology has expanded to the direct-to-consumer market for general commercial use.
- Application of molecular pathology to high-throughput automation and multiplex analysis has provided unprecedented support for evolving omics platforms toward personalized medicine.

The history of medicine aligns with the history of humanity. The Bible recounts Rachel's request of *da'aduim* (mandrakes) from her sister as putative means of promoting fertility[1] and the prophet Isaiah states to "bring a cake of figs, and let them take and lay it on the boil, that he may recover"[2] as a remedy for king Hezekiah's ailment. The maturation of medicine, disease diagnosis, and patient treatment has progressed over millennia, transcended religion and gender and developed in various spheres of people, culture, class, and geography. The Israelite priest diagnosed leprosy and cured it.[3] Egyptian doctors used powdered charcoal as a medicine to

Disclosure: The author has nothing to disclose.
[a] Department of Pathology, Wayne State University School of Medicine, 540 East Canfield Street, Detroit, MI 48201, USA; [b] Pathology Laboratories, Michigan Surgical Hospital, 21230 Dequindre Road, Warren, MI 48091, USA
E-mail address: mbluth@med.wayne.edu

Clin Lab Med 38 (2018) 209–213
https://doi.org/10.1016/j.cll.2018.03.001
labmed.theclinics.com

absorb poisons and cure food poisoning, and women physicians including Merit Ptah (c. 2700 BCE) and Peseshet (c. 2500 BCE) served as the common day Chief of Service.[4,5] Hippocrates (c. 400 BCE) described the four humors as representing ones personality, and Galen (c. 130 BCE) further applied this concept to body fluids defining mood and temperament ("sanguine," "choleric," "melancholy," and "phlegmatic"), which related to disease when out of balance.[6] Saint Basil of Caesarea (CE 369) founded the first 300-bed large-scale hospital for the seriously ill and disabled,[7] and Maimonides and Ibn al-Nafis (circa CE 1100 and 1200, respectively), deduced that the heart sends blood to the lungs to get air.[5]

Innovation is often slow to gain acceptance. The germ theory of disease confirmed and proven by Pasteur and Lister was previously proposed by Ignaz Semmelweis years earlier. However, his suggestion to wash one's hands in clinical practice and before a procedure was met with ridicule and mockery.[8] Kary Mullis, who received the Nobel Prize in chemistry for polymerase chain reaction technology, initiated a technology that was time consuming and laborious. Fortuitously, the alignment of thermostable *Taq* polymerase enzyme with automation yielded the prototype of the polymerase chain reaction technology, which gave rise to molecular pathology used today.

To this end, the success of the Human Genome Project has expanded molecular biology in an exponential manner.[9] It has facilitated the identification of numerous novel genes whose functions can now be determined and whose expressions can be monitored in different disease states. Whereas the discipline of pathology often refers to the rubric of the study of disease in general, molecular pathology refers to the submicroscopic analysis of nucleic acids and proteins to diagnose disease, predict the occurrence of disease, predict the prognosis of diagnosed disease, and guide therapy.

Furthermore, recent advances in molecular pathology have positively affected the practice of medicine, especially diagnostic medicine. These changes result from abilities to clone disease-causing genes and the proteins that they encode and to detect the presence of these genes and proteins in the serum and other body fluids and tissues of patients, even though they may be present in minute quantities. This detection has been made possible by a veritable explosion of new, highly sensitive techniques involving amplification methods, such as polymerase chain reaction, branched DNA, fluorescence in situ hybridization, next-generation sequencing, and mass spectroscopy, among others.[10] The ability to streamline testing in a high-throughput manner, many of which have been automated, enables a single patient sample to be analyzed for multiple genes or proteins.

Molecular pathology has afforded physicians the ability to drill down and interrogate disease states for causes related to chromosomal abnormalities, point mutations, polymorphisms, and the like, which can provide a personalized medicine approach to diagnose a wide spectrum of diseases. To this end, genes that encode drug-metabolizing enzymes, activating and inactivating, and genes that encode ligands and receptors may show polymorphisms that either decrease or increase the therapeutic effectiveness or toxicity of drugs already in clinical use, thus accounting for some idiosyncratic responses previously not understood or predictable.[11] As such, there have been major advances in testing patients for genetic expression of selective enzyme isoforms, allowing prediction of which drugs would be the most effective ones for use in a personalized manner.[12]

As more polymorphisms are identified and correlated with individual patient response to treatment, pathologists will be called on increasingly to profile common polymorphisms in patients who are beginning therapy for common diseases, such as coronary artery disease, congestive heart failure, diabetes, thrombosis, hypertension, cancer, and infections. Mutations in select genes, produced by mutational events associated with, for instance, carcinogens and oncogenic viruses, often result in abnormal activation or overexpression of their encoded proteins. A laboratory's definition of an individual patient's genotype/ phenotype, therefore, may determine the specific drugs and doses suitable for the patient. This evolution has placed pathologists in a more definitive position to determine appropriate therapy than traditional prediction of disease behavior based on morphology of lesions or culture characteristics of infectious organisms.[13]

Cancer is a major area where the differential expression of specific genes characterizes particular tumors.[14] New advances in molecular pathology related to gynecology (see Eman Abdulfatah and colleagues' article, "Gynecologic Cancers: Molecular Updates 2018," in this issue.), gastroenterology (see Amarpreet Bhalla and colleagues' article, "Molecular Diagnostics in Colorectal Carcinoma: Advances and Applications for 2018," in this issue.), dermatology (see Katrin Kiavash and colleagues' article, "An Update Regarding the Molecular Genetics of Melanocytic Neoplasms and the Current Applications of Molecular Genetic Technologies in Their Diagnosis and Treatment," in this issue.), and hematology (see Radhakrishnan Ramchandran and colleagues' article, "Molecular Diagnosis of Hematopoietic Neoplasms: 2018 Update," in this issue.) disciplines among others have provided unprecedented insight into the diagnosis of and screening for several different types of tumors. Similar advances have been accomplished in the disciplines of infectious disease (see Marilynn Ransom Fairfax and colleagues' article, "Diagnostic Molecular Microbiology: A 2018 Snapshot," in this issue.) and transfusion medicine (see Matthew B. Elkins and colleagues' article, "Molecular Pathology in Transfusion Medicine: New Concepts and Applications," in this issue.). Clinical laboratories will likely be called on to perform such in-depth types of analyses with increasing frequency in the near future. A poignant example of this phenomenon is the diagnosis of leukemias and lymphomas. Morphologically and even immunophenotypically, it may prove difficult to distinguish among different types of each disease. Specific gene rearrangements and patterns of gene expression, however, now enable distinction of different types of disease in this regard, which affect treatment approaches. In addition, the relationships among diseases are also more sharply defined, and sometimes radically changed, by comparisons among the diseases' gene expression profiles.

As with all laboratory methods, excellent quality-assurance programs are required to ensure that molecular pathologic results are accurate and useful. Standardized methods for performance of the most common clinical molecular pathologic tests are published by the Clinical and Laboratory Standards Institute (formerly called the National Committee for Clinical Laboratory Standards). Use of these guidelines ensures that the data generated in molecular pathology laboratories are produced by methods that are the standard of excellent practice. Furthermore, interlaboratory comparison of test performance proficiency is provided by the College of American Pathologists (www.cap.org). Applying established standards of quality assurance and using molecular pathologic techniques with a thorough understanding of their respective strengths and weaknesses, pathologists continue to capitalize on the opportunities these techniques offer for improved patient care and the understanding of basic pathobiology.

Financial costs inherent in operations pertaining to a molecular pathology laboratory need to be considered. Although molecular pathology tests can often incur higher costs than conventional testing approaches, there are proponents who argue that molecular testing may actually facilitate a decrease in unnecessary, less-sensitive, and less-specific tests, thereby perpetuating more targeted and appropriate therapy for patients in the long run.[15,16] Recent application of molecular pathology and pharmacogenomics to pharmacovigilance (drug safety) has demonstrated its value to identify patients that may have an increased probability of suffering an adverse event for a trialed drug.[17,18] Incorporation of such pharmacogenomics testing approaches may decrease costs of such adverse events, which result from class action lawsuits, recalls, or other postmarket concerns.

Molecular pathology has also reached the mainstream direct-to-consumer marketplace.[19,20] Numerous companies offer the ability to test selective gene panels, prognosticate disease, elucidate ancestry, and determine the relative risk of future maladies in oneself or one's offspring, often easily obtained by online or drug store purchase. The integrity of such direct-to-consumer offerings is not always clear regarding the presence or proficiency of medical directorship, method validation, accuracy, and degree of interpretative license as one's results relates to actual disease. The term "buyer beware" cannot be overemphasized in this domain because a concerning result can have far reaching social and psychological consequences.

Application of molecular pathology to various health care–centric enterprises has also flourished. The evolving new disciplines of "omics" data mining for biomarkers and profiling of biosignatures is becoming vogue and interfacing with all aspects of conventional health care.[21] Nutrigenomics, metabolomics, lipidomics, glycomics, and transcriptomics represent salient expansions of the original genomics construct while drilling down into the substrata of select biologic processes. The ideal was to apply the "omics" interrogation to the tried and true model of tissue- and blood-based immunohistochemical marker interrogation to avail unparalleled precision for unique biomarker discovery and application. However, the pathology biomarker paradigms of immunohistochemical marker and blood biomarker have not always applied well to the "omics" realm, mainly because of their own specificities and limitations and the disconnect caused by disease heterogeneity. Such heterogeneity can occur within an individual (specimen heterogeneity), and the other can occur between different individuals (disease heterogeneity). Ongoing approaches to better interrelate immunohistochemical marker and "omics" applications and limitations will likely identify disease spaces for best fit with respect to diagnostic discovery, adaptation, and reproducibility.

In summary, molecular diagnostic techniques provide new insights into disease that were never before possible. These techniques, however, must often be used in coordination with traditional laboratory tests while being mindful to the limitations of each approach. In cases of tissue pathology, the morphologic skills involved in histopathology and cytopathology must be used to ensure that appropriate cells and tissues are analyzed via molecular means. Otherwise, analysis of other than targeted cells/tissues, despite high-quality technical methods interpreted with skill and experience, can lead to erroneous, sometimes dangerously misleading, results. In concert with classical pathology algorithms, molecular pathology affords unprecedented potential for refined, highly sensitive, rapid, and patient-specific characterization of disease. To this end, molecular pathologists are situated to serve as proverbial "molecular shepherds"[22] (diagnostic gatekeepers) to ascertain and affirm that the evolution of molecular medicine is handled, processed, and interpreted appropriately for optimal patient care. Continued progress in this discipline will undoubtedly uncover new molecular, epigenetic, and genetic biorealities that can be applied to the human condition in health and disease with the ideal of improving humanity in any era.

REFERENCES

1. Genesis 30:14.
2. 2 Kings 20:7.
3. Leviticus 14:3–5.
4. Available at: https://www.ancient.eu/article/49/female-physicians-in-ancient-egypt/. Accessed November 23, 2017.
5. Available at: https://quatr.us/egypt/doctors-medicine-ancient-egypt.htm. Accessed November 23, 2017.
6. Available at: https://sites.google.com/site/psychologyofpersonalityperiod6/home/type-and-trait-theories/galen-s-personality-theory. Accessed November 23, 2017.
7. Available at: http://admin.cmf.org.uk/pdf/helix/spr00/11history.pdf. Accessed November 23, 2017.
8. Bauer J. The tragic fate of Ignaz Philipp Semmelweis. Calif Med 1963;98:264–6.
9. Venter JC, Adams MD, Myers EW, et al. The sequence of the human genome. Science 2001;291:1304–51.
10. Bluth MJ, Bluth MH. Molecular pathology techniques. Clin Lab Med 2013;33: 753–72.
11. Schwarz DA, George MP, Bluth MH. Precision medicine in toxicology. Clin Lab Med 2016;36:693–708.
12. Li J, Bluth MH. Pharmacogenomics of drug metabolizing enzymes and transporters: implications for cancer therapy. Pharmgenomics Pers Med 2011;4: 11–33.
13. Tozzi V. Pharmacogenetics of antiretrovirals. Antiviral Res 2010;85:190–200.
14. Gabali AM, Czuchlewski DR, Viswanatha DS, et al. Molecular diagnosis of hematopoietic neoplasms. In: McPherson RA, Pincus RM, editors. Henry's clinical diagnosis and management by laboratory methods. 23rd edition. New York: Saunders Publishing; 2016. p. 1465–91.
15. Ross JS. The impact of molecular diagnostic tests on patient outcomes. Clin Lab Med 1999;19:815–31.
16. Ross JS. Financial determinants of outcomes in molecular testing. Arch Pathol Lab Med 1999;123:1071–5.
17. Committee for Medicinal Products for Human Use (CHMP). Guideline on key aspects for the use of pharmacogenomics in the pharmacovigilance of medicinal products EMA/CHMP/281371/2013. 2015.
18. Farahani P, Levine M. Pharmacovigilance in a genomic era. Pharmacogenomics J 2006;6:158–61.
19. Covolo L, Rubinelli S, Ceretti E, Gelatti U. Internet-based direct-to-consumer genetic testing: a systematic review. J Med Internet Res 2015;17:e279.
20. Myers MF. Health care providers and direct-to-consumer access and advertising of genetic testing in the United States. Genome Med 2011;3:81.
21. Abu-Asab MS, Chaouchi M, Alesci S, et al. Biomarkers in the age of omics: time for a systems biology approach. OMICS 2011;15:105–12.
22. Bluth MH. Molecular pathology in the modern era: revisiting Jacob's spotted sheep. Clin Lab Med 2013;33:xi–xiii.

Molecular Pathology
Techniques: Advances in 2018

Mark J. Bluth, PhD[a],*, Martin H. Bluth, MD, PhD[b,c]

KEYWORDS

- Molecular pathology • Methodology • RT-PCR • FISH • RFLP • SNP
- Hybrid capture • Mass spectrometry

KEY POINTS

- Polymerase chain reaction (PCR) remains the cornerstone methodology for nucleic acid amplification. Improvements in nucleic acid detection methodologies (for example PCR) have increased the detection sensitivity by using fluorescent and bead array–based technologies.
- Single base-pair lesions can be detected via sequencing and related techniques to discern point mutations in disease pathogenesis.
- Novel technologies, such as high-resolution melting analysis, provide fast, high-throughput post-PCR analysis of genetic mutations or variance in nucleic acid sequences.
- Infectious disease can now be detected by fluorophore or chemiluminescent detection assays, such as hybrid capture hybridization technology, allowing for rapid diagnosis.

POLYMERASE CHAIN REACTION

Polymerase chain reaction (PCR) is a chemical reaction that facilitates the in vitro synthesis of potentially unlimited quantities of a targeted nucleic acid sequence. Basically, the reaction consists of a target DNA molecule, an excess of the forward and reverse oligonucleotide primers (typically 15–30 nucleotides long), a thermostable DNA polymerase (typically *Taq* or *Pfu*), an equimolar mixture of deoxyribonucleotide triphosphates (dATP, dCTP, dGTP, and dTTP), Mg^{21} or Mn^{21} (depending on the type of polymerase used), KCl, and an appropriate Tris-HCl buffer.

The reaction consists of 3 steps: denaturation, annealing, and extension, which taken together are referred to as a *cycle*. To begin, the reaction mixture is heated (usually to 95°C) to separate the 2 strands of target DNA (denaturation) and then cooled to

Disclosure: The authors have nothing to disclose.
This article has been updated from a version previously published in Clinics in Laboratory Medicine, Volume 33, Issue 4, December 2013.
[a] Bluth Bio Industries, Southfield MI, 48034, USA; [b] Department of Pathology, Wayne State University, School of Medicine, 540 East Canfield Street, Detroit, MI 48201, USA; [c] Pathology Laboratories, Michigan Surgical Hospital, 21230 Dequindre Road, Warren, MI 48091, USA
* Corresponding author.
E-mail address: mark.bluth72@gmail.com

Clin Lab Med 38 (2018) 215–236
https://doi.org/10.1016/j.cll.2018.03.004
0272-2712/18/© 2018 Elsevier Inc. All rights reserved.

a temperature at which the primers bind to the target DNA in a sequence-specific manner (annealing). Immediately after primer annealing, the DNA polymerase binds (as the temperature is raised to 72°C) and initiates polymerization, resulting in the extension of each primer at its 3' end (extension). During the following cycle, the primer extension products are subsequently heated to dissociate from the target DNA. Each new extension product, as well as the original target, can serve as a template for subsequent rounds of primer annealing and extension. In doing so, at the end of each cycle, the PCR products are theoretically doubled.[1,2]

The whole procedure is carried out in a programmable thermocycler that precisely controls the temperature at which the steps occur, the length of time that the reaction is held at the different temperatures, and the number of cycles. Ideally, after 20 cycles of PCR, a million-fold amplification is achieved and, after 30 cycles, the replicons approach a billion-fold.

REVERSE TRANSCRIPTION–POLYMERASE CHAIN REACTION

As described previously, PCR is suitable for the amplification of DNA targets because DNA polymerase does not recognize DNA-primed RNA templates. Reverse transcription (RT)-PCR helps overcome this problem by using the enzyme reverse transcriptase to first synthesize a strand of complementary DNA (cDNA) using the RNA as a template. Because thermolabile RNA is often referred to as the message transcribed from the DNA template, this process provides a thermostable mirror image of the RNA transcript. Typically, recombinant RT is added to a reaction mixture identical to the one for PCR and is incubated at between 37°C and 42°C for 30 minutes, during which time the first-strand cDNA synthesis occurs. Subsequently, the reaction proceeds much like a regular PCR reaction for the appropriate number of cycles at the appropriate temperatures. This method can, however, present problems in terms of both the nonspecific primer annealing and inefficient primer extension due to formation of RNA secondary structures. A secondary RNA structure is a direct consequence of the low temperature at which the reaction is carried out, due to the heat labile nature of most RTs. These problems have been largely overcome by the development of a thermostable DNA polymerase derived from *Thermus thermophilus* (for example Taq polymerase), which, under the proper conditions, can function efficiently as both an RT and a DNA polymerase.[2]

REAL-TIME POLYMERASE CHAIN REACTION

Real-time PCR (also called quantitative PCR or quantitative Real-time PCR, or kinetic PCR or kinetic RT-PCR) is a closed-system assay that can be used to determine the relative quantity of gene expression as well as genotyping by detection of single-nucleotide polymorphisms (SNPs).

In principle, the method works much like the PCR discussed previously; however, real-time PCR also uses an additional oligonucleotide probe. This probe is target message specific and contains a fluorochrome at one end and a quencher molecule at the other. When unhybridized, the probe forms a hairpin structure that brings the fluorochrome in proximity with and binds the quencher, effectively muting its fluorescence. When hybridized, however, the quencher molecule is cleaved, and the bound fluorochrome is now unencumbered and can be detected by a fluorescence absorption assay. Single-nucleotide differences like SNPs can be detected in PCR products by the sequence-specific hybridization of the probe. Because it is possible to have different colored fluorochromes, the probes can be differentially labeled, allowing both alleles of an SNP to be typed in the same tube. These molecules can be used in a closed system for allelic discrimination of PCR products. Both assays can be read in real time or endpoint formats, using a fluorescent thermocycler. This PCR-based assay can be consolidated by combining an amplification primer and the fluorescent detection component in the same molecule to enable real-time genotyping.

Once suitable oligonucleotides are designed, the genotyping of a sample is straight-forward. The instrument is programmed to amplify the DNA and to perform a melting curve analysis. A perfect match has a higher melting temperature than a mismatch. In this way, the fluorescent thermocycler directly genotypes a sample after amplification with no additional handling. With dual-color detection, it is possible to simultaneously genotype 2 different mutations in 1 PCR run.[3-5]

MULTIPLEX POLYMERASE CHAIN REACTION

Multiplex PCR (mpPCR) consists of multiple primer sets within a single PCR mixture to produce amplicons of differing sizes that specifically identify different DNA se-quences. Primer sets are designed so that their annealing temperatures are optimized to work correctly within a single reaction. The resultant amplicons are different enough in size to form distinct bands when visualized by gel electrophoresis. By its original design, this assay is typically efficient for elucidating the presence and relative con-centrations of 2 to 20 distinct messages and is limited by the resolution capacity of electophoretic gel separation.[6]

xTAG TECHNOLOGY

xTAG technology (Luminex Corp, Austin, Texas) is a next-generation form of multi-plexing that overcomes the resolution limits of mpPCR by combining the methods of multiplex amplification with particle-based flow cytometry. Like mpPCR, multiple reactions can be carried out in a single reaction; however, because of the added flow component, many more tests can be run and resolved at the same time.

Using a viral panel as an example, after obtaining a biologic sample, the mRNA is reverse transcribed to cDNA. The cDNA is then amplified using a panel of primers that can specifically amplify many different pathologic/pathogenic nucleic acid se-quences at the same time. Each pathogen-specific primer used is tagged with a unique oligonucleotide sequence (called the tag) as well as a fluorophore. After the multiplex amplification step is completed, the reaction is mixed with microscopic beads that are internally tagged with varying amounts of fluorescent molecules at the time of production. Each different type of bead is also labeled with a unique oligo-nucleotide sequence that is complementary to the unique tag on the pathogen-specific primer (called the antitag). If both the tag and the antitag are present, then hybridization occurs, binding the fluorophore-labeled amplicon to its appropriate fluorophore-labeled bead. The beads are then processed and placed in a special flow-enabled luminometer equipped with 2 lasers for reading. The first of the 2 lasers identifies the bead based on its internal dye content and the second laser detects how much, if any, tagged amplicon is bound to its surface.[7]

This technology allows for the resolution of 100 or more tests from 1 sample at 1 time in 1 tube. It is adaptable to perform tests on nucleic acids, peptides, and proteins in a variety of sample matrixes.

STRAND DISPLACEMENT AMPLIFICATION

Strand displacement amplification method allows for rapid isothermal amplification of target nucleic acid molecules using a series of primers, DNA polymerase (exo-*Bst*), and a restriction endonuclease (*Bso*BI), to amplify a unique nucleic acid sequence exponentially.[8] *Bso*BI recognizes the nucleic acid sequence: 5′ C-(C or T)-C-G-(A or G)-G 3′. One of the primers called the strand displacement amplification primer (SDA), also commonly called the "bump" primer, contains a sequence complimentary to a unique target sequence but also contains a 5′ linker with a built-in *Bso*BI restriction site. Strand displacement amplification can be thought of as occurring in 2 segments: a target generation phase and an exponential amplification phase. In the target generation phase after the heat denaturation of the native nucleic acid, primers anneal (**Fig. 1**) and the polymerization reaction occurs in both directions in the presence of modified dCTPαS (**Fig. 2**), which results in the production of a double-stranded product with a *Bso*BI restriction site 5′ to the target sequence. Next, the *Bso*BI restriction site within the primer is digested with *Bso*BI. Because the newly polymerized DNA strands (the strands complementary to and extended from the bump primer) were synthesized with dCTPαS, however, only 1 side of the *Bso*BI site is sensitive to digestion, resulting in the production of 1 nicked strand (**Fig. 3**). Next, the exo-*Bst* polymerase binds to the nicked strand, on the 5′ side of the nick, and polymerizes a new strand extending from the nick site, displacing the previous strand in the process. The strand is nicked again with *Bso*BI and the process repeats (**Fig. 4**). The newly displaced strand serves as a template in following rounds of amplification. The exponential amplification phase describes the continuous repetition of this process and can produce copies in excess of a million-fold within 2 hours.[9,10]

The reaction can be performed with real-time analysis if coupled with a fluorescent probe and multiplexed via an initial purifying step in which the bumper primer is covalently linked to magnetic or fluorescently labeled beads.

TRANSCRIPTION-MEDIATED AMPLIFICATION

Transcription-mediated amplification (TMA) is an isothermal nucleic acid–based method that can amplify RNA or DNA targets a billion-fold in less than 1 hour (**Fig. 5**). This system is useful for detecting the presence of *Mycobacterium tuberculosis* and *Chlamydia trachomatis*.

Developed at Gen-Probe now (Hologic, San Diego, California), TMA technology uses 2 primers and 2 enzymes: RNA polymerase and RT. One primer contains a promoter sequence for RNA polymerase. In the first step of amplification, this primer hybridizes to the target RNA at a defined site. RT creates a DNA copy of the target RNA

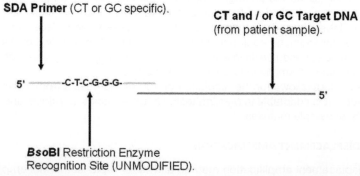

Fig. 1. Primer hybridization. (*Courtesy of* Becton, Dickinson and Company.)

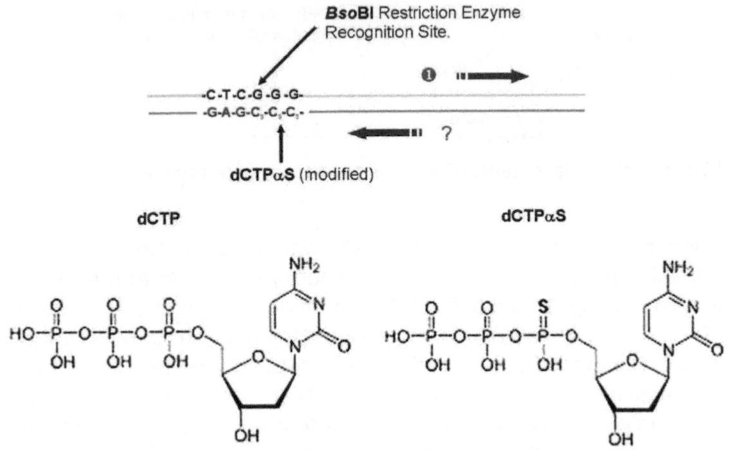

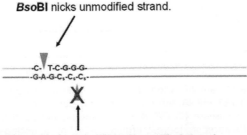

BsoBI Restriction Enzyme
Recognition Site.

❶ ▪▪➡

-C -T -C -G -G -G-
-G -A -G -C₃-C₅-C₅-

◀▪▪ ?

↑
dCTPαS (modified)

dCTP   **dCTPαS**

Fig. 2. Primer extension. (*Courtesy of* Becton, Dickinson and Company.)

by extension from the 3′ end of the promoter primer. The RNA in the resulting RNA:DNA duplex is degraded by the RNase activity of the RT. Next, a second primer binds to the DNA copy. A new strand of DNA is synthesized from the end of this primer by RT, creating a double-stranded DNA (dsDNA) molecule. RNA polymerase recognizes the promoter sequence in the DNA template and initiates transcription. Each of the newly synthesized RNA amplicons re-enters the TMA process and serves as a template for a new round of replication. The amplicons produced in these reactions are detected by a specific gene probe via hybridization protection assay followed by a chemiluminescence detection protocol.[11,12]

DNA SEQUENCING

DNA sequencing using the enzymatic extension reaction makes use of the difference between normal deoxyribonucleotides and dideoxyribonucleotides. Deoxyribonucleotides contain a hydroxyl group at position 3 on the pentose sugar ring, allowing DNA polymerase to join it with the phosphate group of the next nucleotide. A dideoxynucleotide can be incorporated into a growing chain, but because it does not contain a hydroxyl group at position 3, no additional nucleotides can be added, effectively terminating polymerization of that chain at that point.

BsoBI nicks unmodified strand.

/

▼
-C- T-C-G-G-G-
-G-A-G-C₃-C₅-C₅-

✗
↑
BsoBI unable to nick **dCTPαS** modified strand.

Fig. 3. Single-strand digestion. (*Courtesy of* Becton, Dickinson and Company.)

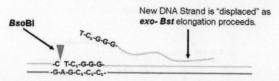

Fig. 4. Nicked-strand displacement. (*Courtesy of* Becton, Dickinson and Company.)

The reaction is the same as a standard PCR with the exception of the supplementation of a small concentration of a labeled dideoxynucleotide to the reaction mix in addition to the regular quantities of the normal deoxynucleotide triphosphates (dATP, dTTP, dCTP, and dGTP). Using dideoxythymidine triphosphate (ddTTP) as an example, the DNA to be sequenced is denatured, complementary primers anneal, and primer extension occurs as normal. When ddTTP is incorporated instead of dTTP, however, DNA polymerization on that molecule terminates. When the reaction is carried out in the presence of the optimal concentrations of both dTTP and ddTTP, there are molecules synthesized that stop at each of the thymidine nucleotides in the sequence. The fragments generated can then be separated out by size via gel electrophoresis and the tag on the ddNTP allows the fragment to be visualized. In the beginning, the reaction was carried out using 4 different tubes, each one containing a different ddNTP. The reaction uses radiolabeled nucleotides (for example S^{35}), and,

Transcription-Mediated Amplification

- One primer contains a T7 promoter sequence for RNA polymerase that hybridizes to the target RNA

- RT creates a cDNA of the target RNA by extension from the 3' end of the promoter-primer

- The RNA of the resulting RNA:DNA duplex is degraded by the RNAse H activities of the RT

- A second primer then binds to the cDNA containing the promoter sequence from the T7 promoter-primer

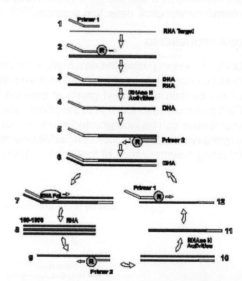

Fig. 5. The TMA RNA amplification technology. (*From* Origoni M, Cristoforoni P, Carminati G, et al. E6/E7 mRNA testing for human papilloma virus-induced high-grade cervical intraepithelial disease (CIN2/CIN3): a promising perspective. ecancer 2015;9:533. Available at: https://ecancer.org/journal/9/full/533-e6-e7-mrna-testing-for-human-papilloma-virus-induced-high-grade-cervical-intraepithelial-disease-cin2-cin3-a-promising-perspective.php; with permission.)

when completed, the reactions were separated in parallel lanes of a gel (1 lane per ddNTP), which was then exposed to film, yielding a staggered pattern of bands each with a 1 nucleotide base difference in size from the next. When the order of the bands from all 4 lanes is read in size order from bottom to top, it corresponds to the sequence of the DNA fragment that was amplified from the primer onward (**Fig. 6**).

This method is excellent for sequencing fragments up to 600 base pairs. As a result, the method can get costly for the time and reagents necessary to perform multiple reactions required to verify the sequence of longer DNA fragments. Today, however, the same reaction can be performed using ddNTPs labeled with different fluorophores in 1 tube, run in 1 lane of a capillary gel, and read with a laser detector. This advance allows for more accurate sequence reading while using less time and reagents (**Fig. 7**).

PYROSEQUENCING

Pyrosequencing is a method of DNA sequencing based on sequencing by the principle of synthesis. First, a sequencing primer is hybridized to a single-stranded DNA template in the presence of the enzymes, DNA polymerase, ATP sulfurylase, luciferase, and apyrase, and the substrates, adenosine 5' phosphosulfate (APS) and luciferin.[13–15]

The first of 4 dNTPs are then added to the reaction and DNA polymerase incorporates it only if it is complementary to the base in the template strand. Each incorporation event is accompanied by the release of pyrophosphate in a quantity equimolar to the amount of incorporated nucleotide (**Fig. 8**, step 2).

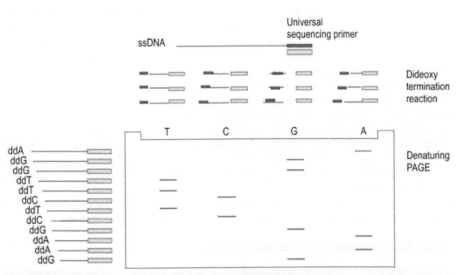

Fig. 6. DNA Sequencing by Dideoxynucleotide (ddNTP) Chain Termination (Sanger). Copying of the DNA by the polymerase is terminated at specific positions when a ddNTP is incorporated. The ddNTP is mixed with deoxynucleotides (dNTPs) so that in each reaction, only some new strands terminate, whereas others continue through to the next complementary nucleotide. The sequencing products can be visualized by autoradiography or by laser scanning in an automated sequencer. (*From* Belmont JW. Molecular methods. In: Rich RR, Fleisher TA, Shearer WT, et al, editors. Clinical immunology: principles and practice. Philadelphia: Elsevier; 2018; p. 1297–1310; with permission.)

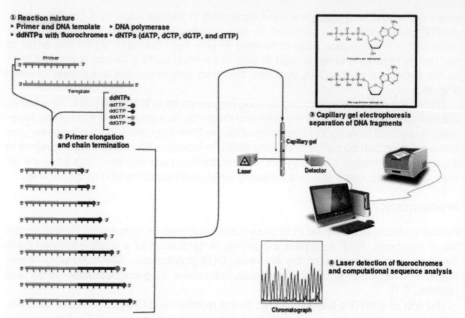

Fig. 7. Next-generation Sanger sequencing using only 1 tube and fluorescent-labeled ddNTPs. (*From* Bluth MJ, Bluth MH. Molecular pathology techniques. Clin Lab Med 2013;33(4):760; with permission.)

ATP sulfurylase quantitatively converts pyrophosphate to ATP in the presence of APS. This ATP drives the luciferase-mediated conversion of luciferin to oxyluciferin, which generates visible light in amounts proportional to the ATP generated. The light produced in the luciferase-catalyzed reaction is detected by a charge-coupled device camera and seen as a peak in a pyrogram. The height of each peak is proportional to the number of a specific nucleotide incorporated (see **Fig. 8**, step 3).

Apyrase, a nucleotide degrading enzyme, continuously degrades ATP and unincorporated dNTPs. Apyrase switches off the light-promoting reaction and regenerates the reaction solution. The next dNTP is then added (see **Fig. 8**, step 4).

The addition of dNTPs is performed one at a time (G then C then T then A then G then C then T, and so forth). As the process continues, the cDNA strand is built up and the nucleotide sequence is determined from the signal peaks in the Pyrogram (see **Fig. 8**, Step 5).

Deoxyadenosine alpha-thiotriphosphate is used as a substitute for dATP because it is used efficiently by DNA polymerase but is not recognized by luciferase.

DENATURING GRADIENT GEL ELECTROPHORESIS

Denaturing gradient gel electrophoresis (DGGE) is a widespread technique that can be used to separate similar-sized fragments of DNA or RNA based on the composition of the double-stranded fragments. The melting temperature (for example the temperature at which base pairs in a dsDNA fragment lose their bond) depends on the base-pair composition of a fragment. Even in the case of a 1 base-pair substitution, the fragment melts at a different temperature.[16]

By adding a GC-rich tail (called a GC clamp) to one of the primers for the amplification, a fragment is produced that only partially melts when it is run into a denaturing

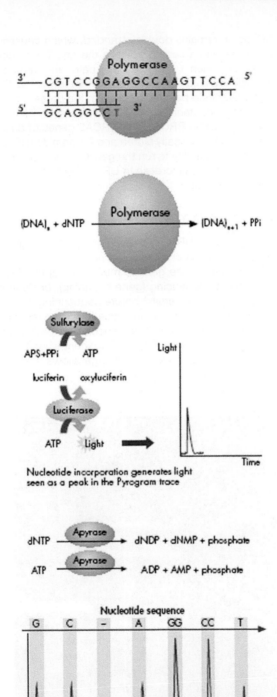

Fig. 8. Stepwise illustration of the pyrosequencing method. (*Courtesy of* QIAGEN.)

gradient gel. The GC clamp remains double stranded, which causes the fragment to stop migrating when it reaches a certain point in the gel. This process occurs at a different position in the gel when 1 or more base pairs are substituted, deleted, or inserted. Therefore, allelic variation or mutation can be detected (**Fig. 9**) using this method.[17] Clinically, DGGE could be used to confirm the presence of and distinguish between which types of mycobacteria are present in a sample.[18] It can also be used to determine what mutations exist in BRCA1 and BRCA2 genes of an individual.[19]

In this method, the gradient is typically a urea and formamide (UF) gradient. The use of the UF gradient results in the ability to run the gel at a much lower temperature than without, using the gradient. A 10% increase in UF concentration has the same effect as a 3.2°C increase in temperature.

HIGH-RESOLUTION MELTING ANALYSIS

High-resolution melting analysis (HRM) is a technique for fast, high-throughput post-PCR analysis of genetic mutations or variance in nucleic acid sequences. It enables researchers to detect and categorize genetic mutations rapidly (eg, SNPs), identify new genetic variants without sequencing (gene scanning), or determine the genetic variation in a population (eg, viral diversity) before sequencing.

The first step of the HRM protocol is the amplification of the region of interest, using standard PCR techniques, in the presence of a specialized dsDNA binding dye (such as SYBR Green). This specialized dye is highly fluorescent when bound to dsDNA and poorly fluorescent in the unbound state. This change allows the user to monitor the DNA amplification during PCR (as in real time PCR).

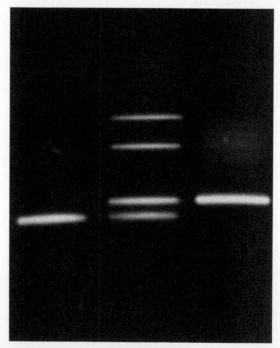

Fig. 9. Illustration of DGGE. Lane 1: homozygous GC. Lane 2: heterozygous sample. Lane 3: homozygous AT. (*Courtesy of* Dr R.W.M. Hofstra, Groningen, The Netherlands.)

After completion of the PCR step, a HRM curve is produced by increasing the temperature of the PCR product, typically in increments of 0.008°C to 0.2°C, thereby gradually denaturing an amplified DNA target. Because SYBR Green is only fluorescent when bound to dsDNA, fluorescence decreases as duplex DNA is denatured, which produces a characteristic melting profile; this is termed melting analysis. The melting profile depends on the length, GC content, sequence, and heterozygosity of the amplified target. When set up correctly, HRM is sensitive enough to allow the detection of a single base change between otherwise identical nucleotide sequences.[20,21]

SOUTHERN AND NORTHERN HYBRIDIZATIONS

Both Southern and Northern hybridizations combine electrophoretic separation of test nucleic acid with transfer to a solid support and subsequent hybridization. These assays, therefore, not only give information about the presence of hybridization but also permit determination of the molecular weight of the hybridizing species.

The original procedure was termed Southern blot hybridization or Southern blotting, after its inventor, E.M. Southern. In this assay, the sample is DNA. Northern blotting was named by analogy for the technique using RNA samples. (Extending the analogy even further, the Western blot is a similar procedure in which proteins are subjected to electrophoresis and transfer; a Southwestern blot has been described for a technique separating and blotting DNA followed by incubation with protein solutions to permit evaluation of specific DNA-binding proteins.)

Sample preparation is time-consuming and labor intensive for both of these techniques. Degradation of sample nucleic acids is not tolerated by the assays, and a relatively large amount of starting material is required. For Southern hybridizations, the DNA must be purified with minimal shearing because sizing of the DNA fragments is achieved through digestion with 1 or more restriction enzymes. Shearing and degradation introduce random breaks in the sample, reducing the quantity available to be cut specifically at appropriate recognition sequences. Impurities in the sample may interfere with the activity and sequence specificity of the restriction enzyme. Partially or improperly digested samples can produce spurious band sizes or result in such a reduced concentration of the specific band that it is no longer detected during hybridization. For Northern hybridizations, the starting material is RNA, and extreme care must be taken to avoid degradation during sample collection and preparation because of the ubiquitous nature of RNases. RNA is composed of fragment sizes determined by transcription and processing of message and ribosomal RNA. It is not digested before electrophoresis but is separated under denaturing conditions to remove secondary structure.

The size-separated fragments in the agarose gel are then transferred to a nylon or nitrocellulose membrane. As originally designed, the transfer occurred passively through capillary action. Most current applications use vacuum or pressure to speed the transfer. After transfer, baking or ultraviolet cross-linking immobilizes the nucleic acids and the entire membrane is then hybridized with labeled probe under stringent conditions.

Hybridization is followed by autoradiographic, colorimetric, or chemiluminescent detection of bands that are bound to the probe. Interpretation involves both detection of a hybridizing species and determination of the molecular weight of the molecule. These technically demanding assays require several days to perform but may be required in clinical applications in which the information cannot be obtained in any other format. The presence of bands at molecular weights different from normal or germline (developmentally unaltered) samples can indicate a change in the genetic material.[22-25]

RESTRICTION FRAGMENT LENGTH POLYMORPHISM ANALYSIS

Restriction fragment length polymorphism (RFLP) analysis is a method that uses restriction endonuclease digestion of DNA and gel electrophoretics separation of the resulting fragments (**Fig. 10**). This technique allows the study of small variances called polymorphisms that occur in the DNA sequences between individuals of the same species. These variances occur in the form of differing numbers of small sequence repeats of DNA—called tandem repeats, minisatellites, and microsatellites—that are normally found in the noncoding regions of DNA. Polymorphisms can occur as a result of mutations—deletions, inversions, additions, substitutions, and translocations—to the DNA sequence.

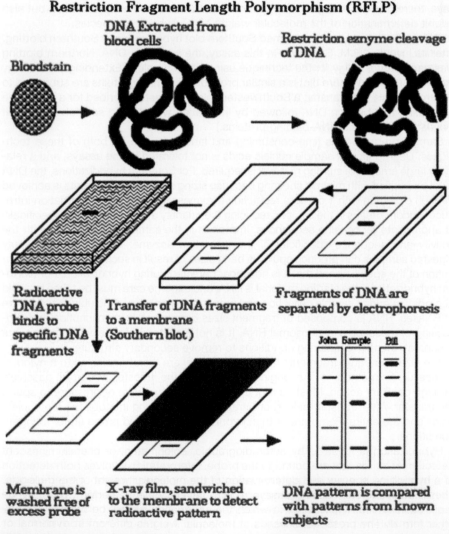

Fig. 10. Process illustrating RFLP analysis. (*Courtesy of* Santa Monica College, Santa Monica, CA.)

Briefly, DNA is carefully isolated (so as to cause as little degradation and mechanical fragmentation as possible) and then digested with a particular endonuclease. The digested DNA is electrophoretically separated in an agarose gel. At this point the separated DNA samples can be viewed using DNA binding dyes, such as ethidium bromide, to compare the banding patterns. Alternatively, the DNA fragments can be Southern blotted (discussed previously), hybridized with labeled probes, and then analyzed.

Therefore, if DNA were digested from 2 individuals (excluding identical twins and clones) and the resulting fragments separated by gel electrophoresis, some differences may be found in the 2 resulting banding patterns because of the differing number of tandem repeats between restriction sites from one individual to another. Analysis of the banding of an individual yields what is commonly known as a "genetic fingerprint." Using RFLP analysis, a difference can also be observed in the RFLP patterns between normal and diseased tissue (for example tumor) from the same individual. If a tumor results from a genetic alteration (mutation), that alteration may result in a change in the size of 1 or more bands as a result of additions or deletions of DNA. In addition, single-nucleotide alterations may be observable via RFLP analysis if the alteration occurs within the sequence of just 1 of the endonuclease restriction sites, rendering that particular site unrecognizable to and uncut by the enzyme, which ultimately changes the banding pattern.[26]

REVERSE LINE BLOT HYBRIDIZATION

Reverse line blot hybridization, also called spacer oligonucleotide typing (spoligotyping),[27] is a method that can detect and identify pathogens based on the presence and comparison of pathogen-specific genes and is useful for confirming the presence of specific pathogens and a proper course of treatment based on possible multidrug resistance. For example, wild-type *M tuberculosis* is a slow-growing bacterium, requiring 2 weeks to 6 weeks to culture, and is sensitive to treatment with rifampicin (RIF). Mutations in the *rpoB* gene can render it resistant to RIF. Using this information, the mutation hot-spot region of the *rpoB* gene is first amplified by mpPCR using as many as 20 different biotinylated primers, which yield labeled amplified products.[28] The PCR products are hybridized to a set of wild-type and mutant oligonucleotide probes, which are covalently bound to a membrane, by reverse line blotting (**Fig. 11**). It is called "reverse" because, in contrast to Southern or Northern blotting, where the sample is transferred onto a membrane and then probed, the probe is first systematically bound to the membrane and the sample is then hybridized to it.

Positive hybridization is detected on film after streptavidin-peroxidase incubation and enhanced chemiluminescence. RIF-sensitive strains only hybridize with the wild-type probes, whereas resistant strains fail to hybridize with 1 or more wild-type probes and show additional hybridization signals for the mutant probes (**Fig. 12**). The resultant hybridization pattern elucidates the genotype of the *M tuberculosis* and thus a proper treatment protocol.

HYBRID CAPTURE

Hybrid capture is a nucleic acid hybridization technology that can precede signal amplification and often uses fluorophore or chemiluminescent detection. To date, human papillomavirus (HPV) cannot be cultured in vitro, and immunologic tests are inadequate to determine the presence of HPV cervical infection. Indirect evidence of anogenital HPV infection can be obtained through physical examination and by the presence of characteristic cellular changes associated with viral replication in

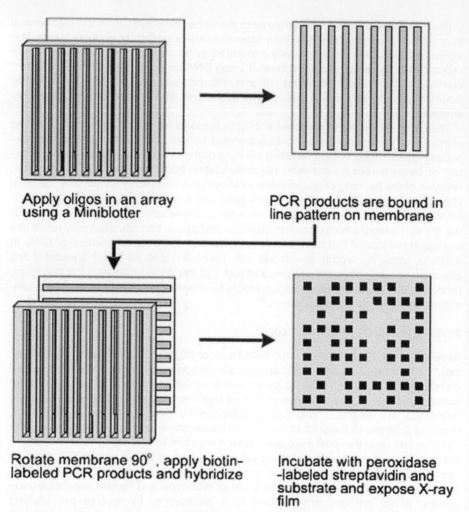

Apply oligos in an array using a Miniblotter

PCR products are bound in line pattern on membrane

Rotate membrane 90°, apply biotin-labeled PCR products and hybridize

Incubate with peroxidase-labeled streptavidin and substrate and expose X-ray film

Fig. 11. Preparation of the probe-labeled reverse line blot hybridization membrane. (*From* Bluth MJ, Bluth MH. Molecular pathology techniques. Clin Lab Med 2013;33(4):766; with permission.)

Papanicolaou smear or biopsy specimens. Alternately, biopsies can be analyzed by nucleic acid hybridization to detect the presence of HPV DNA directly. In cases of modern molecular-based HPV tests, specimens containing the target DNA hybridize with a specific HPV RNA probe cocktail. The resultant RNA:DNA hybrids are captured onto the surface of a solid media (for example a microplate well coated with antibodies specific for RNA:DNA hybrids or covalently linked to beads). Immobilized hybrids are then reacted with alkaline phosphatase–conjugated antibodies specific for the RNA:DNA hybrids and detected with a chemiluminescent substrate. Several alkaline phosphatase molecules are conjugated to each antibody. Multiple conjugated antibodies bind to each captured hybrid, resulting in substantial signal amplification. As the substrate is cleaved by the bound alkaline phosphatase, light is emitted that is measured as relative light units on a luminometer (**Fig. 13**). The intensity of the light emitted denotes the presence or absence of target DNA in the specimen.[29] In the

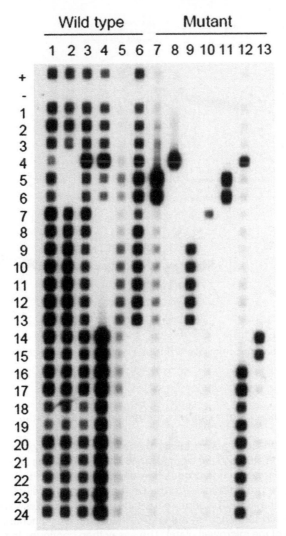

Fig. 12. Results of a reverse line blot hybridization assay. (*From* Bluth MJ, Bluth MH. Molecular pathology techniques. Clin Lab Med 2013;33(4):767; with permission.)

case of HPV, although this technique can elucidate the presence and load of the virus, it cannot determine which specific types of HPV are present. For the identification of the HPV strains present in the sample, PCR with HPV strain–specific primers would be required.[30]

BRANCHED DNA ASSAYS

In contrast with techniques that rely on PCR, the sensitivity of branched DNA (bDNA) methods is achieved by signal amplification on the bDNA probe after direct binding of a large hybridization complex to the RNA target sequence. This series of hybridization steps results in a sandwich complex of probes and target sequence. These unusual synthetic oligonucleotides are composed of a primary sequence and

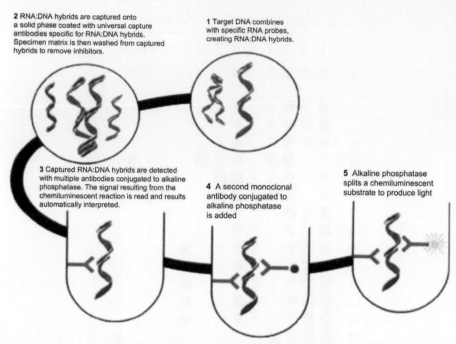

2 RNA:DNA hybrids are captured onto a solid phase coated with universal capture antibodies specific for RNA:DNA hybrids. Specimen matrix is then washed from captured hybrids to remove inhibitors.

1 Target DNA combines with specific RNA probes, creating RNA:DNA hybrids.

3 Captured RNA:DNA hybrids are detected with multiple antibodies conjugated to alkaline phosphatase. The signal resulting from the chemiluminescent reaction is read and results automatically interpreted.

4 A second monoclonal antibody conjugated to alkaline phosphatase is added

5 Alkaline phosphatase splits a chemiluminescent substrate to produce light

Fig. 13. Hybrid capture test principle. (Principles of the hybrid capture test *with permission from* QIAGEN.)

secondary sequences that result in a branched structure extending from the primary sequence.

There is no synthesis reaction taking place. There are 2 steps, however, to this assay: the capturing step and the signal amplification step. In the capturing step, there are 2 capturing oligonucleotide probes: the capture probe and the capture extender probe. The capture probe is linked to the bottom of a microwell plate much like the one used in hybrid capture. The capture extender probe hybridizes to both the capture probe and a specific sequence on the target RNA, effectively anchoring it to the solid medium (bottom of the microwell plate). The assay then continues to the signal amplification step whereby label extender probes are hybridized to specific sequences at precise distances from each other on the target RNA. The label extender probes are designed to serve as platforms for hybridization to preamplifier probes, which only remain attached if hybridized to 2 adjacent label extender probes. Next, amplifier probes, oligonucleotides labeled with alkaline phosphatase, are hybridized to the preamplifier probes. Finally, the assay is treated with a chemoreactive substrate that facilitates the chemiluminescent reaction and is read by a luminometer. This assay can be multiplexed by linking the capture probe to beads instead of the surface of a microwell (**Fig. 14**).

The signal in the bDNA assay is proportional to the number of alkaline phosphatase–labeled probes that hybridize to bDNA secondary sequences. As such, the target RNA can be blocked with blocking probes to increase the stringency of the primary probes bound to it. As with all chemiluminescent-based assays of this type, quantification is achieved by establishing a standard curve as well as negative and positive controls for each run.[31]

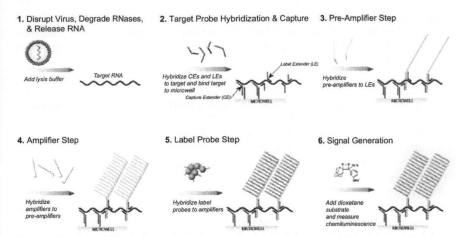

1. Disrupt Virus, Degrade RNases, & Release RNA

Add lysis buffer Target RNA

2. Target Probe Hybridization & Capture

Hybridize CEs and LEs
to target and bind target
to microwell

Capture Extender (CE)

Label Extender (LE)

3. Pre-Amplifier Step

Hybridize
pre-amplifiers to LEs

MICROWELL

4. Amplifier Step

Hybridize
amplifiers to
pre-amplifiers

MICROWELL

5. Label Probe Step

Hybridize label
probes to amplifiers

MICROWELL

6. Signal Generation

Add dioxetane
substrate
and measure
chemiluminescence

MICROWELL

Fig. 14. Illustration of virus detection using the Qauntiplex 3.0 assay via bDNA technology developed by the Bayer Corporation. (*From* Campàs M, Katakis I. DNA biochip arraying, detection and amplification strategies. Trends Analyt Chem 2004;23(1):59; with permission.)

IN SITU HYBRIDIZATION

In situ hybridization is simply the detection of specific genetic information within a morphologic context.[32] In situ hybridization facilitates simultaneous detection, localization, and quantification of individual DNA or RNA molecules at the cellular level in a fixed sample using labeled oligonucleotides or peptides as probes. This specialized type of solid-support assay involves taking morphologically intact tissue, cells, or chromosomes affixed to a glass microscope slide through the hybridization process. Briefly, after a tissue sample is fixed, it is permeabilized and labeled probes are added and allowed to hybridize to target molecules. The samples are then washed and viewed using bright-field or fluorescent microscopy.

Autoradiographic in situ hybridization, chromogenic in situ hybridization[33] (CISH), and fluorescence in situ hybridization (FISH) methods of detection have been applied. Evaluation of the final product is analogous to evaluation of immunohistochemistry and requires experience in histopathology. The strength of the method lies in linking microscopic morphologic evaluation with detection via hybridization.

The method also has applications in cytogenetic analysis of metaphase chromosome spreads or of interphase nuclei. In this context, the detection is usually accomplished via FISH. Detecting numerical aberrations or translocations of chromosomes can be achieved rapidly using probes for specific targets. FISH avoids some of the difficulties of conventional cytogenetics and may have greater sensitivity for some targets. Although FISH cannot completely replace karyotyping, it can complement and reduce the need for the frequency of cytogenetic analysis.[34]

Newer variations of FISH and CISH are exploiting the possibilities of automation (fast-FISH) and expanding the information that can be obtained in a single assay. Fluorescence immunophenotyping and interphase cytogenetics as a tool for investigation of neoplasms (FICTION) combines immunophenotyping with FISH, gold-facilitated in situ hybridization (GOLDFISH) is a gold-enhanced bright field chromogenic in situ gene amplification assay,[35] and fiber FISH makes it possible to detect and map chromosomal break points simultaneously. In situ hybridization can be labor intensive and tedious and, because of the extremely labile nature of mRNA, gives inconsistent results for molecular diagnostic purposes. Recent improvements, however, resulting in automated processing of slides through the assay, hold much promise for more widespread adoption of this technique.

Mass Spectrometry

Mass spectrometry (MS) is a technique that allows for the characterization/identification and quantification of molecules based on their mass and their ability to be positively ionized using a mass spectrometer.[36] Briefly, a molecule or mixture of molecules is first solubilized and then subsequently vaporized by a heat source. The vaporized molecules are simultaneously positively ionized by bombardment with high-speed electrons, causing electrons resident to the molecules to get displaced, resulting in molecules with a net positive charge. The ionized particles are then accelerated, typically along a U-shaped channel, which is sequentially lined by positively electrocharged deflector plates (some devices also use magnetic plates as well) until the particles collide with a detector plate, which records both the mass and charge of the colliding particle. The device then generates a spectrum of whole and fragmented particles based on mass and charge, which can be used for further analysis (**Fig. 15**).

Although this technique is powerful in its ability to help us analyze and quantify molecules, it alone is limited by the fragmentation it causes to larger molecules like proteins and strands of DNA.[37]

Chromatography-Coupled Mass Spectrometry

In an effort to cut down on the background that can result from a mass spectrograph composed of numerous different molecules and their fragments, MS can be coupled with either liquid chromatography or gas chromatography, which can fractionate

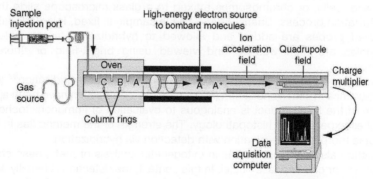

Fig. 15. A schematic view of the components of gas chromatography–mass spectroscopy instrumentation. On the left of the figure is the gas chromatographic system, where a volatilized compound is moved by an inert gas over a column consisting of rings coated with a liquid. Compounds C, B, and A separate on this column and are maintained in the gas phase by the oven that surrounds the column. The separated compounds then enter the mass spectrometer on the right side of the figure, where they are subjected to bombardment by electrons, resulting in molecule ion species. These ionic species then are accelerated in a field and are passed through an electric quadrupole field. Only those ions with a narrow range of mass/charge ratios pass through the tuned field so that they strike the detector. The electric currents that result are digitalized and stored in a computer that analyzes the data. (*From* Pincus MR, Bluth MH, Abraham NZ. Toxicology and therapeutic drug monitoring. In: McPherson RA, Pincus MR, editors. Henry's clinical diagnosis and management by laboratory methods. 23rd edition. New York: Saunders; 2017. p. 329; with permission.)

mixtures of molecules into purer samples before being fed directly into the mass spectrometer. Similar limitations exist, however, for the analysis of larger molecules.

Matrix-Assisted Laser Desorption/Ionization Mass Spectrometry

As discussed previously, the fragmentation of larger molecules, which results from their ionization via bombardment with high-speed electrons, is largely the reason why basic MS is unsuitable for analysis of biomolecules, such as proteins, peptides, or polymerized DNA. A newer methodology, however, for the ionization of molecules called matrix-assisted laser desorption/ionization (MALDI) has eliminated this shortcoming. Briefly, in MALDI, molecules in solution are applied to a crystalline matrix and allowed to dry. The sample and matrix material are then pulsed with a laser, vaporizing the sample from the matrix. Finally, the vaporized sample is ionized by protonation or deprotonation and is subsequently propelled through the apparatus (discussed previously).[38] This method of ionization results in far less fragmentation of these larger molecules. This allows for the analysis of mixtures of biomolecules found in cells.

Matrix-Assisted Laser Desorption/Ionization Time of Flight

For the study of larger molecules, such as biomolecules, an additional variation in the methodology has evolved where instead of simply analyzing the charge and mass of the molecules that strike the detector, the MS apparatus is outfitted with ion reflectors, which significantly increase the time of flight (TOF) of the molecules.[39] The differences in TOF are used in the analysis of the molecules resulting in a much greater sensitivity in identifying and quantifying the types of biomolecules present in the sample. This methodology has become increasingly more common in identifying the presence, numbers, and types of microorganisms in clinical samples[40–42] (Fig. 16).

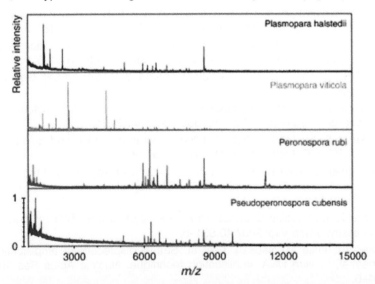

Fig. 16. Positive ion MALDI linear TOF mass spectra of intact spores of *Plasmopara halstedii*, *Plasmopara viticola*, *Peronospora rubi*, and *Pseudoperonospora cubensis*. The microorganisms were used in a concentration of 2 to 5 × 10⁹ spores per mL. All experiments were performed on a Microflex LRF20 MALDI-TOF mass spectrometer (Bruker Daltonik, Bremen, Germany). (*From* Chalupová J, Raus M, Sedlářová M, et al. Identification of fungal microorganisms by MALDI-TOF mass spectrometry. Biotechnol Adv 2014;32(1):236; with permission.)

Desorption Electrospray Ionization Mass Spectrometry

Another method by which to desorb and ionize the sample is by desorption electrospray ionization (DESI), in which the sample is dissolved in a fast-moving, ionic solvent, which causes ionization of the sample molecules but in a much gentler way than MALDI. This results in a greater maintenance of molecular integrity, allowing for the analysis of such things as protein-protein interactions, pharmacokinetics, and the molecular profiling of oncological biomarkers from living tissue in real time.[43] DESI can also be combined with MALDI and TOF analysis for MALDESI-TOF.

OTHER TECHNOLOGIES

Microarray-based technologies have the capacity to interrogate tens of thousands of genes at one time. As such, although array-based algorithms have been Food and Drug Administration approved in selective cases (p450 cytochrome oxidase), the application of the clinical marketplace is not well defined. General array–based and allele-specific (AS) methods, including AS oligonucleotide hybridization (ASOH) (for example dot blot analysis), AS-PCR, oligonucleotide ligation assay (OLA), pyrosequencing with applications to detection of cystic fibrosis CFTR (AS-PCR and OLA), α_1-antitrypsin deficiency, phenylketonuria mutations (AS-PCR), and low-resolution HLA typing (ASOH), KRAS, BRAF, LINE1 methylation mutations in multiple tumor types (pyrosequencing), among others, can be found elsewhere.[44,45] Time will determine, however, how such methods are to be interpreted, reported to physicians, and ultimately used for effective patient management.

REFERENCES

1. Saiki RK, Gelfand DH, Stoffel S, et al. Primer-directed enzymatic amplification of DNA with a thermostable DNA polymerase. Science 1988;239:487–91.
2. Myers TW, Gelfand DH. Reverse transcription and DNA amplification by a Thermus thermophilus DNA polymerase. Biochemistry 1991;30:7661–6.
3. Heid CA, Stevens J, Livak KJ, et al. Real time quantitative PCR. Genome Res 1996;6:986–94.
4. VanGuilder HD, Vrana KE, Freeman WM. Twenty-five years of quantitative PCR for gene expression analysis. Biotechniques 2008;44(5):619–26.
5. Spackman E, Suarez DL. Type A influenza virus detection and quantitation by real-time RT-PCR. Methods Mol Biol 2008;436:19–26.
6. Chamberlain JS, Gibbs RA, Ranier JE, et al. Deletion screening of the Duchenne muscular dystrophy locus via multiplex DNA amplification. Nucleic Acids Res 1988;16(23):11141–56.
7. Merante F, Yaghoubian S, Janeczko R. Principles of the xTAG respiratory viral panel assay. J Clin Virol 2007;40:S31–5.
8. Walker GT, Little M, Nadeau J, et al. Strand displacement amplification—an isothermal, in vitro DNA amplification technique. Nucleic Acids Res 1992;20: 1691–6.
9. Walker GT, Little MC, Nadeau JG, et al. Isothermal in vitro amplification of DNA by a restriction enzyme/DNA polymerase system. Proc Natl Acad Sci U S A 1992;89: 392–6.
10. Walker GT. Empirical aspects of strand displacement amplification [review]. PCR Methods Appl 1993;3(1):1–6.

11. Down JA, O'Connell MA, Dey MS, et al. Detection of Mycobacterium tuberculosis in respiratory specimens by strand displacement amplification of DNA. J Clin Microbiol 1996;34(4):860–5.

12. Available at: https://rokabio.com/technology/transcription-mediated-amplification/. Accessed April 5, 2018.

13. Ronaghi M, Uhlén M, Nyrén P. A sequencing method based on real-time pyrophosphate. Science 1998;281(5375):363.

14. Nyrén P. The history of pyrosequencing. Methods Mol Biol 2007;373:1–14.

15. Nordstrom T, Ronaghi M, Forsberg L, et al. Direct analysis of single-nucleotide polymorphism on double-stranded DNA by pyrosequencing. Biotechnol Appl Biochem 2000;31:107–12.

16. Fischer SG, Lerman LS. DNA fragments differing by single base-pair substitutions are separated in denaturing gradient gels: correspondence with melting theory. Proc Natl Acad Sci U S A 1983;80(6):1579–83.

17. Available at: http://www.ingeny.com/htdocs/DGGE.html. Accessed April 5, 2018.

18. McAuliffe L, Ellis Richard J, Lawes Jo R, et al. 16S rDNA PCR and denaturing gradient gel electrophoresis; a single generic test for detecting and differenti- ating mycoplasma species. J Med Microbiol 2005;54:731–9.

19. van der Hout Annemarie H, van den Ouweland Ans MW, van der Luijt Rob B, et al. A DGGE system for comprehensive mutation screening of BRCA1 and BRCA2: application in a Dutch cancer clinic setting. Hum Mutat 2006;27(7):654–66.

20. Ririe K, Rasmussen RP, Wittwer CT. Product differentiation by analysis of DNA melting curves during the polymerase chain reaction. Anal Biochem 1997;245:154–60.

21. Introduction to high resolution melt analysis guide. Available at: http://www.kapabiosystems.com/public/pdfs/kapa-hrm-fast-pcrkits/Introduction_to_High_Resolution_Melt _Analysis_Guide.pdf. Accessed April 5, 2018.

22. Alberts B, Johnson A, Lewis J, et al. Molecular biology of the cell. 5th edition. New York: Garland Science, Taylor & Francis Group; 2008. p. 538–9.

23. Southern EM. Detection of specific sequences among DNA fragments separated by gel electrophoresis. J Mol Biol 1975;98(3):503–17.

24. Alwine JC, Kemp DJ, Stark GR. Method for detection of specific RNAs in agarose gels by transfer to diazobenzyloxymethyl-paper and hybridization with DNA probes. Proc Natl Acad Sci U S A 1977;74(12):5350–4.

25. Kevil CG, Walsh L, Laroux FS, et al. An improved, rapid northern protocol. Biochem Biophys Res Commun 1997;238:277–9.

26. Rosetti S, Englisch S, Bresin E, et al. Detection of mutations in human genes by a new rapid method: cleavage fragment length polymorphism analysis (CFLPA). Mol Cell Probes 1997;11:155–60.

27. Molhuizen HO, Bunschoten AE, Schouls LM, et al. Rapid detection and simultaneous strain differentiation of Mycobacterium tuberculosis complex bacteria by spoligotyping. Methods Mol Biol 1998;101:381–94.

28. Cowan LS, Diem L, Brake MC, et al. Transfer of a Mycobacterium tuberculosis genotyping method, spoligotyping, from a reverse line-blot hybridization, membrane-based assay to the luminex multianalyte profiling system. J Clin Microbiol 2004;42(1):474–7.

29. Poljak M, Brenc-ic A, Seme K, et al. Comparative evaluation of first- and second-generation digene hybrid capture assays for detection of human pap- illomaviruses associated with high or intermediate risk for cervical cancer. J Clin Microbiol 1999;37(3):796–7.

30. Available at: http://www.thehpvtest.com/patient/how-the-hpv-test-works/. Accessed April 5, 2018
31. Collins ML, Zayati C, Detmer JJ, et al. Preparation and characterization of RNA standards for use in quantitative branched DNA hybridization assays. Anal Biochem 1995;226:120–9.
32. Gall JG, Pardue ML. Formation and detection of RNA-DNA hybrid molecules in cytological preparations. Proc Natl Acad Sci U S A 1969;63(2):378–83.
33. Tautz D, Pfeifle C. A non-radioactive in situ hybridization method for the localization of specific RNAs in Drosophila embryos reveals translational control of the segmentation gene hunchback. Chromosoma 1989;98(2):81–5.
34. Jin L, Lloyd RV. In situ hybridization: methods and applications. J Clin Lab Anal 1997;11(1):2–9.
35. Tubbs R, Pettay J, Skacel M, et al. Gold-facilitated in situ hybridization: a brightfield autometallographic alternative to fluorescence in situ hybridization for detection of HER-2/neu gene amplification. Am J Pathol 2002;160:1589–95.
36. Downard K. Mass spectrometry - a foundation course. Royal Society of Chemistry; 2004.
37. Fenn JB, Mann M, Meng CK, et al. Electrospray ionization for mass spectrometry of large biomolecules. Science 1989;246(4926):64–71.
38. Karas M, Krüger R. Ion formation in MALDI: the cluster ionization mechanism. Chem Rev 2003;103(2):427–40.
39. Guilhaus M. Principles and instrumentation in time-of-flight mass spectrometry. J Mass Spectrom 1995;30:1519–32.
40. Leggieri N, Rida A, Francois P, et al. Molecular diagnosis of bloodstream infections: planning to (physically) reach the bedside. Curr Opin Infect Dis 2010;23: 311–9.
41. La Scola B. Intact cell MALDI-TOF mass spectrometry-based approaches for the diagnosis of bloodstream infections. Expert Rev Mol Diagn 2011;11:287–98.
42. Liesenfeld O, Lehman L, Hunfeld K-P, et al. Molecular diagnosis of sepsis: new aspects and recent developments. Eur J Microbiol Immunol (Bp) 2014;4(1):1–25.
43. Zhang J, Rector J, Lin JQ, et al. Nondestructive tissue analysis for ex vivo and in vivo cancer diagnosis using a handheld mass spectrometry system. Sci Transl Med 2017;406:9.
44. Bluth MH. Hybridization array technologies in McPherson and Pincus: Henry's clinical diagnosis and management by laboratory methods. 23rd edition. New York: Saunders Publishing; 2017. p. 1328–36.
45. Best DH, Dames SA, Wooderchak-Donahue W, et al. Molecular pathology methods. Molecular pathology in clinical practice 2016;19–52.

Clinical Implication of MicroRNAs in Molecular Pathology: An Update for 2018

Seema Sethi, MD[a],*, Sajiv Sethi, MD[b], Martin H. Bluth, MD, PhD[c,d]

KEYWORDS

- miRNAs • Fine-needle aspirates • Serum • Pancreatic cancer • Prostate cancer

KEY POINTS

- The microRNAs (miRNAs) have immense potential in the clinical arena because they can be detected in the blood, serum, tissues (fresh and formalin-fixed paraffin-embedded), and also, fine-needle aspirate specimens. Recently novel in situ hybridization techniques have been described to detect miRNAs in tissues, which enables direct miRNA and histomorphologic correlation.
- Identification of novel molecular miRNAs and their target oncogenomic signatures have the potential to significantly impact clinical management.
- Incorporating miRNA expression profiling on tissue samples in the future may not only confirm diagnosis categorizing diseases and their subtypes but also may predict drug response in helping clinicians define the precise therapy to each individual.
- Increasing the knowledge of disease progression and tumor recurrence might also improve the development of personalized therapies.
- The most attractive feature of miRNA-based therapy is that a single miRNA could be useful for targeting multiple genes that are deregulated in cancers, which can be further investigated through systems biology and network analysis that will allow designing cancer-specific personalized therapy.

INTRODUCTION

In this era of personalized medicine, a plethora of molecular markers are emerging to be used as novel tools in molecular pathology. The role of the pathologist is no longer

The authors have nothing to disclose.
This article has been updated from a version previously published in Clinics in Laboratory Medicine, Volume 33, Issue 4, December 2013.
[a] Department of Pathology, University of Michigan and VA Hospital, E300, 2215 Fuller Road, Ann Arbor, MI 48105, USA; [b] Department of Gastroenterology, University of South Florida, 12901 Bruce B. Downs Boulevard, MDC 82, Tampa, FL 33612, USA; [c] Department of Pathology, Wayne State University, School of Medicine, 540 East Canfield Street, Detroit, MI 48201, USA; [d] Pathology Laboratories, Michigan Surgical Hospital, 21230 Dequindre Road, Warren, MI 48091, USA
* Corresponding author.
E-mail address: drsethi7@gmail.com

confined to being behind the glass slide. Rapid advances in the fields of molecular biology and medicine have led to the development of the newly maturing field of molecular pathology, which has ramifications for the therapeutic management of patients. This field incorporates the use of cellular molecules in the clinical arena for early and accurate diagnosis, determining prognosis and risk stratification of disease, as therapeutic targets for designing molecular therapies, disease surveillance, and more recently prevention of disease progression and metastasis.

The field of molecular pathology has revolutionized clinical medicine. It further directs to the development of a novel branch of molecular pharmacotherapeutics. This is a newly developed branch of pharmacology that evaluates the impact of human genetic variations that affect individual drug responses and further analyzes mechanisms to overcome drug resistance and tailor pharmacologic drug response based on molecular alterations within cells. It includes the potential and challenges of drug optimization, the implications for drug development and regulation, ethical and social aspects of pharmacogenomics, signal transduction, the use of knockout mice, and informed consent process in pharmacogenetic research. Based on gene expression patterns seen in different tumors in individualized patients, the tumor is classified into different genotypes and treated based on an independent set of molecular and genetic characteristics.[1] This molecular tumor profile is then used to select specific targeted treatment approaches for patients with specific types of cancer.[2] Furthermore, the response to molecular-based therapy is then evaluated, taking into consideration the patients' individual drug response and drug resistance of the tumor cells if any, and methods to overcome the same are explored.[3]

Recent literature reveals a deluge of several small molecule inhibitors with possible clinical use in future clinical trials.[4,5] However, before they can be brought into the clinical arena, there is an ongoing process of drug evaluation in vitro and in animal models. This has resulted in significant expansion of the responsibilities of the pathologist in identifying druggable targets, prognostic biomarkers, histopathologic risk predictors, and further assisting in developing molecular targeted therapies. It is in the realm of the pathologist to identify these small molecules, which can be targeted through these small molecule inhibitors. After the small molecular alterations are identified in a subset of tumor types, these are stratified by the pathologist into those that develop early in the course of carcinogenesis, making them relevant biomarkers of disease identification for early and accurate diagnosis. Additionally, the pathologist evaluates whether these small molecules can be used in risk stratification and to determine prognosis in specific tumors. Furthermore, the pathologist can assist in the drug trials in determining the efficacy of small molecule inhibitors in reducing the size of the tumor, reducing the number of tumor cells, and the overall tumor burden leading to pathologic and microscopic identification of druggable target molecules.

One recently described class of molecule that is showing far-reaching clinical effects in molecular pathology is that encompassing microRNA (miRNA) biology and technology.[6,7] These are small, noncoding endogenous single-stranded RNAs comprising only 19 to 25 nucleotides in length but on average of approximately 22 nucleotides in length.[6,7] First described in 1993, these molecules are actively comprised in the regulation of multiple physiologic and pathologic procedures in humans, animals, and plants. They regulate the physiologic embryonic stem cell differentiation,[7,8] and recent studies have also demonstrated their key roles in the pathogenetic evolution, progression, and metastasis of carcinomas.[9–11]

The proposed mechanism of action of miRNAs is through the posttranscriptional gene expression regulation through the 3′ untranslated region binding of target mRNAs.[7,8] This causes mRNA degradation or suppression of their translation to functional proteins.[4] Transcripts complementary to the 3′ untranslated region govern the translation by the RNA-RNA interaction. This results in the translational suppression or cleavage of the targeted mRNA because of the damaged complementarity between miRNA and mRNA. The miRNA genes transcript occurs by RNA polymerase II or III, which then yield primary miRNA. The location of maximum miRNA genes is in intergenic regions approximately 1 kilobase away from annotated genes.[7,8]

In addition to general transcriptional regulation of mRNA expression and translation, miRNAs also influence the development, progression, and metastasis of cancers.[6–8,12–14] Their functional effect may differ depending on their expression levels. They have either an oncogenic potential or tumor-suppressor effect depending on their downstream impact on target genes and thereby controlling the biologic manifestations of cancers.

Emerging evidence suggests that cancer stem cells (CSCs) and epithelial-to-mesenchymal transition phenotypic cells are regulated by the expression of miRNAs, implicating their role in chemo resistance and cancer metastasis.[15–17] There is evidence that these molecules are critical in the formation of CSCs, making them potential targets for overcoming drug resistance. Additionally, they have been proposed to have a part in the epithelial-to-mesenchymal transition phenomenon with implications in cancer drug resistance and metastasis.[17]

CLINICAL PERSPECTIVE

Cancers are a common clinical problem worldwide, leading to immense mortality, morbidity, and escalating health care costs. Despite rapid technologic and clinical advances, the cancer-related mortality and morbidity remain high, which also impacts patients' quality of life. Recent advances in the imaging and diagnostic modalities have resulted in early diagnosis of many cancers wherein select treatments have led to miraculous results with significant reduction in patient anguish. However, many malignancies remain occult until they have reached the late stages of the disease or have metastasized. The best of treatment options, including multimodal therapeutic approaches, have yielded minimal success in such instances. This underlines the need to use novel technologic advances in molecular biology from bench to patient bedside for clinical patient management. Moreover, the molecular mechanism of carcinogenesis, progression, and metastasis in some cancers is still largely unknown despite the "omics" revolution, which clearly suggests that further development in the areas of molecular signatures of disease aggressiveness is urgently needed.

Rapid progress occurring in technology and knowledge of molecular pathology has prompted a paradigm shift in the therapeutic patient management in the clinical arena. There is evidence of increasing integration of molecular markers with clinical and morphologic disease criteria to yield clinically relevant diagnostic, prognostic, and therapeutic algorithms for patient management. Moreover, selection of molecular targeted therapies and determination of prognosis and risk stratification of patients are being based on genomic and proteomic molecular diagnostic and prognostic signatures for patient care.

There is a unique opportunity to think outside the box and look at clinical problems in an analytical manner to solve cancer research dilemmas for the ultimate benefit of patients. Newly developed high-throughput, quantitative image-based methodologies for analysis and subcellular identification of alteration in cancers hold extreme promise in this regard. However, before these can be clinically applicable, they need to be correlated with the morphologic and clinical findings.

Cellular molecules, such as miRNAs, have an immense potential in the clinical realm of molecular pathology. Furthermore, one particular miRNA may target multiple genes in a context-dependent manner, suggesting that targeted deregulation of 1 miRNA will have effects on multiple targets, which seems to be an attractive attribute for cancer therapy. Therefore, modulating activity of miRNAs may provide openings for novel cancer interventions. They have widespread clinical application in various aspects of patient care because their expression levels vary in different tumors and also alter with the disease progression.

Several miRNAs with oncogenic potential have been demonstrated to be upregulated in cancers and miRNAs with tumor-suppressive effect are downregulated in malignancies. Translating the application of miRNAs in clinical context has been enhanced by the applicability of several novel high-throughput multiplex technologies on a wide variety of patient samples, including blood, serum, tissues (fresh and formalin-fixed paraffin-embedded [FFPE]), and cerebrospinal fluid.[12,13,18–20] Apart from being able to decipher small molecules, these technologies lower laboratory costs, increase operational productivity, and enhance yield.[21–24] These are an integral part of the clinical armamentarium of the new-age pathologist, which has strengthened diagnostic capabilities in the move forward into the era of precision medicine.

Therapeutic decision-making and patient clinical management in the current clinical practice is being dictated more by alterations occurring in the tumor microenvironment at the molecular level, namely genetic, epigenetic, miRNA, and multispectral protein levels than by the histomorphology spectrum alone. This has led to a multisystem approach to a patient that includes a team composed of several clinicians with expertise in medical, surgical, pathology, molecular biology, and pharmacotherapeutics working together in synergy for the maximum benefit of the patient, minimizing the side effects and using drugs with targeted approach to achieve the goal of personalized medicine.

USE OF MOLECULAR PATHOLOGY PRACTICE

Molecular diagnostic applications are now an integral part of the management algorithms of several solid tumors. With the use of molecular diagnostics in oncology, pathologists hope to assist early and accurate diagnosis of malignant disease processes during initial workup. Molecular diagnostics also can help in risk stratification based on molecular parameters. Additionally, one can use the molecular biomarkers for disease surveillance during treatment and follow-up. Emerging evidence directed to the complex molecular changes involved in the development and progression of different malignancies produced innovative diagnostic molecular tools leading to the introduction of targeted therapies. In lung cancer, miR-27a regulation of MET, EGFR, and Sprouty2 is being explored for targeted therapies.[25] The promising therapeutic targets for patients with osteosarcoma include integrin, ezrin, statin, NOTCH/HES1, matrix metalloproteinases, and miR-215.[26] The miR-205BP/S3 is a possible promising therapeutic modality for melanoma.[27] The miR-34a may act as a tumor-suppressor miRNA of hepatocellular carcinoma, and current efforts are under way to evaluate strategies to increase miR-34a level as a critical targeted therapy for hepatocellular carcinoma.[28]

Promising candidate biomarkers are being discovered that may soon switch to the realm of clinical management of malignancies. There is a need for new and improved molecular-based treatment options to improve on the modest outcome in patients with cancer. Prognostic molecular biomarkers require validation, which may be challenging at times, to help clinicians classify patients in need of early diagnosis. Recognizing predictive biomarkers that will stratify response to developing targeted therapeutics is additionally required in arenas of cancer research and patient management. Furthermore, there is a need to identify clinically strong molecular tests to classify patients who are further responsive to certain drugs, in the early treatment design based on well-certified molecular prognosticators.

Scientific discoveries of molecular markers are often prematurely highlighted before the completion of clinical trials to establish appropriate application to disease. Before clinicians can use the molecular findings for clinical patient use, there is a need for evidence-based guidelines established by knowledgeable clinicians to communicate emerging molecular clinical standards.

ROLE OF microRNAs IN CLINICAL SPECIMENS

miRNA research has advanced within a decade from one publication to thousands of publications describing their role in gene regulation. miRNA expression profiling has been recently evaluated as a reliable diagnostic biomarker for differentiating between normal and tumor specimens.[6–8,12,29,30] It has shown to be deregulated in multiple cancers in human and mouse models, and has proved to play a critical role in the development and progression of the tumor.[6,7,12,29,30] Most of the miRNAs are differentially expressed, whereas some of them discriminate totally between normal and tumorigenic samples. The miRNA expression enhances (oncogenic miRNA) or reduces (tumor suppressor) as the tumor progresses and was found to be associated with drug resistance.[31]

This discovery of miRNA a decade ago, as a diagnostic and prognostic marker, has now led to miRNA-based targeted therapy in vitro, and may selectively predict better treatment outcome for patients with cancer. In addition, classification of an unknown tumor may be possible by the alteration of tumor-specific miRNA.[32] The nomenclature for assigning names to novel miRNAs for publication in peer-reviewed journals is done by miRBase, which is the central repository for miRNA sequence information.[33] It has an online database with all published miRNA sequences with links to the primary literature and to other secondary databases. Although some miRNAs are tumor specific,[32] miR-21 has proved to be the global oncogenic miRNA in many solid tumors.[34–39] The miRNAs with oncogenic potential include miR-155, miR-17 to 92, and miR-21,[7] but it is not limited to these alone. The level of expression of miR-155 is upregulated in various carcinomas.[40–42] However, they are specifically significant in pancreatic cancers where they have prognostic relevance.[12,40,42,43]

Similarly, miRNA let-7 family and miR-200 family is frequently downregulated in many types of cancer, suggesting their role as a general tumor suppressor.[29,44–48] Low levels of let-7 miRNA[49] have been shown to have poorer prognosis with shorter postoperative survival in human lung cancer.[50] The tumor-suppressor miR-34 is directly transactivated and induced by p53 signaling in the inhibition of human pancreatic cancer tumor-initiating cells.[51] Based on a recent literature review, it has been suggested that modulation of miRNAs is a novel molecular targeted therapeutic approach for cancer in vivo.[52] This has led to the development of an emerging field of miRNA pharmacotherapeutics, which involves altering the expression of miRNAs, which can inhibit cancer growth.[44] The therapeutic strategies suggested using miRNAs include the inhibition of upregulated miRNAs and reexpression of tumor-suppressor miRNAs. They have also been shown to affect CSCs in overcoming drug resistance.[14] Regulation of miRNA levels in patients with ongoing cancer therapies would likely enhance the efficacy of their ongoing therapies.

Several synthetic small molecule inhibitors of miRNAs, such as chemically modified antisense oligonucleotides called "antagomiRs," are currently in use in vitro, targeting against specific oncogenic miRNAs. These antagomiRs silence the overexpressed oncogenic miRNAs in cancers by blocking their function.[7,30] In animal experiments, antagomiRs against miR-16, miR-122, miR-192, and miR-194 were found to be efficacious in reducing the levels of miRNA in the liver, lung, kidney, and ovaries.[52] Reexpression of tumor-suppressor miRNA, such as let-7, is another proposed miRNA therapeutic strategy to upregulate tumor-suppressor miRNA by exogenously transfecting with pre-let-7 that led to the inhibition of growth in vitro and in vivo.[15,44] These characteristics of miRNA suggest their potential role as novel biomarkers for diagnostic, prognostic, and therapeutic targets (**Fig. 1**).

METHODOLOGY AND CLINICAL IMPLICATIONS
Purification of microRNA from Human Plasma

The discovery of circulating miRNAs and their stability in plasma and serum is an interesting characteristic that could be used as noninvasive biomarkers for a variety of cancers, providing valuable tools to observe the changes during tumor progression.[29] Isolating miRNA of appropriate quality and quantity from blood is critical. Exosome RNA seems to be the richest source of miRNA in the serum or plasma. We have successfully isolated RNA from plasma samples,[29] and the detailed methodology is described next. Initially, the steps are carried out on ice, but later at room

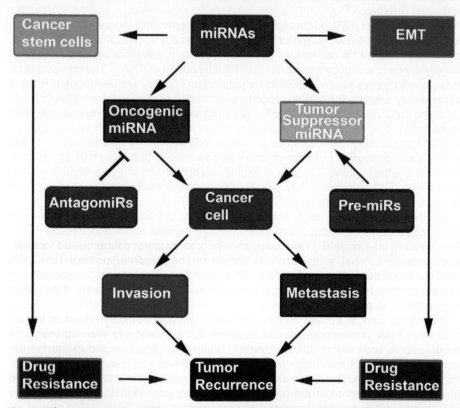

Fig. 1. Schematic representation on the relationship between CSCs and miRNAs with tumor aggressiveness, and the role of antagomiRs and pre-miRNAs on oncogenic and tumor-suppressive miRNAs. EMT, epithelial-to-mesenchymal transition. (*From* Sethi S, Ali S, Kong D, et al. Clinical implication of microRNAs in molecular pathology. Clin Lab Med 2013;33(4):778; with permission.)

temperature. Approximately 250 mL of plasma from each sample is centrifuged at 1000 *g* for 5 minutes to remove debris. The plasma is then transferred (200 mL) into a new tube along with 750 mL of QIAzol master mix containing 800 mL of QIAzol and 1 mg of MS2 RNA, and incubated for 5 minutes at room temperature. To this, 200 mL of chloroform is added, mixed well, and incubated for 5 minutes at room temperature, followed by centrifugation at 12,000 *g* for 15 minutes. All the subsequent steps are carried out at room temperature (20–25°C). The upper aqueous phase is moved into a new microtube containing a 1.5 volume of ethanol. After mixing well, the solution is then transferred onto the RNeasy Mini Spin Column with approximately 750 mL each time, and centrifuged at 13,000 *g* for 30 seconds. The flow-through is discarded, and the steps are repeated until the entire sample is used. The RNeasy Mini Column is then washed once with 700 mL of RWT, and 3 times with 500 mL RPE provided with the kit, and centrifuged for 13,000 *g* for 1 minute. The flow-through is discarded each time. The RNA (containing miRNA) is eluted with approximately 25 mL of water in a new collection tube by centrifugation and stored at 80°C.

The amount of RNA obtained from blood is usually too low a yield compared with RNA obtained from tissue samples to be quantified using single-drop spectrophotometry technology (ie, NanoDrop). However, there are several miRNAs that are detectable in plasma or serum samples thus displaying the presence of miRNAs. One such miRNA is miR-21, which can be detected by conventional real-time reverse-transcriptase polymerase chain reaction (RT-PCR) methodology, and is described next with significant modification using Exiqon-Universal cDNA synthesis kit (Exiqon, Woburn, MA).[12]

Reverse-Transcriptase Reaction

The RT reaction is performed by using Exiqon-Universal cDNA synthesis kit. The cDNA for standard curve is synthesized by reverse transcription using the template mature miRNAs, which can be prepared by diluting it with water. The RT reaction is set up with 20 mL of sample containing 4 mL of 5x RT buffer, 2 mL of enzyme mixture, 10 mL of water, and 4 mL of either the plasma miRNA or 250 nM of standard miRNA for 1 hour at 42°C, and 5 minutes at 95°C. The cDNA samples can be stored at −20°C.

Polymerase Chain Reaction

Multiple housekeeping genes are used in triplicate for data normalization and for analysis by the standard C_t method of quantification using StepOnePlus Real-Time PCR (Applied Biosystems, Foster City, CA). They also serve as controls for variability in sample loading. The sample testing is performed in equivalent with standards to evade batch effects as described next.

The miRNA standard cDNA is diluted in water. The standard curve is set up in triplicate with 5 points starting at 10,000, 5000, 2500, 1250, and 625 copy number. The plasma cDNA is diluted to 20-fold. The real-time PCR reaction is set up with a total volume of 10 mL containing 5 mL of SYBR Green (Applied Biosystems), 1 mL of PCR primer mix, and 4 mL of either the diluted cDNA from miRNA standard or the plasma cDNA, using standard curve model. The plasma miRNA concentration is calculated in 10^{-2} pM units using the Quantity value *3.125/6.02/1000. The reproducibility of the quantitative RT-PCR (qRT-PCR) assay data confirms the efficient extraction of miRNAs from plasma samples.

The method described previously has no limitations or interferences with respect to miRNA extraction and RT-PCR.

METHODOLOGY USING THE MAIN RESOURCES OF FORMALIN-FIXED TISSUES

Because the availability of fresh or frozen tissue is typically limited, archival collections of FFPE tissues are highly desirable and provide a rich source for the study of human disease. Tissue blocks are available worldwide from nearly every patient with well-documented clinical data including histopathologic reports, which makes it ideal to carry out research studies. The summarized methodology of plasma and fine-needle aspirate (FNA) samples is shown in **Fig. 2**. Of interest is that miRNA, because of its strong structure and smaller size, remains protected from degradation during the fixation process, and requires only a small amount to perform miRNA expression profiles or RT-PCR. A recent study using clinical specimens from prostate cancer has demonstrated the use of this in the clinical context.[6] The following section highlights the collection of FNA from tumor mass and the fixation method.

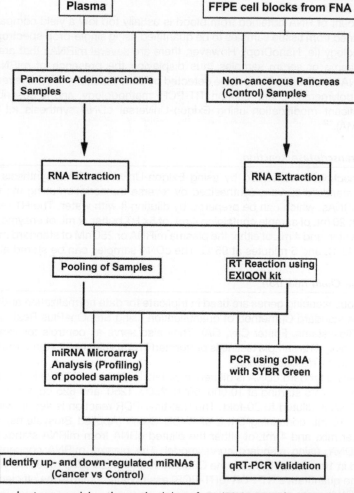

Fig. 2. Flow chart summarizing the methodology for miRNA research using plasma and FFPE cell blocks of FNA samples. (*From* Sethi S, Ali S, Kong D, et al. Clinical implication of micro-RNAs in molecular pathology. Clin Lab Med 2013;33(4):780; with permission.)

Fine-Needle Aspiration Tissue Collection

Diagnostic FNAs from tumor mass can be collected using a 20-gauge to 23-gauge needle from patients with pancreatic cancer (or other cancers) who underwent computerized tomography or endoscopic ultrasound–guided biopsy. Diagnostic smears are stained using Diff-Quick staining (Mercedes Medical, Sarasota, FL). The aspirates are put in fixative fluid, centrifuged, and embedded in paraffin using standard protocol, and are stained by hematoxylin-eosin for the presence of tumor cells. Approximately 50 cells are required to obtain excellent quality and quantity of total RNA (consisting of miRNA) to perform qRT-PCR. For the comparative purpose, normal pancreatic tissues that are farther away from the pancreatic tumor (typically obtained from surgical specimens) also can be similarly fixed to serve as controls.

RNA Isolation

The miRNA is isolated from FFPE tissue using RNeasy Kit (QIAGEN, Valencia, CA) following the manufacturer's protocol with a few modifications, which are described next. Four 10-mm thick and approximately 1 cm in diameter tissue curls are placed in 1 mL of xylene, mixed, and centrifuged for 2 minutes at room temperature. One milliliter of ethanol is added to the pellet and centrifuged for 2 minutes, and mixed with 240 mL of Buffer PKD along with 10 mL of proteinase K and incubated at 55°C, and then at 80°C for 15 minutes each. The mixture is then centrifuged, and the collected flow-through is mixed with 500 mL of buffer RBC to adjust binding conditions. The solution is mixed with ethanol and applied to the RNeasy column, and washed with buffer solution. The total RNA containing miRNA is eluted with RNase-free water. The purity of RNA is measured by the absorption ratio at 260/280 nm and quantified using Nano-Drop 2000 (Thermo Scientific, Pittsburgh, PA). The ratio of 260/280 typically ranges between 1.8 and 2.1.

Real-Time Reverse-Transcriptase Polymerase Chain Reaction

The RT reaction is performed with SYBR Green miRNA-based assay using Exiqon-Universal cDNA synthesis kit (Exiqon). The RT reaction is set up with 10 mL of sample containing 2 mL of 5 RT buffer, 1 mL of enzyme mixture, 2 mL of water, and 10 ng of total RNA in 5 mL for 1 hour at 42°C and 5 minutes at 95°C. All reactions for PCR are carried out in triplicate using StepOnePlus Real-Time PCR (Applied Biosystems). The expression level of miRNAs is analyzed using C_t method.

microRNA Profiling

The prognosis of patients with cancer remains poor. Hence, new biomarkers are essential for early detection of cancer progression. The miRNA profiling can be useful as biomarkers for differentiating tumor from normal samples from plasma, FNA, or surgical tissue samples as discussed in many recent reports.[6,12,29,38,53] For example, equal amount of RNA containing miRNA and combined separately from control and patient samples can be analyzed for miRNA microarray profiling (LC Sciences, Houston, TX). The data are normalized using multiple housekeeping genes. Differentially regulated miRNAs between normal and cancer samples are analyzed using various statistical methodologies (eg, hierarchical clustering). Network analyses are accomplished using World Wide Web–based bioinformatics software programs, such as Ingenuity Pathway Analysis software (Ingenuity Systems, Redwood City, CA) functional network analysis. Pathway analysis is a new innovative tool that reveals the expression of deregulated[12] miRNAs and their putative targets in a signaling pathway.[6,54] Because each miRNA may have more than 1 target, miRNA-based therapy can be beneficial to target multiple signaling pathways, which include inhibition of oncogenic miRNAs by antisense oligonucleotides or by overexpression of tumor-suppressor miRNA by precursor miRNAs.[6,30,44]

ADVANCES MADE IN CHARACTERIZING microRNA PROFILING

Because there is an urgent need to investigate potential biomarkers for early detection of malignancies in a fast and straightforward way, miRNA research has made a significant impact on many types of cancer research, revealing basic gene expression changes toward identifying major signaling pathways involved in biomedical research. It empowers efficient profiling of deregulated miRNAs in plasma, serum, FFPE, and many other sample types because of their stability, which enables their detection and analysis, thus leading to a potentially reliable biomarker. Profiling of miRNAs not only provides access to hundreds of expressed miRNAs in the sample, but also differentiates between healthy and diseased state. Some of the miRNAs are substantially upregulated or downregulated in cancer cells or tumor tissues relative to normal cells or normal tissues, permitting the identification of miRNA signature. Differential expression of lead candidate miRNAs can be individually further validated by RT-PCR; however, it is unlikely that any one of the conventional housekeeping genes will be sufficient to normalize the data. Hence, the use of multiple housekeeping genes for data normalization using the standard method of quantification may be the ideal way of performing miRNA profiling. Overall, miRNA profiling is one of the most current methods to differentiate abnormally expressed miRNAs in a set of samples.

DIAGNOSTIC AND PROGNOSTIC IMPLICATIONS OF microRNAs

Biomarkers that are predictive, prognostic, and diagnostic can be a valuable tool to clinicians in making important decisions about patient care.[6] The discovery of circulating miRNAs in plasma and serum, because of their noninvasive nature, are excellent biomarkers for a variety of cancer detection and prognostic purposes. We have previously shown circulating miRNAs as biomarkers in pancreatic cancer. A previous report by Ali and colleagues[29] has identified a group of 7 miRNAs including 2 oncogenic and 5 tumor-suppressor miRNAs that were recognized and validated as a diagnostic marker in 50 plasma samples from patients with pancreatic cancer in comparison with healthy control subjects. Similar reports on FNA from FFPE cell blocks in patients with pancreatic cancer also identified 7 miRNAs that were differentially expressed in tumor cells compared with normal tissues.[12] These 7 miRNAs both from plasma and FNA showed substantial differences in their expression level and hence may serve as diagnostic biomarkers in the detection of cancer. In addition, the Ingenuity networking pathway analysis in FNA study provided a unique strategy to study various signaling pathways, which revealed 15 biofunctional network groups relating to cancer, genetic disorder, and gastrointestinal disease that are expected to improve prognosis and response to certain therapies.[12] Other investigators also performed miRNA profiling in various other solid tumors to discover a differentially expressed panel of miRNAs in pooled samples that reached excellent diagnostic properties to classify them as biomarkers for cancer detection.[34,38,53,55] Novel high-throughput multiplex technologies hold immense promise in this regard. However, before these can be clinically applicable, these need to be correlated with the morphologic and clinical findings to decipher those that are clinically relevant. Additional studies are needed to edify miRNA biomarkers to reduce patient mortality, morbidity, and introduce early diagnosis, thereby reducing health care costs and applying these approaches to patient care.

RECENT ADVANCES IN THE FIELD OF microRNAs

miRNAs are rapidly evolving as significant molecular markers in the fields of oncology, clinical diagnostics, and therapeutics. Rapid advances in the diagnostic technologies of miRNAs have led to identification of these molecules in several body fluids as circulating biomarkers of disease.[56] This has led to markedly increased potential of miRNAs in the clinical arena.[57] miRNA therapeutics is currently evolving with clinical applications in several disease conditions, including cardiac disorders[58] and malignancies.[59] Recent techniques describing purification and detection of miRNAs in the urine specimens has tremendously increased the noninvasive clinical potential of this molecule in early diagnosis, prognosis, and surveillance of different malignancies, especially urothelial carcinomas.[60] Not only are the miRNAs being used for oncology but also have wide-ranging potential applications in several clinical conditions, including sepsis,[61] hepatic diseases,[62] including drug-induced liver injury,[63] atherosclerosis,[64] and Parkinson disease,[65] among others. Prior knowledge of the action of miRNAs targeting CSCs is now being used in the field of oncotherapeutics as a new paradigm for cancer treatment and prevention of tumor recurrence.[59] miR-17 miRNA family is currently being evaluated as a therapeutic strategy against vulvar carcinoma.[66] miRNAs are also being used to predict response to therapy in patients with malignancies, including prediction of response to radiation therapy in non–small-cell lung carcinoma.[67] Overall, miRNAs hold great promise as molecular biomarkers with immense potential in early diagnosis, prognosis, and therapeutics in wide-ranging malignancies including ovarian cancer,[68] prostate carcinoma,[69] head and neck carcinomas,[70] and breast carcinomas[71] in this area of personalized medicine.

SUMMARY

The miRNAs have immense potential in the clinical arena because they can be detected in the blood, serum, tissues (fresh and FFPE), and FNA specimens. Identification of novel molecular miRNAs and their target oncogenomic signatures has the potential to significantly impact clinical management. The discovery of miRNAs and their expression profile in a wide variety of cancers has led investigators to understand the key role of miRNAs as biomarkers during cancer progression. Incorporating miRNA expression profiling on tissue samples in the future may not only confirm diagnosis categorizing diseases and their subtypes, but also may predict drug response in helping clinicians define the precise therapy to each patient. Moreover, increasing the knowledge of disease progression and tumor recurrence might also improve the development of personalized therapies. The most attractive feature of miRNA-based therapy is that a single miRNA could be useful for targeting multiple genes that are deregulated in cancers, which can be further investigated through systems biology and network analysis that allows designing cancer-specific personalized therapy. In summary, miRNAs are poised to provide diagnostic, prognostic, and therapeutic targets for several diseases, including malignancies for precision medicine.

REFERENCES

1. Lei Z, Tan IB, Das K, et al. Identification of molecular subtypes of gastric cancer with different responses to PI3-kinase inhibitors and 5-fluorouracil. Gastroenterology 2013;145:554–65.
2. Elghannam DM, Ibrahim L, Ebrahim MA, et al. Association of MDR1 gene polymorphism (G2677T) with imatinib response in Egyptian chronic myeloid leukemia patients. Hematology 2014;19(3):123–8.

3. Tan J, Yu Q. Molecular mechanisms of tumor resistance to PI3K-mTOR targeted cancer therapy. Chin J Cancer 2013;32(7):376–9.

4. Lv X, Ma X, Hu Y. Furthering the design and the discovery of small molecule ATP-competitive mTOR inhibitors as an effective cancer treatment. Expert Opin Drug Discov 2013;8(8):991–1012.

5. Rai G, Vyjayanti VN, Dorjsuren D, et al. Small Molecule Inhibitors of the Human Apurinic/apyrimidinic Endonuclease 1 (APE1) 2010 [Updated 2013]. In: Probe Reports from the NIH Molecular Libraries Program [Internet]. Bethesda (MD): National Center for Biotechnology Information (US); 2010. Available at: https://www.ncbi.nlm.nih.gov/books/NBK133448/. Accessed March 27, 2018.

6. Sethi S, Kong D, Land S, et al. Comprehensive molecular oncogenomic profiling and miRNA analysis of prostate cancer. Am J Transl Res 2013;5:200–11.

7. Sethi S, Sarkar FH. Evolving concept of cancer stem cells: role of micro-RNAs and their implications in tumor aggressiveness. J Carcinogene Mutagene 2011;(S1):005.

8. Hassan O, Ahmad A, Sethi S, et al. Recent updates on the role of microRNAs in prostate cancer. J Hematol Oncol 2012;5:9.

9. Bao L, Yan Y, Xu C, et al. MicroRNA-21 suppresses PTEN and hSulf-1 expression and promotes hepatocellular carcinoma progression through AKT/ERK pathways. Cancer Lett 2013;337(2):226–36.

10. Lei H, Zou D, Li Z, et al. MicroRNA-219-2-3p functions as a tumor suppressor in gastric cancer and is regulated by DNA methylation. PLoS One 2013;8:e60369.

11. Shen SN, Wang LF, Jia YF, et al. Upregulation of microRNA-224 is associated with aggressive progression and poor prognosis in human cervical cancer. Diagn Pathol 2013;8:69.

12. Ali S, Saleh H, Sethi S, et al. MicroRNA profiling of diagnostic needle aspirates from patients with pancreatic cancer. Br J Cancer 2012;107:1354–60.

13. Qazi AM, Gruzdyn O, Semaan A, et al. Restoration of E-cadherin expression in pancreatic ductal adenocarcinoma treated with microRNA-101. Surgery 2012; 152:704–11.

14. Ahmad A, Sarkar SH, Bitar B, et al. Garcinol regulates EMT and Wnt signaling pathways in vitro and in vivo, leading to anticancer activity against breast cancer cells. Mol Cancer Ther 2012;11:2193–201.

15. Kong D, Heath E, Chen W, et al. Loss of let-7 up-regulates EZH2 in prostate cancer consistent with the acquisition of cancer stem cell signatures that are attenuated by BR-DIM. PLoS One 2012;7:e33729.

16. Ahmad A, Aboukameel A, Kong D, et al. Phosphoglucose isomerase/autocrine motility factor mediates epithelial-mesenchymal transition regulated by miR-200 in breast cancer cells. Cancer Res 2011;71:3400–9.

17. Kong D, Banerjee S, Ahmad A, et al. Epithelial to mesenchymal transition is mechanistically linked with stem cell signatures in prostate cancer cells. PLoS One 2010;5:e12445.

18. Baraniskin A, Kuhnhenn J, Schlegel U, et al. MicroRNAs in cerebrospinal fluid as biomarker for disease course monitoring in primary central nervous system lymphoma. J Neurooncol 2012;109:239–44.

19. Brunet VA, Pericay C, Moya I, et al. microRNA expression profile in stage III colorectal cancer: circulating miR-18a and miR-29a as promising biomarkers. Oncol Rep 2013;30:320–6.

20. Ulivi P, Foschi G, Mengozzi M, et al. Peripheral blood miR-328 expression as a potential biomarker for the early diagnosis of NSCLC. Int J Mol Sci 2013;14: 10332–42.

21. Bi S, Cui Y, Li L. Dumbbell probe-mediated cascade isothermal amplification: a novel strategy for label-free detection of microRNAs and its application to real sample assay. Anal Chim Acta 2013;760:69–74.
22. Gu LQ, Wanunu M, Wang MX, et al. Detection of miRNAs with a nanopore single-molecule counter. Expert Rev Mol Diagn 2012;12:573–84.
23. Guan DG, Liao JY, Qu ZH, et al. mirExplorer: detecting microRNAs from genome and next generation sequencing data using the AdaBoost method with transition probability matrix and combined features. RNA Biol 2011;8:922–34.
24. Luo S. MicroRNA expression analysis using the Illumina microRNA-Seq Platform. Methods Mol Biol 2012;822:183–8.
25. Acunzo M, Romano G, Palmieri D, et al. Cross-talk between MET and EGFR in non-small cell lung cancer involves miR-27a and Sprouty2. Proc Natl Acad Sci U S A 2013;110:8573–8.
26. Yang J, Zhang W. New molecular insights into osteosarcoma targeted therapy. Curr Opin Oncol 2013;25:398–406.
27. Noguchi S, Iwasaki J, Kumazaki M, et al. Chemically modified synthetic microRNA-205 inhibits the growth of melanoma cells in vitro and in vivo. Mol Ther 2013;21:1204–11.
28. Dang Y, Luo D, Rong M, et al. Underexpression of miR-34a in hepatocellular carcinoma and its contribution towards enhancement of proliferating inhibitory effects of agents targeting c-MET. PLoS One 2013;8:e61054.
29. Ali S, Almhanna K, Chen W, et al. Differentially expressed miRNAs in the plasma may provide a molecular signature for aggressive pancreatic cancer. Am J Transl Res 2010;3:28–47.
30. Ali S, Banerjee S, Logna F, et al. Inactivation of Ink4a/Arf leads to deregulated expression of miRNAs in K-Ras transgenic mouse model of pancreatic cancer. J Cell Physiol 2012;227:3373–80.
31. Ali S, Ahmad A, Banerjee S, et al. Gemcitabine sensitivity can be induced in pancreatic cancer cells through modulation of miR-200 and miR-21 expression by curcumin or its analogue CDF. Cancer Res 2010;70:3606–17.
32. Liang Y, Ridzon D, Wong L, et al. Characterization of microRNA expression profiles in normal human tissues. BMC Genomics 2007;8:166.
33. Griffiths-Jones S. miRBase: microRNA sequences and annotation. Curr Protoc Bioinformatics 2010;29:12.9.1–12.9.10.
34. Gall TM, Frampton AE, Krell J, et al. Blood-based miRNAs as noninvasive diagnostic and surrogative biomarkers in colorectal cancer. Expert Rev Mol Diagn 2013;13:141–5.
35. Hermansen SK, Dahlrot RH, Nielsen BS, et al. MiR-21 expression in the tumor cell compartment holds unfavorable prognostic value in gliomas. J Neurooncol 2013;111:71–81.
36. Si H, Sun X, Chen Y, et al. Circulating microRNA-92a and microRNA-21 as novel minimally invasive biomarkers for primary breast cancer. J Cancer Res Clin Oncol 2013;139:223–9.
37. Sicard F, Gayral M, Lulka H, et al. Targeting miR-21 for the therapy of pancreatic cancer. Mol Ther 2013;21(5):986–94.
38. Tang D, Shen Y, Wang M, et al. Identification of plasma microRNAs as novel noninvasive biomarkers for early detection of lung cancer. Eur J Cancer Prev 2013;22(6):540–8.
39. Yang SM, Huang C, Li XF, et al. miR-21 confers cisplatin resistance in gastric cancer cells by regulating PTEN. Toxicology 2013;306:162–8.

40. Liu R, Liao J, Yang M, et al. Circulating miR-155 expression in plasma: a potential biomarker for early diagnosis of esophageal cancer in humans. J Toxicol Environ Health A 2012;75:1154–62.
41. Yang M, Shen H, Qiu C, et al. High expression of miR-21 and miR-155 predicts recurrence and unfavourable survival in non-small cell lung cancer. Eur J Cancer 2013;49:604–15.
42. Zhang Y, Roccaro AM, Rombaoa C, et al. LNA-mediated anti-miR-155 silencing in low-grade B-cell lymphomas. Blood 2012;120:1678–86.
43. Yabushita S, Fukamachi K, Tanaka H, et al. Circulating microRNAs in serum of human K-ras oncogene transgenic rats with pancreatic ductal adenocarcinomas. Pancreas 2012;41:1013–8.
44. Ali S, Ahmad A, Aboukameel A, et al. Increased Ras GTPase activity is regulated by miRNAs that can be attenuated by CDF treatment in pancreatic cancer cells. Cancer Lett 2012;319:173–81.
45. Bhutia YD, Hung SW, Krentz M, et al. Differential processing of let-7a precursors influences RRM2 expression and chemosensitivity in pancreatic cancer: role of LIN-28 and SET oncoprotein. PLoS One 2013;8:e53436.
46. Hu X, Guo J, Zheng L, et al. The heterochronic microRNA let-7 inhibits cell motility by regulating the genes in the actin cytoskeleton pathway in breast cancer. Mol Cancer Res 2013;11:240–50.
47. Kang HW, Crawford M, Fabbri M, et al. A mathematical model for microRNA in lung cancer. PLoS One 2013;8:e53663.
48. Zaman MS, Maher DM, Khan S, et al. Current status and implications of microRNAs in ovarian cancer diagnosis and therapy. J Ovarian Res 2012;5:44.
49. Jusufovic E, Rijavec M, Keser D, et al. let-7b and miR-126 are down-regulated in tumor tissue and correlate with microvessel density and survival outcomes in non–small-cell lung cancer. PLoS One 2012;7:e45577.
50. Xia XM, Jin WY, Shi RZ, et al. Clinical significance and the correlation of expression between Let-7 and K-ras in non-small cell lung cancer. Oncol Lett 2010;1:1045–7.
51. Vogt M, Munding J, Gruner M, et al. Frequent concomitant inactivation of miR-34a and miR-34b/c by CpG methylation in colorectal, pancreatic, mammary, ovarian, urothelial, and renal cell carcinomas and soft tissue sarcomas. Virchows Arch 2011;458:313–22.
52. Krutzfeldt J, Rajewsky N, Braich R, et al. Silencing of microRNAs in vivo with 'antagomirs'. Nature 2005;438:685–9.
53. Callari M, Dugo M, Musella V, et al. Comparison of microarray platforms for measuring differential microRNA expression in paired normal/cancer colon tissues. PLoS One 2012;7:e45105.
54. Azmi AS, Ali S, Banerjee S, et al. Network modeling of CDF treated pancreatic cancer cells reveals a novel c-myc-p73 dependent apoptotic mechanism. Am J Transl Res 2011;3:374–82.
55. Lang MF, Yang S, Zhao C, et al. Genome-wide profiling identified a set of miRNAs that are differentially expressed in glioblastoma stem cells and normal neural stem cells. PLoS One 2012;7:e36248.
56. Jung HJ, Suh Y. Circulating miRNAs in ageing and ageing-related diseases. J Genet Genomics 2014;41(9):465–72.
57. Rocci A, Hofmeister CC, Pichiorri F. The potential of miRNAs as biomarkers for multiple myeloma. Expert Rev Mol Diagn 2014;14(8):947–59.
58. Bernardo BC, Ooi JY, Lin RC, et al. miRNA therapeutics: a new class of drugs with potential therapeutic applications in the heart. Future Med Chem 2015;7(13):1771–92.

59. Osaki M, Okada F, Ochiya T. miRNA therapy targeting cancer stem cells: a new paradigm for cancer treatment and prevention of tumor recurrence. Ther Deliv 2015;6(3):323–37.
60. Channavajjhala SK, Rossato M, Morandini F, et al. Optimizing the purification and analysis of miRNAs from urinary exosomes. Clin Chem Lab Med 2014;52(3): 345–54.
61. Dumache R, Rogobete AF, Bedreag OH, et al. Use of miRNAs as biomarkers in sepsis. Anal Cell Pathol (Amst) 2015;2015:186716.
62. Zhou B, Li Z, Yang H, et al. Extracellular miRNAs: origin, function and biomarkers in hepatic diseases. J Biomed Nanotechnol 2014;10(10):2865–90.
63. Wang Y, Chen T, Tong W. miRNAs and their application in drug-induced liver injury. Biomark Med 2014;8(2):161–72.
64. Toba H, Cortez D, Lindsey ML, et al. Applications of miRNA technology for atherosclerosis. Curr Atheroscler Rep 2014;16(2):386.
65. Hesse M, Arenz C. miRNAs as novel therapeutic targets and diagnostic bio-markers for Parkinson's disease: a patent evaluation of WO2014018650. Expert Opin Ther Pat 2014;24(11):1271–6.
66. de Melo Maia B, Ling H, Monroig P, et al. Design of a miRNA sponge for the miR-17 miRNA family as a therapeutic strategy against vulvar carcinoma. Mol Cell Probes 2015;29(6):420–6.
67. Sun Y, Hawkins PG, Bi N, et al. Serum MicroRNA signature predicts response to high-dose radiation therapy in locally advanced non-small cell lung cancer. Int J Radiat Oncol Biol Phys 2018;100(1):107–14.
68. Mandilaras V, Vernon M, Meryet-Figuière M, et al. Updates and current challenges in microRNA research for personalized medicine in ovarian cancer. Expert Opin Biol Ther 2017;17(8):927–43.
69. Souza MF, Kuasne H, Barros-Filho MC, et al. Circulating mRNAs and miRNAs as candidate markers for the diagnosis and prognosis of prostate cancer. PLoS One 2017;12(9):e0184094.
70. Hess AK, Müer A, Mairinger FD, et al. MiR-200b and miR-155 as predictive bio-markers for the efficacy of chemoradiation in locally advanced head and neck squamous cell carcinoma. Eur J Cancer 2017;77:3–12.
71. Xie X, Tan W, Chen B, et al. Preoperative prediction nomogram based on primary tumor miRNAs signature and clinical-related features for axillary lymph node metastasis in early-stage invasive breast cancer. Int J Cancer 2018;142(9): 1901–10.

Diagnostic Molecular Microbiology: A 2018 Snapshot

Marilynn Ransom Fairfax, MD, PhD[a,b,]*, Martin H. Bluth, MD, PhD[a,c],
Hossein Salimnia, PhD, D(ABMM)[a,b]

KEYWORDS

- Molecular microbiology • PCR • Probe tests
- Rapid molecular diagnosis of infections • MALDI-TOF • Nuclear magnetic resonance
- Next gen sequencing • Time lapsed imaging

KEY POINTS

- Molecular biological techniques have evolved expeditiously and in turn have been applied to the detection of infectious disease.
- Maturation of these technologies and their coupling with technological advancements have afforded clinical medicine additional tools toward expedient identification of infectious organisms at concentrations and sensitivities previously unattainable.
- These advancements have been adapted in select settings toward addressing clinical demands for more timely and effective patient management.

INTRODUCTION

When Kary Mullis developed the polymerase chain reaction (PCR) in 1983, its potential benefits were obvious to clinical microbiologists: faster, cheaper, more accurate detection and enumeration of all organisms in a specimen, without waiting for a culture. The discipline of infectious disease also sought the opportunity for simultaneous antimicrobial susceptibility testing. These dreams have slowly matured into realities. Multiplex arrays are approved or in development for the diagnosis of respiratory and gastrointestinal infections direct from patient specimens with results obtained in under an hour. An array was cleared by the US Food and Drug Administration (FDA) in August, 2013 that can detect common bacterial and fungal agents of bloodstream infections, as well as several important antibiotic-resistant genes, within about an hour after the culture bottle turns positive. Approaches are being made to organism identification and susceptibility testing directly from a blood sample without the

[a] Department of Pathology, Wayne State University School of Medicine, 540 East Canfield Street, Detroit, MI 48201, USA; [b] Clinical Microbiology Laboratories, DMC University Laboratories, 4201 St. Antoine Street, Detroit, MI 48201, USA; [c] Pathology Laboratories, Michigan Surgical Hospital, 21230 Dequindre Road, Warren, MI 48091, USA
* Corresponding author.
E-mail address: mfairfax@dmc.org

Clin Lab Med 38 (2018) 253–276
https://doi.org/10.1016/j.cll.2018.02.004
0272-2712/18/© 2018 Elsevier Inc. All rights reserved.

labmed.theclinics.com

necessity for culture. Microbiology lines are available, starting with automated plate streakers and ending with molecular identification of organisms grown on solid media. Despite these molecular and technological advancements, humans must still view the culture plates, perhaps on a television screen, and select colonies to analyze.

Furthermore, although cost containment is of paramount importance in today's medical marketplace, "cheaper" is an ambiguous target. Microbiology laboratories are diagnostic facilities that drive subsequent therapy. Increased laboratory costs for more rapid microbial identification have been shown to result in the earlier use of appropriate antibiotics, shorter durations of hospital stay, better outcomes, and decreasing overall health care costs.[1–3]

The diagnosis of persistent human papilloma virus (HPV) infections followed by appropriate therapeutic interventions should decrease the incidence of cervical carcinomas, the cost of treatment, and the attributable morbidity and mortality.

New technologies have enabled microbiologic investigations that were not included in our original diagnostic approaches. Next-generation sequencing (NGS) can detect and quantify populations of organisms in patient specimens. This raises the possibility of distinguishing pathogenic organisms, present in high numbers, from colonizers that are generally presumed to be present in lower numbers. Certain colonic organism profiles seem to correlate with the development of cardiovascular disease.[4] A patient's colonic flora could be analyzed, and if the profile were unfavorable, the bacteria could be eradicated and replaced.

Tests in use in 2018 have evolved significantly from those cited in our 2013 review[5] and will continue to do so. Thus, this article is a snapshot of rapidly changing diagnostic microbiology laboratory techniques and its clinical applications. Emphasis has been placed on tests with high market share in diagnostic microbiology and on those with technologies that are personally regarded by the authors as particularly interesting. The role of specimen processing in concentrating nucleic acid targets and removing inhibitors of amplification is largely neglected, despite its important role in the sensitivity of the assay. However, many new procedures are automated and include specimen processing as part of a hands-off procedure. Most techniques mentioned here involve real-time PCR (RT-PCR), unless otherwise specified. Because most RT-PCR platforms are closed systems, they decrease the incidence of amplicon contamination in the laboratory, and have allowed many nucleic acid amplification techniques to become commercially available. The authors have also attempted to select current citations to support salient points, and these selections are arbitrary. Failure to mention a publication, technique, or trade name should not be construed as denigrating that article, technique, or manufacturer.

PROBE TECHNIQUES

The first molecular diagnostic tests approved by the FDA were probe techniques. Many probe tests are still in wide use today because they fill important niches. Some involve novel detection methodologies.

Hybridization Protection Assays

Among the first FDA-approved molecular tests were the Gen-Probe ([San Diego, CA], which became a wholly owned subsidiary of Hologic [Bedford, MA] in 2012). Pace 2 probe hybridization protection techniques are used for the diagnosis of *Chlamydia trachomatis* and *Neisseria gonorrhoeae* from patient specimens. They have been largely replaced by more sensitive amplification tests. A number of their AccuProbe culture confirmation tests remain available. Among the most useful are *Mycobacterium tuberculosis* complex, *Mycobacterium avium, Mycobacterium intracellulare* (separately or together), *Mycobacterium kansasii*, and *Mycobacterium gordoni*. These and other tests available from the same manufacturer all use most of the same reagents and instrumentation, which facilitates the use of multiple assays in the same laboratory.

These tests succeed because they target ribosomal RNA (rRNA), which is present in up to 10^5 copies per organism. In bacterial ribosomes, there are common sequences, as well as genus-specific and species-specific sequences. The culture confirmation tests remain viable because they are intended to detect organisms in visible colonies or in liquid medium with detectable growth. Thus, 2 amplification steps have already been performed by nature. Sensitivities reported in the Hologic/Gen-Probe package inserts range from 98% to 100%.

At development, these assays were novel; they were nonradioactive and performed totally in solution, with 1 sample transfer step and no nucleic acid extraction. The hybridization protection assays are based on the differential sensitivity of the acridinium ester, which is used to distinguish the relatively labile ester on nonhybridized probes from the more stable form in DNA–RNA hybrids. This detection system is also used in this manufacturer's nucleic acid amplification tests (NAATs). All the AccuProbe assays are similar, but the nucleic acid release steps are variable, depending on the ease of disruption of the organism.[6]

The mycobacterial probe tests are particularly valuable when used in conjunction with liquid medium or 7H11 thin-plate techniques[7] used for the rapid detection and identification of mycobacteria required by the College of American Pathologists (Northfield, IL). Thin-plate colonies can be probed the day they are detected, and their morphology can be used as a guide to selection of the appropriate probe. This represents significant time and money savings, although it does not eliminate the need to grow *M tuberculosis* for susceptibility testing. Cultures in Middlebrook 7H9 broth must be AFB stained to confirm the presence of mycobacteria[8] and then probed with all 4 probes. The probe techniques described are also used to detect amplification products in amplification assays developed by GenProbe/Hologic for sexually transmitted diseases and blood bank testing (discussed elsewhere in this article).

Hybrid capture technique

Since the 1940s, Pap smears have contributed to great advances in the prevention and diagnosis of cervical carcinoma. In the 1980s and 1990s, it was recognized that infection with HPV is necessary but not sufficient for the development of cervical carcinoma. More than 100 HPV genotypes exist, of which 13 are associated with a high risk of cervical carcinoma (16, 18, 31, 33, 35, 39, 45, 51, 52, 56, 58, 59, and 68). More than 70% of sexually active women become infected with HPV. Most infections, even with high-risk organisms, resolve without apparent sequalae. Why others progress is still unknown.[9] The Digene Hybrid Capture 2 (hc2; Qiagen, Gaithersburg, MD) is FDA approved for primary screening, and to determine whether women with atypical squamous cells of undetermined significance should be subjected to culposcopy. It may be used with the Cytyc PreservCyt Solution for the Cytyc ThinPrep Pap Test (Hologic).[10] In the first step, the patient specimen is allowed to react with a pool of RNA probes designed to hybridize specifically to the DNA of high-risk HPV strains. Antibody to RNA/DNA hybrids coats the wells of a microtiter plate and captures any hybrids. After washing away unbound specimen and reagents, detector antihybrid antibodies, each conjugated with multiple molecules of alkaline phosphatase, bind to each capture target, thereby amplifying the signal. A colorless substrate for the alkaline phosphatase is added and chemiluminescence develops proportional to the amount of second antibody bound.

More sensitive tests, typically involving target amplification, have been devised, but most clinical outcomes data are available with hc2. The need for more sensitivity has been questioned, because hc2 has already been shown to be sensitive, but not highly specific, for the development of cervical intraepithelial neoplasia or overt malignancy. The presence of high-risk DNA below the detection limit of hc2 seems to be associated with a low risk for malignancy.[9] However, new information suggests that infections acquired in the early years of sexual activity may reactivate with aging.[11] If this is supported by further studies, more sensitive assays might be indicated. There is also a suggestion that unusual HPV strains may cause cervical carcinoma or precursor lesions in restricted populations.[12] Thus, the strains included in the assay may need periodic review. Amplification techniques are now available which can distinguish HPV-16 and HPV-18 from the other high-risk organisms, which has facilitated targeted follow-up algorithms, and outcomes data are increasing so that this unique probe technique is becoming less common. The use of hybrid capture as the basis a detection system in amplification assays is still possible, and used in some assays; however, it is not considered a method with high sensitivity.

Peptide nucleic acid fluorescence in situ hybridization
Peptide nucleic acid fluorescence in situ hybridization (PNA-FISH; AdvanDx, Inc, Woburn, MA, now owned by OpGen) accelerated the diagnosis of sepsis. Common agents of sepsis can be identified in about an hour after the blood culture bottle has been gram stained. Although behaving like a standard FISH assay, the PNA-FISH probes consist of an uncharged peptide backbone to which the bases are attached. This is thought to allow the probes to enter the permeabilized bacterial cell more easily and then bind more tightly to the negatively charged rRNA target. Numerous publications confirm that the use of this technique for rapid identification of the common organisms growing in the blood culture bottles improves antibiotic stewardship and shortens length of stay.[1,2] Depending on the patient, identification of a coagulase-negative *Staphylococcus* may facilitate discontinuation of antibiotics and early discharge.

Our high-throughput laboratory (>200 blood cultures per day) was an early adapter of the staphylococcal, enterococcal, and candida probes, although we do not currently use those for bacteria owing to the availability of more sensitive platforms with the ability to detect a great number of pathogens involved in bacteremia and sepsis. Multiple PNA-FISH assays received FDA clearance, including the assay for the detection of *Staphylococcus aureus*/coagulase-negative *Staphylococcus*, *Enterococuus fecalis/E faceium*, gram-negative traffic light (identification of *E coli*, *Klebsiella penumoniae*, and *Pseudomonas aeruginosa*) and yeast traffic light (identification of *Candida albicans*, *C krusei*, *C tropicalis*, *C glabrata*, and *C parapsilosis*). Our laboratory has been involved in clinical trials of AdvanDx PNA-FISH products and our data showed high sensitivity and specificity of these products as well as the ease of use.[13–16] Although the popularity of PNA-FISH as a diagnostic test in large laboratories is declining, the FISH technique is being used by Accelerate Diagnostics (Tucson, AZ) to facilitate organism identification in positive blood culture bottles.

Affirm VPIII microbial identification test The VPIII probe test (Becton Dickinson, Franklin Lakes, NJ) is intended for the diagnosis of vaginitis/vaginosis, conditions causing millions of physician visits annually. Affirm detects rRNA from *Gardnerella vaginalis*, used as an indicator for bacterial vaginosis (BV), *C albicans*, and *Trichomonas vaginalis*. The sensitivity has been adjusted to avoid giving positive results with low concentrations of *G vaginalis* and *C albicans*, which often colonize the normal vagina using a lateral flow immunochromatographic enzyme assay. This assay maintains low sensitivity (requiring about 5000 copies of trichomonas nucleic acid to give a positive result), which may be ideal for *Gardnerella* but bad for *Trichomonas* species. It is formatted to be performed in a cassette superficially resembling the lateral flow tests used for the serologic detection of influenza or rotavirus antigens and was the first FDA-approved molecular test based on lateral flow. The methodology for lateral flow is as follows: after collection on a proprietary swab, the specimen is lysed to release the nucleic acids, buffered to stabilize the nucleic acids and establish stringency, and added to the cassette, which is incubated at the proper temperature for nucleic acid hybridization. The cassette contains 5 "beads," each coupled to a capture probe: 1 for each of the 3 analytes, plus positive and negative controls. Next, enzyme-linked detector probes bind to specific sequences on the target organism's rRNA. Unbound sample components and probes are washed away. A colorless substrate is converted to a blue product if sufficient target and detector probe have bound. A blue "bead" indicates a positive result.[17]

Numerous publications have revealed that health care providers are significantly less accurate than VPIII for the diagnosis of significant candidiasis and *T vaginalis*. The Affirm test has highlighted the fact that multiple infections are common. The role of the VPIII in the diagnosis of BV is the subject of debate, however, because the use of *G vaginalis* alone as an indicator of BV is not optimal. In addition, there have been criticisms of the limit of detection (LOD) of the assay, particularly for *T vaginalis*, and of the inability of the assay to highlight the presence of drug-resistant *Candida* spp. Automated NAAT assays (including the MAX Vaginal Panel assay by Becton Dickinson) resolve many of these problems. Becton Dickinson now suggests that the Affirm assay may be appropriate for smaller laboratories, whereas larger laboratories may wish to transition to its NAAT assay.

The Becton Dickinson MAX Vaginal Panel is the first FDA cleared, microbiome-based, PCR assay that directly detects the 3 most common infectious causes of vaginitis: BV, vulvovaginal candidiasis, and trichomoniasis. The MAX Vaginal Panel performed on the Becton Dickinson Max instrument is fully automated and diagnoses BV using a unique algorithm that quantitates the presence of *Lactobacillus spp.* (good bacteria) as compared with *G vaginalis, Atopobium vaginae,* BV-associated bacteria, and *Megasphaerae* (BV-associated bacteria). It separately determines the presence of *T vaginalis*, as well as the presence of the *Candida* group (*albicans, tropicalis, parapsilosis,* and *dublinensis*), and of *C glabrata* and *C krusei*, which are more antibiotic resistant.[18]

Advances in Sexually Transmitted Disease Testing

Culture, immunoassay, and probe tests for both *N gonorrhoeae* also known as *Gonococci* and *C trachomatis* are less sensitive than NAATs, and NAATs have been the standard of care since the late 1990s, although certain jurisdictions still require culture for legal cases. In this text *N gonorrhoeae* and *Gonococci* are used interchangeably.

C trachomatis and gonococcal infections of the female genital tract present a diagnostic challenge because many patients with *C trachomatis* and *Gonococci* are asymptomatic. Sexually transmitted diseases are becoming more prevalent even in the United States and Europe. This has led to the implementation of widespread screening, using urine or self-collected swabs, collection procedures with increased patient acceptance. All of these tests are also available for physician-collected vaginal swabs and for male urethral swabs and urines.

Commercial qualitative NAATS for diagnosis of *C trachomatis* and *Gonococci* have been available for about 20 years. The first PCR assay, the semiautomated Amplicor *C trachomatis/N gonorrhoeae* test, was developed by Roche (Basel, Switzerland). It was closely followed by the Abbott LCX assay (Abbott Laboratories, Chicago, IL) for the simultaneous detection of *C trachomatis* and *N gonorrhoeae*, which used ligase chain reaction technology to amplify the targets. In 2003, the Abbott LCX assay for *C trachomatis/Gonococci* was withdrawn abruptly from the market. In the late 1990s, other amplification assays became available, a strand-displacement amplification assay from Becton Dickinson, the ProbeTec ET, and a transcription-mediated amplification test from GenProbe were introduced. Both of these evolved over the years and additional tests were also FDA approved. Other testing approaches include the Becton Dickinson ProbeTec *C trachomatis/Gonococci* Qx assay performed on the Viper XTR, Hologic/Gen-Probe Aptima Combo 2 assay performed on both the Panther and Tigris instruments, the Abbott Real-Time *C trachomatis/N gonorrhoeae* assay, and the Roche Diagnostics Cobas *C trachomatis/N gonorrhoeae* assay run on the Cobas 4800 instrument.

A current problem with all molecular diagnostic tests for *C trachomatis/Gonococci* is the inability to test for antibiotic resistance. *N gonorrhoeae* has inexorably developed resistance to each antibiotic regimen that became widely used, and the question of antimicrobial resistance in *C trachomatis* has hardly been considered, although treatment failures are well-known. Because the transport systems for *C trachomatis* and *Gonococci* are not compatible with culture and susceptibility testing, it seems inevitable that molecular susceptibility testing must be developed, but we are unaware of any such development.

Hologic/Gen-Probe Aptima Combo 2 assay

This assay is performed on either the Tigris or the Panther instruments. It targets a region of the 23S rRNA of *C trachomatis* and one from the 16S rRNA from *Gonococci*. They are amplified via DNA intermediates by using transcription-mediated amplification, a technique that uses both a reverse transcriptase enzyme and a phage-derived RNA-dependent RNA polymerase. The detection of the amplicons is achieved using the hybridization protection assay described herein in the section on probe tests. Briefly, single-strand chemiluminescent DNA probes bind to their complementary target, protecting the labile acridinium ester. After hydrolysis of the esters on unbound probes, light emitted from the ester that had been protected within the target-probe hybrids is measured and reported as relative light units. Assay results are determined by a cutoff based on the total relative light units and the curve type.[19,20]

Becton Dickinson ProbeTec C trachomatis/Gonococci Qx assay on the Viper XTR

This assay uses the isothermal DNA nick translation technique called strand-displacement amplification for the detection of target sequences in the patient sample. It targets a sequence in the cryptic *C trachomatis* plasmid and a sequence of *Gonococci* genomic DNA, respectively. Extraction of DNA from clinical samples is based on pH-dependent binding of the DNA to ferric oxide particles followed by binding of the combination to paramagnetic beads. After removing the contaminants, the purified DNA is released and amplified by real-time strand-displacement amplification in the presence of a fluorescently labeled detector probe. The presence of the target DNA is determined by comparing the peak fluorescence with a cutoff value. Many articles have discussed the performance of this assay to detect the targets in clinical specimens, such as urine or vaginal/cervical samples. This assay is not evaluated for pregnant women as well as patients younger than 18 years of age.[21–23]

The Abbott RealTime C trachomatis/N gonorrhoeae assay

This RT-PCR assay targets 2 sequences within the cryptic plasmid of *C trachomatis*. This plasmid is found in all serovars of *Chlamydia* to date. The dual targets allow detection of both the wild-type *C trachomatis* and the variant, which has a deletion in one of the target sequences. The *Gonococci* target is found within the organism's Opa gene. Cheng and colleagues[24] evaluated the Abbott RealTime *C trachomatis/Gonococci* assay in comparison with the Roche Cobas Amplicor *C trachomatis/N gonorrhoeae* assay. They showed high agreement between the 2 assay. However, their data demonstrated that the Abbott assay was more sensitive than the Roche assay for both *C trachomatis* and *N gonorrhoeae* with enhanced ability to detect dual infections.

Roche Cobas 4800 instrument and C trachomatis/N gonorrhoeae assay

This multiplex PCR assay simultaneously detects 2 independent DNA targets for *C trachomatis*, one in the cryptic plasmid and the other on the *C trachomatis* genome. This assay can detect infections caused by the wild-type *C trachomatis*, in addition to other *Chlamydia* strains that may have deletions in the cryptic plasmid, or those that might not carry the cryptic plasmid at all. DR-9, a direct repeat region, is the target of the *N gonorrhoeae* assay. The use of this target makes the assay highly specific to *N gonorrhoeae*. This target does not cross-react with sequences found in commensal *Neisseria*, a feature that hampers the use of some other *Gonococci* assays for oropharyngeal and rectal samples.

Chernesky and colleagues[25] performed a direct comparison of 4 second-generation *C trachomatis/Gonococci* assays to obtain information about their relative sensitivities and specificities. They used both first void urine and self-collected vaginal swabs. The sensitivities for *C trachomatis* using self-collected swabs were: Aptima Combo 2 run on the Tigris, 98.1%, and on the Panther, 96.2% (Hologic/GenProbe): RealTime assay on the m2000, 98.0% (Abbott): ProbeTec Q^X assay on the Viper, 90.6% (Becton Dickinson), and the Cobas assay tested on the Cobas 4800, 84.6% (Roche).

Other qualitative assays

Hologic-Gen-Probe manufactures several widely used qualitative, transcription-mediated amplification-based microbiology tests; included among these are a direct test for *M tuberculosis* and the Procleix Ultrio Plus assay (Ultrio), which has also been licensed to Novartis (Emoryville, CA). The first assay (without the Plus) has long been approved for detection of human immunodeficiency virus (HIV) and hepatitis C virus (HCV) in specimens from blood donors and from organ donors, both living and deceased, but is not intended for the diagnostic workup of the diseases in the general population. Testing a pool of samples from up to 16 blood donor units is approved for blood bank testing. Recently, the FDA approved the inclusion of hepatitis B virus in this assay, and it has been renamed Ultrio Plus. It contains several HIV targets that allow it to detect HIV-1 (several strains) and HIV-2. Because test results are generally negative and high sensitivity is necessary, the inclusion of an internal control is essential. Components of positive pools are retested individually and then by assays for each individual analyte.[26]

Other published data contain a listing of more than 135 published RT-PCR assays developed for the detection of 32 species of bacteria.[27] This list does not include multiplexed tests or assays for viruses. The publication acknowledged that the list is incomplete and commented that most are laboratory-developed tests, with only 35 (counted from the list) being commercially available, whether FDA approved or not. This finding emphasizes the need for more rapid commercial development and FDA approval methods.

Although cyber green, a nonspecific detector, is still used occasionally, 3 main molecular detection systems are used: dual hybridization (fluorescent resonance energy transfer), TaqMan, and molecular beacon.

The fluorescent resonance energy transfer detector consists of 2 different probes, complementary to adjacent sequences on the target amplicon, and each attached to a different fluorophore. When activated by incident ultraviolet light, the first fluorophore emits energy at an unmonitored wavelength. If the second probe is bound adjacent to it, the energy is transferred to the second fluorophore, which then emits light at the wavelength monitored by the sensor. At the end of the PCR assay, a melting curve for the amplicon–probe complex can be generated. The melting temperature is characteristic of each amplicon–probe combination. If there is a mismatch between the probe and the amplicon, the melting temperature decreases.[28] The melting temperature difference has been exploited in a test that distinguishes between herpes simplex 1 and 2 (Roche). The PCR primers bind sequences common to both viruses within the HSV DNA polymerase gene. The amplicon detector probes match the HSV-2 sequence, which differs from that of HSV-1 by 2 bp. Melting curve analysis reveals a reproducible melting temperature for HSV-2 that is about 10°C higher than that exhibited by HSV-1.[29] Occasional mutant HSV strains have been detected that have intermediate melting temperatures. These tests can be reported as positive for HSV, but the type is not clear. Types 1 and 2 could be distinguished by sequencing the amplicons, by using an assay using a different target sequence, or by the melting temperature of the amplicon, which is said to be 0.9°C higher for the HSV-2 variant than the type 1 variant.[30]

The MultiCode RTx system uses an unusual PCR amplification technique in which no detector probe is used and in which the fluorescence actually decreases as amplification progresses. It was developed by EraGen BioSciences, Inc (Madison, WI; acquired by Luminex Corporation [Austin, TX] in 2011). Their MultiCode-RTx herpes simplex virus 1 and 2 kit was FDA approved in 2011. MultiCode RTx assays use 2 unusual nucleotide bases iC (2-deoxy-5-methylisocytidine) and iG (2-deoxyisoguanoside) that base pair only to one another and that are efficiently incorporated into PCR products. iG is put at the 5′ end of the RTx primers along with its linked fluorophore. The reaction mix contains iC covalently linked to a quencher. In the initial cycle amplification, the iG, with its attached fluorophore, appears at the 5′ end of the primer and hence at the 5′ end of the nascent amplicon strands. When these serve as templates for copying in the other direction, an iC, with its attached quencher is added to the 3′ end of the new strand, opposite the iG and its fluorophore. The approximation of fluorophore and quencher decreases the fluorescence. In melting curve analysis, fluorescence increases as the amplicons melt, and the melting temperature allows determination of the nature of the analyte.[31]

QUANTITATIVE TECHNIQUES

Quantitative PCR in clinical microbiology are confined mainly to NAATs used for HIV viral load testing, although there are also FDA-approved quantitative RT-PCR assays for HCV, hepatitis B virus, and recently for cytomegalovirus. The trend is to make the assays referable to a World Health Organization international standard. Quantitative techniques have advanced significantly since the early days when Alice Huang first demonstrated that quantitative PCR was possible (for a detailed discussion and review of the literature, see Fairfax and Salimnia[28]).

RT-PCR is inherently semiquantitative. Theoretically, one can construct a standard curve of copy number versus cycle threshold—and determine the quantity of analyte in a patient specimen by referring to the curve. However, variations in extraction efficiency and the presence of inhibitors can introduce significant errors, particularly at low levels of analyte, when one is attempting to distinguishing "only a few" from "none." One relatively straightforward method to overcome this problem includes the addition of a control target or quantitation standard into the patient sample before extraction. The target and the quantitation standard are extracted, amplified, and detected together, controlling for the extraction and for any inhibitors present.

The ideal quantitation standard should be the same size and base composition as the target to be quantified, with the same primer binding sites. It should differ enough in sequence that the detector probe or probes for the target do not bind to it, and its own detector probe should fluoresce at a different wavelength from that of the target. Then, quantitation should be a simple mathematical calculation.[28] However, at low target concentrations, the standard curve is no longer straight. Roche has incorporated complex mathematical calculations into its recent viral load assays to account for this divergence.

Conversations have recently begun about possible "cures" of HIV infection, and as highly active antiretroviral therapy and improved plasma HIV viral load techniques converge, discussions have ensued about how to evaluate residual virus in well-controlled or possibly cured individuals. The most sensitive assays for determination of low-level infection are likely to be assays for HIV DNA copies in single cells. How to determine which ones are replication competent is crucial to this discussion. Aside from circulating CD4 cells, what cells should be investigated is unclear at this time. This active area of investigation was recently reviewed by Strain and Richman,[32] who discussed very low-level contamination, signal-to-noise ratios in PCR testing, single-cell PCR, and other techniques that are beyond the scope of this article.

With respect to HIV quantification in plasma, further considerations affect testing and result interpretation. The most obvious problem results from the increase in sensitivity as the assays improve. Patients who were told that their virus levels were "undetectable," suddenly have quantifiable virus. Time-consuming correlations between viral load and prognosis have to be redone for each new, more sensitive assay. Sequence differences between the numerous organism strains and the inherent mutability of the organisms also make accurate quantification difficult, especially for RNA viruses, such as HIV and HCV. One must target a stable sequence. However, the viral RNA polymerase enzymes are error prone and lack proofreading activity. Changes in the genetic sequence, particularly in the primer or probe-binding sites, may reduce the detected viral load. Minority quasi-species also cause problems (discussed elsewhere in this article). It seems that more than 1 target will be necessary for future assays.

Because approval and release of diagnostic tests by different manufacturers are not coordinated, it is difficult to find articles comparing the performance of the latest offerings by different companies. Two current assays for HIV quantification in the United States are the Roche Cobas AmpliPrep Cobas TaqMan HIV viral load version 2.0 (CAP/CTM2) and the Abbott RealTime HIV-1 assay (ART HIV). The 2 assays have different lower limits of quantitation, 20 copies/mL for CAP/CTM2 and 40 copies/mL for ART HIV, which introduces difficulties in comparison. They have, however, been compared in 2 recent articles.[33,34] Sire and colleagues[33] extrapolated the ART HIV curves, and found that 10 of 17 specimens that were quantifiable by the CAP/CTM2 but not by the ART HIV could actually be quantified. The assays correlated well ($r = 0.96$),[32] although CAP/CTM2 was more than 0.5 $\log_{10}$ higher than the ART HIV in 20% of 51 samples, whereas the ART HIV was more than 0.5 $\log_{10}$ higher in only 2 of them.[33] Whose result is more accurate remains to be determined.

HIGHLY MULTIPLEXED POLYMERASE CHAIN REACTION PANELS

This section focuses only on highly multiplexed assays, roughly defined as those detecting more than 10 targets. Although many assays for individual etiology agents of disease are available, testing for individual organisms is often uninformative. Numerous viral and some bacterial agents of respiratory disease cause similar symptoms. It is usually not obvious which agent or agents are infecting a given patient. Even at the peak of an influenza epidemic, an individual may be infected with respiratory syncytial virus instead or concurrently. Furthermore, mixed infections are more common than many had imagined. [35,36] Some virus infections are treatable, and others have different isolation requirements if the patient is hospitalized.[36] Thus, molecular panels that could detect multiple etiologic agents of diseases clearly are desirable. As of December 2017, 6 multiplex respiratory panels are FDA approved: Luminex xTAG RVP (xRVP) and RVP Fast (xRVPF) and Verigene respiratory pathogen flex (LUMINEX corporation); Film Array Respiratory Panel (FARP; BioFire Diagnostics [Now bioMerieux], Salt Lake City, UT), and the eSensor respiratory viral panel, ePlex Respiratory Pathogen Panel (GenMark Diagnostics, Carlsbad, CA). In comparison with other systems, the FARP detects the greatest number of pathogens, including 3 bacteria and 17 viral pathogens. One head-to-head comparison of all 4 test modalities was recently published.[37] The various analytes differ in sensitivity and specificity, but this study found that the eSRP had 100% sensitivity for all analytes compared. The xRVP was second, and more sensitive than the xRVPF, which was similar to the FARP. These results will require confirmation by other researchers; Babady and colleagues[35] found the FARP to be more sensitive than the xRVPF for many analytes. All tests are capable of detecting mixed infections.

Ultimately, the final decision as to which test to implement in one's laboratory may come down to questions of cost, hands-on time, complexity, time to result, and convenience. The FARP provides a result within about 1 hour, requiring only a few minutes of hands-on time, but can handle only 1 sample at a time. It seems ideally suited to a medium-sized laboratory where technologists without specialized molecular expertise can perform the tests. Some larger laboratories have bought multiple instruments or instruments with higher throughput (eg, Torch from BioFire) to facilitate throughput. But surge capacity may be lacking. The other systems test samples in batch mode with high throughput, but they require sample extraction before testing, and amplicon manipulation afterward, which may confine them to a "PCR laboratory." Each handles 21 samples per run. None is suitable for 2 runs per shift, although staggered technologist start times could allow it with the xRVPF. The xRVP and eSRP require 7 to 8 hours for results.[37]

A problem with panels is that they tend to maximize the number of analytes detected in their initial offering, based on instrument constraints. Therefore, adding something new seems to require that something old be removed. FDA reapproval requires significant financial outlays for any change, and new respiratory viruses keep appearing. Newly detected viruses since 2001 include human metapneumoviruses (2001), severe acute respiratory syndrome (2003), human bocavirus (2005), new influenza A viruses (H1N1, 2009; H7N9, 2013), and now, Middle East respiratory syndrome corona virus (2012), the latter 2 of which apparently have not (yet) appeared in the United States. MERS and H7N9 have not been reported in the United States between 2014 and 2017 (source: CDC https://www.cdc.gov/features/novelcoronavirus/index.html) but they apparently have a high mortality rate.[38–40] The human metapneumoviruses and human bocavirus are included in some of the previously mentioned assays. It is not clear whether MERS corona virus can be detected by the coronavirus detector systems in these assays, but if so, it could not be distinguished from those that cause more common respiratory infections. Thus, keeping panels updated may prove difficult.

New multiplex panels have been developed and received FDA clearance for viral, parasitic, and bacterial agents of gastrointestinal diseases, and central nervous system infections. A BioFire assay for usual agents of bloodstream infections was FDA approved in August 2013. The Biofire gastrointestinal panel and meningitis panel also received FDA clearance on May 2014 and November 2015, respectively. In addition to the detection of bacterial pathogens, it detects several antibiotic resistance genes. Another system known as Verigene bloodstream tests (made by Nanoshere, now Luminex Corporation) provides bacterial identification and antibiotic resistance determination directly from positive blood culture bottles. The assay includes 2 cartridges, gram positive and gram negative. A Gram stain of positive blood culture bottle is needed to decide if a gram-positive or a gram-negative cartridge should be used. Luminex and BioFire also offer FDA-cleared gastrointestinal panels that detect and identify viral, bacterial, and toxins such as shiga1/2 directly from stool samples, whereas the blood culture panels should be run from positive culture bottles (which may take up to 5 days to become positive). Some can detect several antibiotic resistance genes as well as infecting bacteria.

Prove-It Sepsis

The Prove-It Sepsis assay can identify bacteria and fungi from positive blood culture in about 3.5 hours. The assay is approved in Europe, but not FDA cleared in the United States. Prove-it Sepsis runs on a strip with 8 wells, each of which can identify 2 sample. Each microarray identifies more than 60 bacteria, mecA, vanA, and vanB resistance markers and 13 fungi in a single assay. Tissari and colleagues,[41] evaluated the clinical performance of this assay using 3300 patient samples and found. Based on their data, Prove-it Sepsis showed 95% sensitivity and 99% specificity.

Quantitative Digital Polymerase Chain Reaction with Increased Accuracy at Low Copy Numbers

Digital PCR (dPCR) is a quantitative method that provides a sensitive and reproducible way of measuring the amount of DNA or RNA present in a sample that is present in low copy numbers. It is similar to quantitative PCR in the reagents and amplification reaction. The method is simple and reproducible, and does not need quantitation standards or standard curves. Before amplification, the initial sample mix is partitioned into multiple individual wells or droplets, many of which end up containing no target sequence. After amplification, the number of positive and negative reactions is determined and the absolute number of target present in the initial reaction mix is calculated using Poisson statistics.

The dPCR is advantageous for applications requiring high sensitivity combined with accurate and reproducible enumeration of small numbers of targets. This method is obviously useful for quantification of viral loads, but can also be used for detection of rare alleles, determination of copy number variations, quantification of NGS libraries, as well as measurements of gene expression heterogeneity and multiplexing. There are currently no FDA-approved, commercially available dPCR systems in United States. However, several companies such as Raindrop Digital PCR System (Raindance Technologies, Lexington, MA), QX200 Droplet Digital PCR System (Bio-Rad, Hercules, CA), BioMark HD System, qdPCR 37K IFC (Fluidigm Corporation, South San Francisco, CA) and QuantStudio 3D Digital PCR System (Life Technologies, Carlsbad, CA) offer dPCR systems for research use. More information on dPCR, can be found in references.[42–45]

Use of Mass Spectrometry and Spectroscopy for the Identification of Pathogens

Matrix-assisted laser desorption/ionization time-of-flight mass spectrometry

Although "molecular diagnostics" is generally assumed to imply nucleic acid–based methods, mass spectroscopy has been used in microbiology since the 1970s. At that time, mass spectroscopy was used almost exclusively for the identification of anaerobes by analysis of volatile or volatilized short-chain organic acids. New mass spectroscopy techniques provide a general tool for the identification of microorganisms growing in colonies on culture plates. This requires 2 to 5 minutes and has the potential to improve significantly the turnaround time for microbiology culture reports and to reduce labor costs, especially when coupled with other laboratory automation that is now becoming available. Up-front costs are high, but the cost per test is low and the rapidity of results and low cost per individual result can impact antibiotic usage and patient outcomes, shortening hospital stays and lowering total costs.[3]

The new technology is matrix-assisted laser desorption/ionization time of flight (MALDI-TOF). Currently, there are 2 FDA-approved MALDI-TOF instruments available in the United States for rapid identification of microorganisms: one developed by Shimadzu Scientific Instruments (Columbia, MD) and licensed to BioMerieux (Durham, NC) and a second, manufactured by Bruker Daltonics (Billerica, MA), and licensed to both Siemens Healthcare Diagnostics (Tarrytown, NY) and to Becton Dickinson (Sparks, MD). The great benefit of quick, easy, and accurate identification of microorganisms has encouraged larger laboratories to implement these systems for routine organism identification despite their initial high instrument cost.

Microorganism identification by MALDI-TOF is based on the observation that each pathogenic organism has its own unique protein signature. Bacterial cells are fixed in a matrix and irradiated by a laser beam that releases and ionizes the proteins. These enter a vacuum column and move toward the detector based on charge and mass. The protein signature is checked for a match against a large and still growing database derived from different genera and species of microorganisms. Different instruments have different databases, and the government has limited laboratory access to databases containing the protein signature of potential agents of bioterrorism, although these are endemic in certain areas of the United States.

MALDI-TOF can identify bacteria, both aerobic and anaerobic, mycobacteria, and fungi. The analysis of organisms with tougher cell walls, such as gram-positive bacteria, yeasts, and fungi, requires slight modifications of procedure.[46] Hundreds of abstracts and articles attest to its ability to rapidly and accurately identify bacteria and fungi to the genus and species level.

MALDI-TOF for the identification of etiologic agents of sepsis generally cannot be performed until the pathogen has first been grown in blood culture bottles and subcultured onto standard solid media. These steps are time consuming and lead to the use of broad-spectrum, empiric antibiotics. To increase speed of identification, protocols have been developed to use MALDI-TOF directly from newly positive blood culture bottles,[47–49] although it should not be used in samples containing multiple organisms Data are also accumulating illustrating the ability of MALDI-TOF to identify some antibiotic-resistant organisms.[50] However, more work is needed in this area before MALDI-TOF could become a valid alternative to routine antibiotic susceptibility testing.

Laser-induced breakdown spectroscopy

Rapid advances in the development of laser-induced breakdown spectroscopy (LIBS) have transformed it from an elemental analysis technique to one that can be used directly for the identification of complex materials, including clinical microbiology specimens. A growing number of recent articles have illustrated the ability of LIBS to rapidly detect and accurately identify various biological, biomedical, or clinical samples. These analyses are sensitive, specific, and rapid, requiring no sample preparation. LIBS can identify microorganisms based on a determination of their elemental compositions. LIBS uses a strong laser pulse to atomize the content of bacterial cells. Light from these "high-temperature sparks" is collected. Analysis of the peaks in the atomic emission spectrum allows the identification and relative quantification of the atoms present in each sample. The "spectral fingerprint" of the peaks and their ratios is compared with a database of LIBS spectra derived from different genera and species of microorganisms to allow identification of bacterial genus and species. As yet, there is no FDA-cleared LIBS system for rapid identification of pathogen microorganisms.[51,52]

Raman spectroscopy

Interest has also recently been generated in the possibility of using Raman spectroscopy for the rapid identification of a variety of bacteria. Raman spectroscopy uses the interaction of light with molecules to measure functional group vibrations. When photons from an incident, focused laser interact with a molecule, they cause the molecule to transition to an excited vibrational state, accompanied by a corresponding energy loss in the photon; this energy loss results in the light undergoing a frequency shift, and hence a change in color, which is measured. The spectrum is unique for each bacterial species. It can be checked against a database for rapid identification of the pathogen. Raman spectroscopy is distinct from other current techniques because of its ease, low cost, and high speed. It provides information on the chemical composition and the structure of biomolecules within the microorganisms. Thus, slight changes in the chemical makeup of organisms can be determined by Raman spectroscopy and used to differentiate genera, species, or even strains. A study by Chouthai and colleagues,[53] showed reliable, rapid, and accurate identification of *Candida* species using Raman spectroscopy. Detection of pathogens is possible from complex matrices, such as soil, food, and body fluids. Further, spectroscopic analysis may allow determination of the effect of antibiotics on bacteria.[53–55]

Multiplexed Automated Digital Microscopy (Time Lapse Imaging): Accelerate Pheno System

The automated Accelerate Pheno technique (AXDX; Accelerate Diagnostics) received FDA approval in February 2017. It performs both bacterial identification and antibiotic susceptibility testing directly from the positive blood culture bottle, without requiring the isolation of purified colonies, cutting almost 40 hours off the time to identification and antibiotic susceptibility testing. The techniques use digital microscopy and allow identification of 1 to 4 bacterial pathogens from a positive blood culture bottle in around 1 hour and antibiotic susceptibility testing about 6 hours later. It succeeds where other techniques fail because it analyzes single cells. Organism identification is performed using multiplexed automated digital microscopy and FISH probes (described elsewhere in this article). Antibiotic susceptibility testing is performed by observing the growth of individual, live, immobilized bacterial cells in the presence of antimicrobial agents. Phenotypic antibiotic susceptibility testing results with a panel of standard antibiotics require about 7 hours after the blood culture bottle turns positive. By guiding appropriate antibiotic therapy this microscopic technique can reduce mortality and morbidity.

AXDX identifies and performs antibiotic susceptibility testing on 6 gram-positive and 8 gram-negative bacterial genera/species and 2 *Candida* species. In this system, bacterial cells are first purified from blood culture growth medium by gel electrofiltration followed by cell immobilization via electrokinetic concentration before FISH and antibiotic susceptibility testing.

Our laboratory has evaluated the performance (accuracy) of Accelerate system. In 2015 and 2016, we tested 300 clinical samples on this system and compared the result with our standard method, which currently consists of a combination of phenotypic, biochemical, and/or MALDI-TOF techniques for pathogen identification combined with antibiotic susceptibility testing via the Becton Dickinson Phenix automated microbiology system. The data revealed high sensitivity (93.8%) and specificity (99.7%) for identification of pathogens as well as high categorical (94.8%) and essential agreement (96.3%) for antibiotic susceptibility testing results. The system was robust and on average provided identification in 1.4 and antibiotic susceptibility testing results in 6.7 hours after bottle positivity.[56]

Marschal and colleagues compared the performance of AXDX with conventional culture-based methods. AXDX correctly identified 88.7% (102 of 115) of all blood stream infections (BSI) episodes and 97.1% (102 of 105) of 28 isolates that are covered by the system's identification panel. The AXDX generated an antibiotic susceptibility testing result for 91.3% (95 of 104) samples in which it identified a gram-negative pathogen. They found the overall category agreement of 96.4%, for sensitive, intermediate, and resistant interpretation between AXDX and culture-based antibiotic susceptibility testing, with the rate for minor discrepancies 1.4% (change between sensitive or resistant and intermediate), major discrepancies 2.3% and 33 very major discrepancies 1.0%.[57]

Resonant mass measurement for determination of antibiotic susceptibility in bacteria
LifeScale biosensor rapid antimicrobial susceptibility LifeScale (Affinity Biosensors, Santa Barbara, CA) uses resonant mass measurement to enumerate and determine the mass of bacteria exposed to antibiotics, allowing it to determine antibiotic susceptibility within approximately 3 hours. A beam suspended at 1 end resonates at a specific frequency. If a mass is added to the beam, the resonant frequency decreases an amount related to the added mass. The beam is suspended in a vacuum and the bacteria, in growth medium, pass through a microchannel in the beam. This technology has been developed into the Life Scale Biosensor, which can make these determinations in a standard 96-well plate, including the minimum inhibitory concentration plates prepared by Sensititre (ThermoScientific, Waltham, MA). Individual bacteria can be enumerated and their individual masses rapidly determined (in femtograms 10^{-15} g) can be determined rapidly as they pass through the microchannel in the beam. Two posters were presented at the 2016 ASM Microbe to demonstrate proof of concept. Antibiotic susceptibility was determined using multiple gram-negative organisms that are generally used in clinical laboratories as antibiotic susceptibility testing control organisms. Resonant mass measurement and standard laboratory antibiotic susceptibility testing results were compared. More than two-thirds of these antibiotics demonstrated 100% essential agreement with the standard results after 3 hours or less, whereas the standard techniques required 16 to 24 hours. Two antibiotics were in less than 90% categorical agreement and required a longer incubation time. The results indicate that a rapid antibiotic susceptibility testing based on resonant mass measurement produces reliable antibiotic susceptibility testing results on gram-negative strains. Ongoing investigations are planned to extend these results to gram-positive strains and to validate the method on clinical samples from positive blood cultures.[58,59]

Colorimetric sensor array: use of volatile organic compounds and color active indicator array for rapid bacterial identification The SpecID (Specific Technologies, Mt. Lakes, CA) blood culture system provides organism detection and identification while the etiologic agent of sepsis is growing in a modified blood culture bottle and does so more rapidly than detection alone can occur in similar comparator blood culture bottles. When bacteria grow, they produce characteristic volatile organic compounds (VOC) that accumulate in the head gasses above the culture medium in the bottle; the spectrum of VOC produced is characteristic of a given genus and species of bacteria. An inexpensive, disposable array can be substituted for the top of a bottle or built into a proprietary bottle. This array consists of chemical indicators that change color differently when exposed to the VOC mixtures, allowing for the determination of the VOCs released. The first instrument using this technique was shown in Amsterdam at European Society of Clinical Microbiology and Infectious Diseases 2016. In a proof-of-principle paper, Lim and colleagues[60] demonstrated that the SpecID fingerprint can detect and identification the VOC fingerprints of organisms in pure culture with a sensitivity and specificity of 91% and 99.4%, respectively. It could distinguish between strains of *S aureus*, suggesting that it may be used for epidemiologic purposes as well. Furthermore, detection was rapid, with organism identification with the arrays detecting growth almost 2 hours faster than the standard system. Whether it will work in mixed infections remains to be determined.

Shrestha and colleagues[61] studied the ability of the SpecID arrays to identify a panel of important yeast pathogens. BacT/Alert bottles modified to contain the arrays were compared with standard bottles, all of which were inoculated with 10 mL of blood either unspiked or spiked with different quantities of the yeast species. Bottles containing no yeast were reported as negative, and the yeast in all positive bottles were detected correctly, regardless of a wide range of inoculum sizes. Growth by colorimetric sensor array was detected 6.8 hours faster than BacT/Alert system. The mean sensitivity for species-level identification by colorimetric sensor array was 74% at the time of growth detection, and increased with time, reaching almost 95% at 4 hours after growth detection.[60,61]

Cultureless systems for rapid detection and identification of pathogens directly from patient's specimen

Magicplex sepsis real-time test (SeeGene) Magicplex screens for more than 90 pathogens that cover more than 90% of sepsis-causing pathogens as well as 3 drug resistance markers for methicillin and vancomycin (mecA, vanA, and vanB) from whole blood sample. Also, this test is able to further identify the pathogens that are detected in the previous screening step with an additional 30 minutes. There are 73 gram-positive, 12 gram-negative, 6 fungi, and 3 antibiotic resistant genes that can also be discriminated. The Magicplex Sepsis Test requires 1 mL of a patient's whole blood and provides test results within 3 hours (after extraction). The microbial DNA enrichment is based on Molzym's MolYsis technology (Bremen, Germany) enabling up to 40,000-fold DNA enrichment over conventional technologies. Automated DNA isolation is performed with Seegene's Seeprep12 (Seoul, Korea) instrument based on Nordiag's "Arrow" technology/system. The pathogens identified by MagicPlex Sepsis assay are Streptococci (*S agalactiae, S pyogenes, S pneumoniae*), Enterococci (*E faecalis, E gallinarum, E faecium*), Staphylococci (*S epidermidis, S haemolyticus, S aureus*), *P aeruginosa, Acinetobacter baumannii, S maltophilia, S marcescens, B fragilis, S typhi, Klebsiella pneumoniae, K oxytoca, P mirabilis, E coli, E cloacae, E aerogenes, C albicans, C tropicalis, C parapsilosis, C glabrata, C krusei,* and *A fumigatus*. The MagicPlex is compatible with AB7500 RT-CR (Lifetime

Technologies, Hanoi, Japan), CFX96 Real-time PCR (Bio-Rad), and SmartCycler II RT-PCR.

In a clinical validation of MagicPlex, Serra and colleagues[62] demonstrated the detection of *Candida* DNA in pediatric patients in which the culture result was negative. However, the assay also had some false-negative results. In this study at least 1 mL of blood sample was inoculated into a VersaTREK REDOX1 bottle, which was incubated at 37°C for 3 hours or longer before DNA extraction. Carrara and colleagues[63] showed the result of a comparative study of MagicPlex and standard blood culture on 267 patients. From 98 positive results, 11% were positive by both system, 11% only by MagicPlex, and 15% only by blood culture. Sensitivity and specificity were 65% and 92%, respectively, for the Magicplex Sepsis Test and 71% and 88%, respectively for blood culture. Denina and colleagues[64] in a study of 89 pediatric patients, found that Magicplex allowed a 143% increase in the detection of septic episodes. However Ziegler and coworkers[65] found that the test detected many organisms suspected to be contaminants and investigated increasing the cut-off value for positive. They concluded that MagicPlex shows a high specificity but changes in design are needed to increase pathogen detection. For viability in clinical laboratories, technical improvements are also required to further automate the process. This product is IVD CE marked and is not available in the United States.

LightCycler SeptiFast test MGRADE SeptiFast (Roche Molecular Systems), provides rapid identification to the species level of 25 common etiologic agents of BSI (bacterial and fungal) in less than 6 hours directly from 1.5 mL of whole blood without prior culture. The assay targets a multicopy region (internal transcribed spacer) to increase sensitivity (the detection limit is approximately 300 colony-forming units [CFU]/mL). Targets include 8 gram-negative bacteria or related groups, 6 gram positives, and 8 fungi including *Aspergillus fumigatus*. The test is designed to be run on the LightCycler2.0 Instrument manufactured by Roche, which combines rapid amplification with melting point analysis for rapid results. A related assay also can detect the mecA gene detection from *S aureus*, in a subsequent run using the LightCycler SeptiFast MecA Test MGRADE. SeptiFast is CE marked but not available in the United States. Markota and colleagues[66] demonstrated a sensitivity of 87.5%, a specificity of 92.6%, and a negative predictive value 97.8% in comparison with standard blood culture and suggested that this system can be used as a supplement to the standard blood culture.

SepsiTest-UMD SepsiTest-UMD (Molzym) can use 1 to 10 mL of whole blood or tissue samples for detection of bacterial pathogens and yeast. After sample preparation and DNA concentration, the PCR assay amplifies 16S and 18S ribosomal sequences. Primers for Sanger sequencing are included in the assay. If positives are detected, they are identified by basic local alignment search tool analysis using an online data base. Additional kits are available for other fluids and swabs, but many are for research use only. Disqué and colleagues[67] compared the SepsiTest with blood culture and found a sensitivity of 60%, a specificity of 98%, a negative predictive value of 91%, and a positive predictive value of 86%. The system is not fully automated, and the results are not available quickly. The test is approved for in vitro diagnostics in Europe but not in the United States.

T2 biosystems sepsis solution The T2 biosystem is recognized in the US market for their FDA-approved assay for the diagnosis of candidemia directly from a blood sample of a patient in about 5 hours. T2-weighted MRI is a small instrument that uses PCR, followed by hybridization on probe-decorated nanoparticle microclusters.

Hybridization will induce changes in magnetic resonance signals, resulting in rapid identification of candida. One of the important features of this technique is direct use of blood samples by the instrument without any prior processing steps. It also benefits from high sensitivity that enables the system to detect a few CFU per milliliter of the target in whole blood. In a report from Mylanakis and colleagues,[68] the performance of T2 system for rapid detection of *Candida* species directly from the bloods of patients with suspected candidemia was evaluated. The report indicates that T2-weighted MRI demonstrated an overall specificity per assay of 99.4% (95% confidence interval [CI], 99.1%– 99.6%) with a mean time to a negative result of 4.2 ± 0.9 hours. Subanalysis yielded a specificity of 98.9% (95% CI, 98.3%–99.4%) for *C albicans/Candida tropicalis*, 99.3% (95% CI, 98.7%–99.6%) for *Candida parapsilosis*, and 99.9% (95% CI, 99.7%–100.0%) for *Candida krusei/Candida glabrata*. The overall sensitivity was found to be 91.1% (95% CI, 86.9%–94.2%) with a mean time of 4.4 ± 1.0 hours for detection and species identification. The subgroup analysis showed a sensitivity of 92.3% (95% CI, 85.4%–96.6%) for *C albicans/C tropicalis*, 94.2% (95% CI, 84.1%–98.8%) for *C parapsilosis*, and 88.1% (95% CI, 80.2%–93.7%) for *C krusei/C glabrata*. The LOD was 1 CFU/mL for *C tropicalis* and *C krusei*, 2 CFU/mL for *C albicans* and *C glabrata*, and 3 CFU/mL for *C parapsilosis*. The negative predictive value was estimated to range from 99.5% to 99.0% in a study population with 5% and 10% prevalence of candidemia, respectively.[68] The T2 bacterial panel is another assay for detection of bacterial pathogens directly from the blood of patients with suspected bacteremia/sepsis. It can detect *Escherichia coli, K pneumoniae, Pseudomonas aeruginosa, A baumannii, S aureus*, and *Enterococcus faecium* and is expected to be FDA cleared by 2018. The usefulness of this system in the clinical setting and its potential impact on patient outcome await data from clinical studies.

Qvella FAST ID BSI panel The Qvella blood pathogen detection system (FAST ID BSI Panel) has been developed to identify bacterial and fungal pathogens directly from blood samples in less than 1 hour. It uses the rRNA as the target in a multiplex PCR for bacterial identification. The system benefits also from a tailored electric field for the lysis of the bacterial cells present in the blood sample, followed by a concentration step to obtain a highly concentrated and purified bacterial genomic materials. The purified nucleic acids are used in the multiplex real time reverse transcriptase PCR for rapid detection and identification of microorganisms directly from blood.

The FAST technology is implemented in the FAST ID BSI Panel, which is an integrated and closed device designed to fully automate the isolation, concentration, and lysis, as well as amplification and detection of nucleic acids from pathogens from whole blood samples. To perform a test, a whole blood tube is inserted into a FAST ID BSI Panel and it is placed into the FAST analyzer. The following processes occur automatically during the processing of a FAST ID BSI Panel by the analyzer: Target cell isolation and concentration, target cell electrical lysis and treatment, and amplification and detection of bacterial and fungal ribosomal targets in a spatially multiplexed array. This assay can detect the majority of sepsis-causing species. The system has been shown to be able to identify polymicrobial infections in spiked samples.

Khine and colleagues[69] presented data at the 27th European Society of Clinical Microbiology and Infectious Diseases regarding the lower LOD of the Qvella FAST system. The LOD was determined to be approximately 1 CFU/mL for the various cell types. This low LOD is consistent with pathogen concentrations typically found in infected whole blood samples. For this dataset, detection was made at 100% of the time for *Klebsiella pneumoniae, Pseudomonas aeruginosa, E faecium, C albicans*, and *C glabrata* down to 1 CFU/mL. For *S aureus*, detection was made at 100% of the time at or greater than 2 CFU/mL and greater than 80% of the time for 1 CFU/mL. However, less than 100% detection of *S aureus* was at least partly attributable to the inherent difficulty and accuracy associated with spiking certain gram-positive bacteria at very low concentrations. The Qvella blood identification system is designed to detect more than 90% of pathogens isolated from patients with sepsis. Clinical trial of this system is expected to start in the second quarter of 2018.

NEXT-GENERATION SEQUENCING

The advances in sequencing technology known as NGS have led to significant advances in basic sciences and clinical laboratory medicine, including microbiology. Currently available NGS techniques are based on using clonal amplicons for parallel multistrand sequencing. The combination of high-speed and high-throughput data analysis has made NGS an excellent tool to take clinical analysis of nucleic acid sequences to a new level. With NGS, it is possible to detect and quantify quasispecies of HIV, HCV, or hepatitis B virus circulating at low levels in the blood of infected patients and to learn more about their roles in the development of resistance and associated treatment failures. This was difficult or impossible by using methods mentioned previously. Despite increasing numbers of articles on the applications of NGS, this system has not found its way into routine clinical microbiology testing because of lack of FDA approval, high cost, and availability of alternative technologies.[28] From the diagnostic microbiology viewpoint, NGS has significantly improved our ability to study the makeup of entire communities of microorganisms without culture. NGS can provide the genetic sequences of the members of entire microbial communities (microbiomes) and determine their relative frequencies. It could also be used to determine gene expression and metabolic pathway use in a microbial community, although this is currently beyond the scope of the clinical microbiology laboratory. Many studies of human microbiomes are focusing on the relationship between microbial communities and health and disease, including for example, the effect of colonic microorganisms on cardiovascular disease.[4] NGS has also been applied to rapid investigations of outbreaks in hospital settings. We discuss herein 2 NGS-based diagnostic microbiology systems that are currently fairly advanced in development. They highlight the potential of NGS to improve detection and identification of pathogens in the clinical laboratory, especially those involving organisms that may be difficult or impossible to identify, or those situations that are otherwise technically demanding.[70–72]

Systems Based on Next-Generation Sequencing for the Identification of Pathogens from Clinical Specimens

Karius digital culture

Karius (Redwood City, CA) has developed an NGS-based test to detect the presence in plasma of cell-free DNA, which is presumably derived from infecting pathogens. After amplification, human DNA is removed by a proprietary technique. NGS is performed on the total nucleic acids, enriching for the microbial sequences. These sequences are aligned with a pathogen sequence bank that consists not only of publicly available genetic information, but also of Karius's internal data. Thus, it can potentially detect thousands of infecting organisms. The system is unique in that it can detect sequences from DNA viruses in addition to those from bacteria and fungi. Like standard organism detection assays, this system can detect bacteremia and fungemia.

In several studies Karius and collaborators have also shown that the system is able to diagnose infections with certain highly fastidious organisms or after antibiotics have rendered the infecting organism nonviable. The system could also detect the infecting organism in infections outside of the bloodstream when organismal DNA is released into the blood, including osteomyelitis, and deep infections that would otherwise require biopsies. In patients with known or suspected bacteremia, their system showed 80.0% positive agreement and 73.8% negative agreement (overall agreement of 76.7%) with standard blood culture. In comparison with the clinical diagnosis, their system showed 82.4% and 79.1% positive and negative agreement, respectively.[73-75]

PathoQuest iDTECT

The iDTECT Blood (PathoQuest, Paris, France) also combines untargeted NGS with their sample preparation process and their genome sequence database, which is said to cover all clinically relevant human pathogens. It is the first CE-marked (October 2016), NGS-based method to detect bacteria and viruses in patients with known or suspected infections directly from patient blood thereby improving pathogen detection in biological samples. PathoQuest's technology combines an NGS platform and a proprietary sample preparation process with a proprietary pathogen genome sequence database and automated analysis software covering all known clinically relevant human pathogens. Parize and colleagues,[76] using a prototype version of iDTECT, identified a relevant pathogen in more patients in a difficult-to-diagnose population than conventional testing.

SUMMARY

The application of molecular testing to the discipline of infectious disease diagnosis, prognosis and management has matured exponentially over the last few years. Future improvements will no doubt avail additional milestones in sensitivity, specificity, cost reduction, and turnaround time from specimen procurement to result for effective and expeditious patient management.

REFERENCES

1. Alexander BD, Ashley ED, Reller LB, et al. Cost savings with implementation of PNA FISH testing for identification of *Candida albicans* in blood cultures. Diagn Microbiol Infect Dis 2006;54:277–82.
2. Forrest GN, Roghmann MC, Toombs LS, et al. Peptide nucleic acid fluorescent in situ hybridization for hospital-acquired enterococcal bacteremia: delivering earlier effective antimicrobial therapy. Antimicrob Agents Chemother 2008;52:3558–63.
3. Perez KK, Olsen RJ, Musick WL, et al. Integrating rapid pathogen identification and antimicrobial stewardship significantly decreases hospital costs. Arch Pathol Lab Med 2013;137(9):1247–54. Accessed September 12, 2013.
4. Karlsson FH, Fak F, Nookaew I, et al. Symptomatic atherosclerosis is associated with an altered gut metagenome. Nat Commun 2012;3:1245. Accessed September 12, 2013.
5. Fairfax MR, Salimnia H. Diagnostic molecular microbiology: a 2013 snapshot. Clin Lab Med 2013;33:787–803.
6. AccuProbe *Mycobacterium tuberculosis* complex culture identification test. Package Insert. Hologic Gen-Probe. Revision 2011-02. Available at: http://www.gen-probe.com/pdfs/pi/102896RevN.pdf. Accessed April 28, 2013.
7. Welch DF, Guruswamy AP, Sides SJ, et al. Timely culture for mycobacteria which utilizes a microcolony method. J Clin Microbiol 1993;31:2178–84.

8. Becton Dickinson. Bacte Myco/F Sputa. Package Insert. Revision 2010/2. Available at: http://www.bd.com/ds/technicalCenter/inserts/PP101JAA(2011002).pdf. Accessed April 20, 2013.

9. Lie AK, Kristensen G. Human papillomavirus E6/E7 mRNA testing as a predictive marker for cervical carcinoma. Expert Rev Mol Diagn 2008;8:405–15.

10. Qiagen. Digene Hybrid Capture 2 High-Risk HPV DNATest. Ref 5199–1220. Package insert. Available at: http://www.qiagen.com/resources/Download.aspx?id5(0A98CB57-25B9-48A9-9C4F-4C66D1CDA47C) &lang5en&ver55. Accessed September 9, 2013.

11. Gravitt E, Rostich AF, Silver MI, et al. A cohort effect of the sexual revolution may be masking an increase in human papillomavirus detection at menopause in the United States. J Infect Dis 2013;207:274–80. Queried on line April 2, 2013.

12. Quiroga-Garza G, Zhou H, Mody DR. Unexpected high prevalence of HPV 90 infection in an underserved population: is it really a low-risk genotype? Arch Pathol Lab Med 2013;137(11):1569–73.

13. Salimnia H, Fairfax MR, Lephart P, et al. An international, prospective, multicenter evaluation of the combination of AdvanDx Staphylococcus QuickFISH BC with mecA XpressFISH for detection of methicillin-resistant Staphylococcus aureus isolates from positive blood cultures. J Clin Micrbiol 2014;52(11):3928–32.

14. Della-Latta P, Salimnia H, Painter T, et al. Identification of Escherichia coli, Klebsiella pneumoniae, and Pseudomonas aeruginosa in blood cultures: a multicenter performance evaluation of a three-color peptide nucleic acid fluorescence in situ hybridization assay. J Clin Microbiol 2011;49(6):2259–61.

15. Morgan M, Marlowe E, Della-Latta P, et al. Multicenter evaluation of a new shortened peptide nucleic acid fluorescence in situ hybridization procedure for species identification of select Gram-negative bacilli from blood cultures. J Clin Microbiol 2010;48(6):2268–70.

16. Abdelhamed AM, Zhang SX, Watkins T, et al. Multicenter evaluation of Candida QuickFISH BC for identification of Candida species directly from blood culture bottles. J Clin Microbiol 2015;53(5):1672–6.

17. Becton Dickinson. BD Affirm VPIII Microbial Identification Test. Package Insert. Revision of 2006/02 Queried on line April 25, 2013. Available at: http://www.bd.com/ds/technicalCenter/inserts/pkgInserts.asp#PF8.

18. BD Max vaginal panel package insert. Available at: http://www.bd.com/resource.aspx?IDX=32632. Accessed December 1, 2017.

19. Andrea SB, Chapin KC. Comparison of Aptima Trichomonas vaginalis transcription-mediated amplification assay and BD Affirm VPIII for detection of T. vaginalis in symptomatic women: performance parameters and epidemiologic implications. J Clin Microbiol 2011;49:866–9.

20. Gen-Probe. Aptima Combo 2 Assay. Package Insert. Version 2011-04. Queried on line: May 20, 2013. Available at: http://www.gen-probe.com/pdfs/pi/501799-EN-RevD.pdf.

21. Taylor SN, Van der Pol B, Lillis B, et al. Clinical evaluation of the BD ProbeTec Chlamydia trachomatis Qx amplified DNA assay on the BD Viper system with XTR technology. Sex Transm Dis 2011;38:603–9.

22. Becton Dickinson. ProbeTec Chlamydia trachomatis (CT) Qx Amplified DNA assay. Package insert. Version 2010/12. queried on line May 12, 2013. Available at: http://www.bd.com/ds/technicalCenter/inserts/8981498(201012).pdf.

23. Wolfe D, Hook EW, Mena L, et al. Evaluation of the BD Viper™ System in Extracted Mode to Detect Chlamydia trachomatis and Neisseria gonorrhoeae in

Male Swab and Urine Specimens Clinical Virology Symposium. Daytona Beach, FL, April 27, 2008.

24. Cheng A, Qian Q, Kirby JE. Evaluation of the Abbott RealTime CT/NG assay in comparison to the Roche Cobas Amplicor CT/NG assay. J Clin Microbiol 2011; 49:1294–300.

25. Chernesky M, Jang D, Gilchrist J, et al. Head-to-head comparison of second-generation nucleic acid amplification tests for detection of *Chlamydia trachomatis* and *Neisseria gonorrhoeae* on urine samples from female subjects and self-collected vaginal swabs. J Clin Microbiol 2014;52(7):2305–10.

26. Gen-Probe Procleix Ultrio Plus Assay. 502432-REG Rev.7, as sub- mitted to the FDA. Queried on line May 20, 2013. Available at: http://www.fda.gov/downloads/ BiologicsBloodVaccines/BloodBloodProducts/ApprovedProducts/LicensedProducts BLAs/BloodDonorScreening/InfectiousDisease/UCM335285. pdf.

27. Maurin M. Real-time PCR as a diagnostic tool for bacterial diseases. Expert Rev Mol Diagn 2012;12:731–54.

28. Fairfax MR, Salimnia H. Quantitative PCR: an introduction. In: Grody WW, Strom C, Kiechle FL, et al, editors. Handbook of molecular diagnostics. London: Academic Press; 2010. p. 3–14.

29. Espy MJ, Uhl P, Mitchell S, et al. Diagnosis of herpes simplex virus in the clinical laboratory by LightCycler PCR. J Clin Microbiol 2000;38:795–9.

30. Issa NC, Espy MJ, Uhl P, et al. Sequencing and resolution of amplified herpes simplex virus with intermediate melting curves as genotype 1 or 2 by light cycler PCR assay. J Clin Microbiol 2005;43:1843–5.

31. Available at: http://www.luminexcorp.com/prod/groups/public/documents/ lmnxcorp/342-multicode-tech.pdf. Accessed May 12, 2013.

32. Strain MC, Richmond DD. New assays for monitoring residual HIV burden in effectively treated individuals. Curr Opin HIV AIDS 2013;8:106–10.

33. Sire JM, Vray M, Merzouk M, et al. Comparative RNA quantification of HIV-1 group M and non-m with the Roche Cobas AmpliPrep/Cobas TaqMan HIV-1 v2.0 and Abbott Real-Time HIV-1 PCR assays. J Acquir Immune Defic Syndr 2011;56(3):239–43.

34. Wojewoda CM, Shalinger T, Harmon ML, et al. Comparison of Roche Cobas Am-pliPrep/Cobas TaqMan HIV-1 test version 2.0 (CAP/CTM v2.0) with other real-time PCR assays in HIV monitoring and follow-up of low-level viral loads. J Virol Methods 2013;187:1–5.

35. Babady NE, Mead P, Stiles J, et al. Comparison of the Luminex xTAG RVP Fast-assay with the Idaho Technology FilmArray RP assay for detection of respiratory viruses in pediatric patients at a cancer hospital. J Clin Microbiol 2012;50: 2282–8.

36. McGrath EJ, Thomas R, Asmar B, et al. Detection of respiratory co-infections in pediatric patients using a small volume polymerase chain reaction array respira-tory panel: more evidence for combined droplet and contact isolation. Am J Infect Control 2013;41:868–73. Queried on line April 1, 2013.

37. Popowich EB, O'Niel SS, Miller MM. Comparison of the Biofire FilmArray RP, Gen-mark eSensor RBP, Luminex xTAG RVPv1, and Luminex xTAG RVP Fast multiplex assays for detection of respiratory viruses. J Clin Microbiol 2013;51(5):1528–33. Accessed May 16, 2012.

38. Mahoney JB. Nucleic acid amplification-based diagnosis of respiratory virus in-fections. Expert Rev Anti Infect Ther 2010;8(11):1273–92. Accessed May 16, 2013.

39. de Groot RJ, Baker SC, Baric RS, et al. Middle East Respiratory Syndrome Coronavirus (MERS-CoV); announcement of the coronavirus study group. J Virol 2013;87:7790–2.

40. Liu D, Shi W, Shi Y, et al. Origin and diversity of novel avian influenza A H7N9 viruses causing human infection: phylogenetic, structural, and coalescent analyses. Lancet 2013;381(9881):1926–32.

41. Tissari P, Zumla A, Tarkka E, et al. Accurate and rapid identification of bacterial species from positive blood cultures with a DNA-based microarray platform: an observational study. Lancet 2010;375(9710):224–30.

42. Huggett JM, Whale A. Digital PCR as a novel technology and its potential implications for molecular diagnostics. Clin Chem 2013;59:1691–3.

43. Sedlak RH, Jerome KR. Viral diagnostics in the era of digital PCR. Diagn Microbiol Infect Dis 2013;75(1):1–4.

44. Laurie MT, Bertout JA, Taylor SD, et al. Simultaneous digital quantification and fluorescence-based size characterization of massively parallel sequencing libraries. Biotechniques 2013;55(2):61–7.

45. Whale AS, Cowen S, Foy CA, et al. Methods for applying accurate digital PCR analysis on low copy DNA samples. PLoS One 2013;8(3):e58177.

46. Theel ES, Schmitt BH, Hall L, et al. Formic acid-based direct, on-plate testing of yeast and corynebacterium species by Bruker Biotyper matrix-assisted laser desorption ionization-time of flight mass spectrometry. J Clin Microbiol 2012;50:3093–5.

47. March-Rosselló GA, Muñoz-Moreno MF, García-Loygorri-Jordán de Urriés MC, et al. A differential centrifugation protocol and validation criterion for enhancing mass spectrometry (MALDI-TOF) results in microbial identification using blood culture growth bottles. Eur J Clin Microbiol Infect Dis 2013;32:699–704.

48. Mestas J, Felsenstein S, Bard JD. Direct identification of bacteria from positive BacT/ALERT blood culture bottles using matrix-assisted laser desorption ionization-time-of-flight mass spectrometry. Diagn Microbiol Infect Dis 2014;80(3):193–6.

49. Mitchell SL, Alby K. Performance of microbial identification by MALDI-TOF MS and susceptibility testing by VITEK 2 from positive blood cultures after minimal incubation on solid media. Eur J Clin Microbiol Infect Dis 2017;36(11):2201–6.

50. Wimmer JL, Long SW, Cernoch P, et al. Strategy for rapid identification and antibiotic susceptibility testing of gram-negative bacteria directly recovered from positive blood cultures using the Bruker MALDI Biotyper and the BD Phoenix system. J Clin Microbiol 2012;50(7):2452–4.

51. Rehse SJ, Salimnia H, Miziolek AW, et al. Laser-induced breakdown spectroscopy (LIBS): an overview of recent progress and future potential for biomedical applications. J Med Eng Technol 2012;36:77–89.

52. Malenfant DJ, Gillies DJ, Rehse SJ. Bacterial suspensions deposited on microbiological filter material for rapid laser-induced breakdown spectroscopy identification. Appl Spectrosc 2016;70(3):485–93.

53. Chouthai NS, Shah AA, Salimnia H, et al. Use of Raman spectroscopy to decrease time for identifying the species of candida growth in cultures. Avicenna J Med Biotechnol 2015;7(1):45–8.

54. Ashton L, Lau K, Winder CL, et al. Raman spectroscopy: lighting up the future of microbial identification. Future Microbiol 2011;6(9):991–7.

55. Smith E, Dent G. A comprehensive but readable introduction to the field of Raman spectroscopy. In: Smith E, Dent G, editors. Modern Raman Spectroscpy, a

Practical Approach. West Sussex (United Kingdom): John Wiley and Sons; 2005. p. 1–21.

56. Lephart P, Kaye KS, Pogue JM, et al. Evaluation of accelerate Pheno™ system in a clinical setting: comparison of identification and antibiotic susceptibility test results of 224 prospective positive blood cultures to standard laboratory methods at Detroit Medical Center. European Congress of Clinical Microbiology and Infectious Diseases, Vienna, Austria, April 22–25, 2017.

57. Marschal M, Bachmaier J, Autenrieth I, et al. Evaluation of the accelerate Pheno system for Fast identification and antimicrobial susceptibility testing from positive blood cultures in bloodstream infections caused by gram-negative pathogens. J Clin Microbiol 2017;55(7):2116–26.

58. Schneider C, Babcock K, Harris P, et al. Rapid antimicrobial susceptibility tests by mass measurement on a 96 well plate. ASM microbe. Boston, June 16–20, 2016.

59. Babcock K, Schneider C, Harris P, et al. Phenotypic response of bacteria to antibiotics at single minute time scales. ASM microbe. Boston, June 16–19, 2016.

60. Lim SH, Mix S, Anikst V, et al. Bacterial culture detection and identification in blood agar plates with an optoelectronic nose. Analyst 2016;141:918.

61. Shrestha NK, Lim SH, Wilson D, et al. The combined rapid detection and species-level identification of yeasts in simulated blood culture using a colorimetric sensor array. PLoS One 2017;12(3):e0173130.

62. Serra J, Rosello E, Figueras C, et al. Clinical evaluation of the Magicplex sepsis real-time test (Seegene) to detect Candida DNA in pediatric patients. Crit Care 2012;16(Suppl 3):P42.

63. Carrara L, Navarro F, Turbau M, et al. Molecular diagnosis of bloodstream infections with a new dual-priming oligonucleotide-based multiplex PCR assay. J Med Microbiol 2013;62:1673–9.

64. Denina M, Scolfaro c, Colombo S, et al. Magicplex sepsis real-time test to improve bloodstream infection diagnostics in children. Eur J Pediatr 2016; 175(8):1107–11.

65. Ziegler I, Fagerstrom A, Stralin K, et al. Evaluation of a commercial multiplex PCR assay for detection of pathogen DNA in blood from patients with suspected sepsis. PLoS One 2016;11(12):e0167883.

66. Markota A, Seme K, Golle A, et al. SeptiFast real-time PCR for detection of blood-borne pathogens in patients with severe sepsis or septic shock. Coll Antropol 2014;38(3):829–33.

67. Disqué C, Kochem AJ, Mühl H, et al. Polymerase chain reaction detection of sepsis-inducing pathogens in blood using SepsiTest™. Crit Care 2008; 12(Suppl 5):P10.

68. Mylonakis E, Clancy CJ, Ostrosky-Zeichner L, et al. T2 magnetic resonance assay for the rapid diagnosis of candidemia in whole blood: a clinical trial. Clin Infect Dis 2015;60:892–9.

69. Khine AA, Parmar V, Talebpour A, et al. Evaluating the analytical sensitivity of Qvella's FAST(TM) ID system for early detection and identification of bloodstream infection in whole blood 27th ECCMID. Vienna, Austria, April 22–25, 2017.

70. Capobianchi MR, Giombini E, Rozera G. Next-generation sequencing technology in clinical virology. Clin Microbiol Infect 2013;19(1):15–22.

71. Song S, Jarvie T, Hattori M. Our second genome-human metagenome: how next-generation sequencer changes our life through microbiology. Adv Microb Physiol 2013;62:119–44.

72. Sherry NL, Porter JL, Seemann T, et al. Outbreak investigation using high-throughput genome sequencing within a diagnostic microbiology laboratory. J Clin Microbiol 2013;51:1396–401.

73. Abril MK, Barnett AS, Wegermann K, et al. Diagnosis of *Capnocytophaga canimorss* sepsis by whole-genome next-generation sequencing. Open Forum Infect Dis 2016;3(3):ofw144.

74. Wanda L, Ruffin F, Hill-Rorie J, et al. Direct Detection and quantification of bacterial cell-free DNA in patients with bloodstream infection (BSI) using the Karius Plasma Next Generation Sequencing (NGS) Test. ID week October 4–8, 2017, San Diego.

75. Benamu E, Gajurel K, Anderson JN, et al. Performance of the Karius Plasma Next Generation Sequencing Test in Determining the Etiologic Diagnosis of Febrile Neutropenia: results from a pilot study. ID week October 4–8, 2017, San Diego.

76. Parize P, Muth E, Richaud C, et al. Untargeted next-generation sequencing-based first-line diagnosis of infection in immunocompromised adults: a multicentre, blinded, prospective study. Clin Microbiol Infect 2017;23(8):574.e1-6.

Molecular Pathology in Transfusion Medicine

New Concepts and Applications

Matthew B. Elkins, MD, PhD[a],*, Robertson D. Davenport, MD[b],
Martin H. Bluth, MD, PhD[c,d]

KEYWORDS

- Genotype • Phenotype • Serology • Antigen • Antibody • Blood donors
- Transfusion • Red blood cells

KEY POINTS

- Virtually all the red blood cell and platelet antigen systems have been characterized at the molecular level and highly reliable methods for red blood cell and platelet antigen genotyping are now available.
- Genotyping is a useful adjunct to traditional serology and can help resolve complex serologic problems.
- Although red blood cell and platelet phenotypes can be inferred from genotype, knowledge of the molecular basis essential for accurate assignment.
- Genotyping of blood donors is an effective method of identifying antigen-negative and/or particularly rare donors.
- Cell-free DNA analysis provides a promising noninvasive method of assessing fetal genotypes of blood group alloantigens.

OVERVIEW

Testing performed in transfusion medicine focuses on detection of antigens expressed on the cell membrane of red blood cells (RBCs) and/or platelets and the detection of antibodies against RBC or platelet antigens in a patient's plasma. Detection of these antigens and antibodies is critical because RBC or platelet units that are positive for a given antigen and that are transfused into a patient who has antibodies

This article has been updated from a version previously published in Clinics in Laboratory Medicine, Volume 33, Issue 4, December 2013.
[a] Department of Pathology, Upstate Medical University, 750 East Adams Street, Syracuse, NY 13210, USA; [b] Department of Pathology, University of Michigan, UH 2g332, 1500 East Medical Center Drive, Ann Arbor, MI 48109-5054, USA; [c] Department of Pathology, Wayne State University, School of Medicine, 540 East Canfield Street, Detroit, MI 48201, USA; [d] Pathology Laboratories, Michigan Surgical Hospital, 21230 Dequindre Road, Warren, MI 48091, USA
* Corresponding author.
E-mail address: ElkinsM@upstate.edu

Clin Lab Med 38 (2018) 277–292
https://doi.org/10.1016/j.cll.2018.02.001
0272-2712/18/© 2018 Elsevier Inc. All rights reserved.

labmed.theclinics.com

against that specific antigen may cause decreased blood product survival, hemolytic transfusion reactions, hyperhemolysis reactions, and even death.

RBCs and platelet antigens and antibodies are traditionally detected using serologic assays. These assays overwhelmingly use hemagglutination principles to indicate the presence of an antibody in the tested serum and the presence of the antigen on the tested RBC or platelet product. For example, forward typing of a patient's RBC antigens is performed by combining the patient's RBCs with known anti-A, anti-B, and anti-D antisera. Any reaction resulting in agglutinated RBCs suggests that the RBCs have that antigen on their surface (eg, agglutination in anti-A reaction suggests the presence of the A antigen on the RBC membrane). To cause agglutination, the assays rely on the agglutination capability of the tested antibodies (eg, ABO testing) for the IgM class and secondary antibodies (eg, antihuman globulin antibodies and anti-C3 antibodies) for the IgG class.

ADVANTAGES OF MOLECULAR TESTING

Molecular testing is complementary to traditional serologic testing used for most transfusion medicine testing.[1] Molecular testing does not replace serologic testing, and serologic testing is still very much the backbone of transfusion medicine testing. Serologic testing is well characterized, sensitive enough to find and identify most clinically significant alloantibodies, and useful for most patient situations. Serologic testing is limited, however, in specific patients and situations, including the following:

- Patients with confounding antibodies (warm or cold autoantibodies or cold agglutinins, and neonates with passive maternal antibodies)
- Patients with antigens or antibodies for which testing antibodies or antisera are not available (partial or variant antigens, rare antigens, and high-incidence antigens)
- Patients with a mixture of circulating RBCs or plasma (recently transfused, after bone marrow transplant, and after plasmapheresis)
- Patients in whom antigen zygosity needs to be determined
- Patients with select diseases (ie, sickle cell) where frequent transfusions increase immunohematological difficulties
- Mass screenings of blood donors

In each of these situations, serologic testing may be of limited sensitivity and specificity or may be prohibitive in time, effort, or cost.

Obscuring autoantibodies or multiple alloantibodies can cause unexpected agglutination in test reactions. This can result in an inability to rule out alloantibody possibilities, making it difficult or impossible to identify any clinically significant alloantibodies in a patient's serum. Antibodies against low-incidence antigens may not be effectively identified because of the limited availability of antisera and antigen-positive test RBCs. Similarly, antibodies to high-incidence antigens may be difficult to identify because of the lack of commercially available antisera or antigen-negative reagent RBCs. In patients who have received multiple RBC transfusions, the transfused RBCs may obscure the presence or absence of antigens of interest on a patient's native RBCs. Likewise, the serum of patients receiving multiple plasma transfusions or automated plasma exchange cannot be evaluated for antibodies from the patient's native immune system because of obscuring or dilution by the transfused plasma. For many RBC or platelet antigens, the phenotypes of homozygous and heterozygous patients are often indistinguishable by serologic means. For example, although there is the concept of "dosing," observing differences in the strength of hemagglutination when reagent

RBCs have homozygous versus heterozygous expression of a given phenotype, RBCs that only have 1 copy of a specific allele can look the same as RBCs with 2 copies. Mass screenings of the antigen status of RBCs or platelets is a daunting task using serologic methods because of the poor scalability, considerable cost, and limited automation options. Thus, each blood component unit must be individually tested for each antigen using labor-intensive techniques.

In contrast, for each of these situations, molecular testing may allow determination of antigens expressed by the patient or donor. Determination of the antigens expressed by a patient also may be used presumptively to predict which alloantibodies can be produced by the patient (because an individual can make alloantibodies only against antigens that the individual lacks). Such predictive approaches have been applied to specific patient populations (those with sickle cell disease, thalassemia, and so forth) where molecular analysis can predict what antibodies could be generated, thereby reducing the risk and clinical relevance of future transfusion incompatibilities and reactivities where blood availability presents an issue.[2]

LIMITATIONS OF MOLECULAR TESTING

There are limitations to the application of molecular testing in transfusion medicine. Primarily, molecular testing provides information on the genotype of the patient and, as such, cannot determine the specificities of any antibodies within a patient's serum. Molecular testing can only determine the antigens that a patient makes and, therefore, which antigen specificities that patient could theoretically make antibodies against. A patient with unknown antibody (or antibodies) may be molecularly typed to express D, C, e, and Jk(a) but not express c, E, and Jk(b). Based solely on this information, antibodies in a patient's serum could be specific to any 1 or multiples of the antigens c, E, Jk(b) or to another RBC antigen not tested by the molecular assay. Serologic testing is required to determine the specificity (or specificities) of the patient's antibody (or antibodies).

Molecular testing is promulgated on the frequency of anticipated polymorphism common within a population. As such, it is limited in detection of genes with an abundance of alleles (eg, ABO system) and antigens for which the coding gene is not known. Furthermore, molecular testing assays performed using allele-specific polymerase chain reaction (PCR) in which amplicon identification is made based on size do not detect point mutations, inversions, or other alterations of the DNA sequence that do not alter either the targeted primer sites or the amplicon size. Most institutions are batching molecular testing, thus increasing turn-around time, with the result that, currently, molecular testing may be significantly slower than serologic testing for uncomplicated patients. Finally, if possible, molecular testing results should be confirmed using serologic testing because genetic determinants outside the gene tested (eg, promoters) may affect the expression of that antigen. This results in a patient or donor labeled "positive" for an antigen when the patient or donor does not actually express that antigen.[3] An example is the D phenotype, in which there is no apparent expression by serologic testing of any of the *RHCE* antigens in a D-positive person despite the presence of the *RHCE* genes. This phenotype is due to a single nucleotide (907C) deletion in exon 6 that introduces a premature stop codon, which results in the silencing of the *RHCE* genes.[4] Similarly, alleles that vary expression depending on their cis or trans orientation may also lead to discrepant results between phenotype and genotype testing approaches.

MOLECULAR TECHNIQUES USED IN TRANSFUSION MEDICINE

The molecular techniques currently used for testing in transfusion medicine are all based on amplification of sequences from the DNA of the patient or donor. The targets of testing are the genes that determine the production of RBC or platelet antigenic determinants. These techniques are used as an adjunct to serologic testing in determining either the antigens expressed on the cell membranes of donated blood products or antigens not expressed on the cell membranes of blood transfusion recipients. These techniques help determine which antigens the recipient may make antibodies against, thereby forecasting possible incompatibilities for future transfusions.

Transfusion testing is particularly amenable to molecular methods because most assays evaluate constitutional genetic expression (germline expression), thus avoiding the sensitivity problems seen in some molecular testing targeted toward somatic mutations within a background of germline genes.

Current testing methodologies include various permutations of PCR, restriction fragment length polymorphism, single-nucleotide polymorphism (SNP) detection, Sanger sequencing, and high-throughput multiplex PCR. The most commonly used testing methods are PCR with allele-specific primers and detection of amplicons by traditional gel or capillary electrophoresis, using either commercially available kits or published or in-house protocols.[5,6] The downside of this approach is that a separate PCR reaction must be set up and a separate detection assay (gel or capillary electrophoresis) must be run for each antigen evaluated. This results in a slow, labor-intensive process. In a practice with a low volume of molecular testing, however, these assays require low investment in supporting technology.

One of the approaches to minimizing the labor required and increasing the information output from a single assay is to multiplex the molecular assays, using multiple PCR primer sets in a single reaction to assay for multiple allele-specific RBC antigen genes. There are various multiplex approaches, each of which uses a specific detection method to report which allelic amplicons are produced by the multiplex PCR. Commercially available systems using multiplexed PCR include the SNaPshot (Applied Biosystems, Foster City, California),[7] the Multiplex Ligation-dependent Probe Amplification (MLPA) system (MRC-Holland, Amsterdam, the Netherlands),[8] the OpenArray Real-Time PCR System (ThermoFisher Scientific, Waltham, Massachusetts),[9] the BioArray HEA BeadChip system and LifeCodes RBC (both Immucor, Norcross, Georgia),[10–12] ID CORE XT (Progenika Biopharma–Grifols, Bizkaia, Spain) using the Luminex platform and xMAP (Luminex, Austin, Texas),[13] the BLOODchip (Progenika, Medford, Massachusetts),[14] and the Hemo ID Blood Group Genotyping Panel using the MassARRAY System (Agena Bioscience, San Diego, California).[15,16] The SNaPshot system provides detection of the products of a multiplexed PCR reaction using allele-specific primers with different lengths of nonsense nucleotide tails (**Fig. 1**).[7] These primers are allowed to hybridize to the PCR products and bind right next to the gene polymorphism resulting in the RBC antigen genotype. These PCR products combined with the primer are incubated with fluorescently labeled dideoxynucleotides (ddNTPs) resulting in extension of only a single nucleotide (similar to what is used in classic Sanger sequencing). The resulting fragments are separated based on the size (imparted by the nonsense primer tail) and the fluorescence of the product (imparted by the labeled ddNTPs) determines the nucleotide at the polymorphism site, which identifies the genotype of each of the interrogated RBC antigen genes. The MLPA system uses an array of primers for diverse RBC antigens, which bind to the unamplified genomic DNA (**Fig. 2**).[8] Primer pairs that are an exact match for the target gene are ligated to form a template for subsequent amplification. Due to differences in length of the original ligation primers, the specific primers that were able to bind to the genomic DNA can be determined using capillary electrophoresis. The OpenArray Real-Time PCR System uses genomic DNA as a template for amplification using the TaqMan enzyme, which releases a fluorescent molecule from the inhibition of a

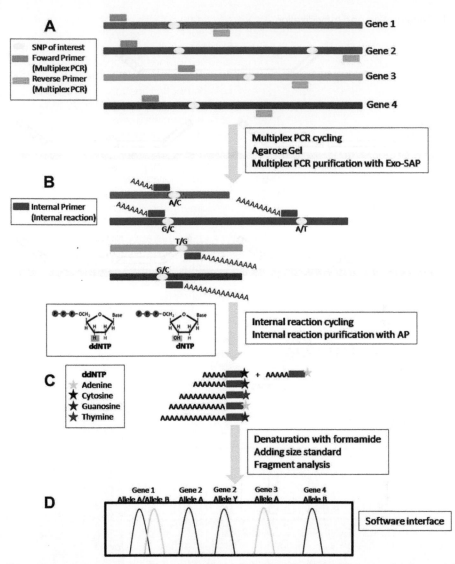

Fig. 1. Schematic representation of SNaPshot. (*A*) Multiplex PCR. (*B*) Internal primers. (*C*) Fragments after internal primer reaction. (*D*) Sample genotype using a specific software: *Gene1*A/Gene1*B, Gene2*A/Gene2*A, Gene2*Y/Gene2*Y, Gene3*A/Gene3*A, Gene4*B/ Gene4*B*. AP, alkaline phosphatase; ddNTPs, dideoxynucleotides; dNTPs, deoxynucleotides; Exo-SAP, exonuclease and alkaline phosphatase; SNPs, single nucleotide polymorphisms. (*From* Latini FRM, Castilho LM. An overview of the use of SNaPshot for predicting blood group antigens. Immunohematology 2015;31(2):53; with permission.)

quencher if the primers are a perfect match (**Fig. 3**).[9] This reaction is multiplexed into multiple wells, each with a different set of TaqMan primers to interrogate a different RBC antigen polymorphism. Evaluation of the pattern of fluorescence provides the RBC antigen genotyping of the sample. In the BeadChip system, multiplex PCR amplicons are hybridized to allele-specific probes bound to fluorescent beads. If the sequences are a match, the probe is extended by PCR and the resultant increase in

1. Denaturation and hybridization

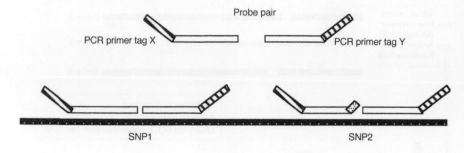

SNP1   SNP2

2. Ligation reaction

3. PCR

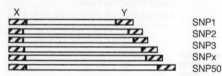

SNP1
SNP2
SNP3
SNPx
SNP50

4. Capillary electrophoresis

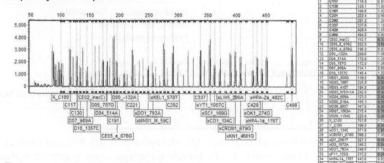

5. Data comparison to reference sample

Fig. 2. The MLPA procedure in 5 steps. (1) A mix containing up to 50 probe pairs is hybridized overnight to produce denatured genomic DNA. Every probe pair has an X and Y tag with PCR primer sequence. (2) Ligation of perfectly hybridized probes. In cases of a mismatch, no ligation takes place. (3) PCR amplification of the ligated product with primer X and Y, resulting in a series of products of unique length. (4) The PCR products are separated by capillary electrophoresis, resulting in a peak pattern. (5) Data are analyzed by comparing the peaks of a test sample with those of a reference sample. Analysis software produces a table with peak ratios compared with a reference sample; from these results, the genotype and the associated phenotype can be inferred manually. (*From* Veldhuisen B, van der Schoot CE, de Haas M. Multiplex ligation-dependent probe amplification (MLPA) assay for blood group genotyping, copy number quantification, and analysis of *RH* variants. Immunohematology 2015;31(2):59; with permission.)

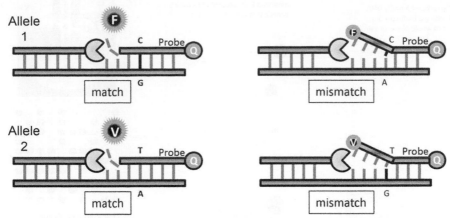

Fig. 3. The principle of the TaqMan assay involves prevention of fluorescence of a fluorophore by the close proximity with a quencher in a nucleotide probe. As the *Taq* polymerase reaches the probe, the 5′ to 3′ exonuclease activity of the polymerase degrades the probe, the fluorophore is released from the quencher, and fluorescence is detected (*left panels*). A typical TaqMan assay has 2 such probes that detect a single nucleotide difference at a specific location between 2 alleles of a given gene. Probes that are not 100% homologous with the DNA sequenced do not bind sufficiently and the *Taq* polymerase cannot degrade the probe to release the fluorophore from the quencher (*right panels*). (*From* Denomme GA, Schanen MJ. Mass-scale donor red cell genotyping using real-time array technology. Immunohematology 2015;31(2):70.)

fluorescence is detected. The pattern of fluorescence of these beads is then interpreted to determine which PCR products are present and, therefore, which genes are present in a patient's DNA. In the BLOODchip system, the multiplex PCR amplicons are fragmented and specifically labeled with fluorophores. The labeled fragments are then hybridized to allele-specific DNA probes bound to an array on a solid substrate and the resultant fluorescence pattern is interrogated to determine the presence of amplicons for each antigen. The LifeCodes system uses multiplexed RBC antigen allele-specific polymorphisms, which are detected using a fluorescent capture bead platform.[12] Using this system, a single multiplexed PCR reaction may be used to determine the genotype for Rh, Kell, Kidd, Duffy, MNS, and Dombrock antigen groups. A second PCR multiplex may be used to determine the genotype for Colton, Dombrock, Scianna, Lutheran, Diego, Landsteiner-Wiener (LW), Cartwright, Knops, and Cromer antigen groups. After PCR, the amplicon products are incubated with fluorescent beads to which oligonucleotide probes are bound. The probes selectively bind the PCR products for each antigen allele. The DNA-bound beads are then detected using a flow cytometer. Using the multiplexed PCR reactions and a single flow cytometer run to detect approximately 25-antigen SNPs greatly increases the efficiency of molecular assays compared with a PCR reaction with a detection assay for each antigen SNP product. The ID CORE X system uses a multiplex PCR of the genomic DNA using biotin-labeled primers (**Fig. 4**).[13] The amplicons are then allowed to bind with microspheres, which have allele-specific DNA probes bound. The biotin is then detected with a streptavidin-phycoerythrin label and the resultant phycoerythrin signal as well as the fluorescent signature of each of the microspheres using the Luminex flow cytometry platform. This allows interrogation of 29 polymorphisms and 37 RBC antigens in a single run. The Hemo ID Blood Group Genotyping Panel uses matrix-assisted laser desorption/ionization, time-of-flight mass spectrometry (MALDI-TOF

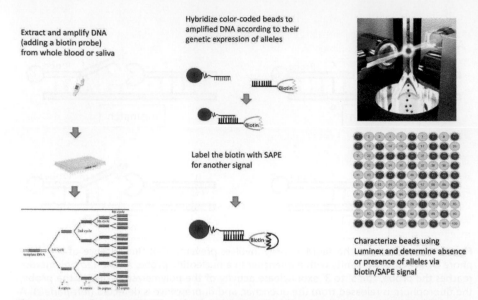

Fig. 4. Progenika ID CORE XT method. SAPE, streptavidin-phycoerythrin. (*From* Goldman M, Nogues N, Castilho LM. An overview of the Progenika ID CORE XT: an automated genotyping platform based on a fluidic microarray system. Immunohematology 2015;31(2):63; with permission.)

MS) to differentiate RBC antigen multiplex PCR products based on the molecular size of the PCR products. RBC genes are amplified using targeted multiplex PCR. The amplicons are then incubated with sequence-specific primers (SSPs) for the target RBC genes and ddNTPs to allow addition of a single nucleotide. The primers are engineered such that the terminal nucleotide added is the determining the RBC antigen phenotype. MALDI-TOF MS is then used to interrogate the products to determine which nucleotide was added to the specific primer.

Most RBC antigens have a limited array of alleles, which make them amenable to allele-specific PCR. Some genes, however, have a larger genetic variation (eg, Rh genes), and DNA sequencing may be used to determine the specific genetic variation present. Typically, Sanger sequencing is used, although next-generation sequencing is being explored for application to transfusion medicine testing. Sanger sequencing is performed using tagged terminating nucleotides in a single-direction PCR. The PCR products are then evaluated using electrophoresis, either gel or capillary, with the length of each product correlating with the position of the terminating base.

TERMINOLOGY AND NOTATION

The results of molecular testing for transfusion medicine may be reported at diverse levels of detail using various notation strategies. Additionally, molecular testing results may be reported either as the expressed phenotype or as the genotype, although current notation does not differentiate phenotype from genotype. For example, molecular testing may be done for the C698T point mutation resulting in the T193M amino acid substitution on the Kell glycoprotein, which results in the antigen commonly referred to simply as *K* or *Kell*.[17] If this testing yields a positive result, the result may be reported as "positive for K," "positive for Kell," "heterozygous for Kell," "positive for C698T," "positive for T193M," and so forth. There are no current widely accepted standards about how this result should be reported. One recent attempt at this standardization has been made by the International Society of Blood Transfusion, most recently referenced by Storry and colleagues[18] in 2011. The society's complete guidelines may be found at http://www.isbtweb.org/working-parties/red-cell-immunogenetics-and-blood-group-terminology/. These guidelines provide suggestions for naming conventions of genotype, phenotype, and antigen status for current RBC antigens as well as guidelines for newly identified antigens.

RED BLOOD CELL ANTIGEN EXPRESSION

The molecular basis of virtually all the known blood group antigens has now been established. Blood group polymorphisms arise from a variety of genetic mechanisms, including SNPs, single-nucleotide deletion, gene deletion, sequence duplication, and intergenic recombination. Most antigens are the result of SNPs. The most commonly tested, clinically significant SNPs are listed in **Table 1**. Deletion of the *RHD* gene is the most common basis for the Rh-negative phenotype. Homozygous deletion of the glycophorin B (*GYPB*) gene also accounts for the S-s-U- phenotype. Deletion of a single

Table 1
Genetic basis of common blood group antigens

Blood Group System	HUGO Gene Name	Antigens	Nucleotide Changes
MNS	*GYPA*	M/N	60C > T
			72G > A
	GYPB	S/s	243T > C
Rh	*RHCE*	C/c	178A > C
			203G > A
			307T > C
		E/e	676C > G
Lutheran	*BCAM*	Lu(a/b)	230G > A
Kell	KEL	K/k	698T > C
		Kp(a/b)	961T > C
		Js(a/b)	1910C > T
Duffy	DARC	Fy(a/b)	125G > A
		Fy(a-b-)	−33T > C
Kidd	SLC14A1	Jk(a/b)	838G > A
Diego	SLC4A1	Di(a/b)	2561T > C
		Wr(a/b)	1972A > G
Cartwright	ACHE	Yt(a/b)	1057C > A
Dombrock	DO	Do(a/b)	378C > T
			624T > C
			79A > G
		Hy(±)	323G > T
		Jo(a+/a-)	350C > T
Colton	AQP1	Co(a/b)	134C > T
LW	ICAM4	LW(a/b)	308A > G
Cromer	CD55	Cr(a+/a-)	679G > C
Knopps	CR1	Kn(a/b)	4681G > A
		McC(a/b)	4768A > G
		Sl(a)	4828T > A

Data from Reid ME, Lomas-Francis C. The blood group antigens fact book. 2nd edition. Waltham (MA): Elsevier; 2004; and Blood group antigen gene mutation database. HUGO, Human Genome Organisation. Available at: http://www.ncbi.nlm.nih. gov/projects/gv/mhc/xslcgi.cgi?cmd5bgmut/home. Accessed April 16, 2013.

nucleotide results in a frame shift that may introduce a stop codon and is responsible for the common O alleles and for the A2 allele of the ABO system. Sequence duplication with introduction of a nonsense mutation is responsible for the inactive *RHD* gene (*RHD*φ) common among Rh-negative African Americans.

Knowledge of RBC phenotype is essential for provision of compatible blood with a recipient who has produced clinically significant antibodies and is an important part RBC antibody identification. RBC phenotype is determined by immunohematologic methods. These methods are limited, however, by availability of reliable antisera, are inherently subjective, and are difficult to perform when a patient was recently transfused or has a positive direct antiglobulin test. In most cases, RBC phenotype can be inferred from genotype and is a valuable adjunct to, or possible substitute for, phenotyping. The most commonly tested blood group genotypes are listed in **Table 1**. Genotyping is highly reliable and can be automated. Phenotyping may still be preferable, however, for some antigens, for instance, those with numerous allelic variations, such as ABO and Rh(D), which can be rapidly determined in most patients using inexpensive, readily available immunohematology methods.

The A and B determinants are carbohydrate structures, present on some RBC membrane glycoproteins and glycolipids, which result from the action of glycosyltransferases. The most common ABO alleles differ at 6 positions with exons 6 and 7, resulting in the A-transferase (N-acetylgalactosaminyltransferase), B-transferase (galactosyltransferase), or a nonfunctional product. More than 180 ABO alleles, however, have been described to date.[19] In addition, the acceptor substrate for the A-transferases and B-transferases is the H antigen, which is produced by transferases encoded by the tissue-specific genes FUT1 and FUT2. Although the H-negative phenotype is rare, it is responsible for a group O phenotype (Oh or Bombay) regardless of the alleles at the ABO locus. For these reasons, the value of ABO genotyping is largely for resolution of unusual ABO types.

Rh is genetically the most complex blood group system. The antigens of the Rh system are encoded by 2 closely linked genes, *RHD* and *RHCE*. *RHD* encodes the many epitopes of the D antigen. The most common genetic bases of the Rh-negative phenotype are deletion of *RHD* and the presence of a frameshift mutation resulting in a premature stop codon. Genotyping for *RHD* is largely reserved for resolution of some weak or partial D phenotypes.

Beyond the ABO and D antigens, most of the common clinically significant RBC antigens result from SNPs (see **Table 1**). The MNS antigens are present on glycophorin A *(GPA)* and glycophorin B *(GPB)*, which are products of 2 closely linked homologous genes, *GYPA* and *GYPB* of the glycophorin gene family, each present in 2 different allelic forms.[20] *GPA* and *GPB* show a high degree of sequence homology. *GPA* carries the epitopes for the MN blood groups, and *GPB* carries the epitopes for the Ss blood groups. Gene rearrangements are a prevailing mechanism for the observed DNA variation, resulting in variant *GPA* and *GPB* alleles.[21] Numerous variant alleles exist that are common in some populations and may be clinically significant.

The Kell system consists of 25 antigens, which include 6 pairs of antithetical antigens. Each Kell antigen is determined by single-nucleotide point mutations of the KEL gene encoding the Kell glycoprotein. There is considerable variation in the incidence of Kell antigens between ethnic populations.[22] On the RBC membrane, the Kell glycoprotein is covalently linked to the XK protein, which carries the Kx blood group. Weak expression of Kell antigens can be inherited or acquired and transient. Inherited weak expression occurs in the McLeod phenotype (absence of XK protein), the Leach phenotype (lack of a portion of glycophorin C), and some Gerbich-negative phenotypes (lack of all or portions of glycophorins C or D).

The Duffy blood group system comprises 2 common antithetical antigens and 2 high-incidence antigens.[22] The Duffy glycoprotein is functionally significant for its ability to bind multiple chemokines, known as Duffy antigen chemokine receptor (DARC). It is also the receptor exploited by *Plasmodium vivax* merozoites for entry into RBCs. Because of selective pressure due to malaria, the Duffy null phenotype is common in some populations. The molecular basis of the Fy(a–b–) phenotype found in African Americans is an SNP in the promoter region (33 T > C), which disrupts a binding site for the erythroid transcription factor GATA-1, with resultant loss of DARC expression on RBCs. Because the erythroid promoter controls expression only in erythroid cells, DARC expression on endothelium is normal. To date, all alleles carrying the mutated GATA box have been shown to carry FYB, therefore Fy(b) is expressed on their nonerythroid tissues. This explains why Fy(a–b–) individuals can make anti-Fy(a) but not anti-Fy(b).

The Kidd blood group system is relatively simple, with 2 antithetical antigens resulting from an SNP. In addition, a high-incidence antigen, Jk3, is absent in the null phenotype. The Kidd null phenotype results from 2 different genetic backgrounds: homozygous inheritance of a silent allele or inheritance of a dominant inhibitor gene In(Jk) unlinked to the Kidd locus SLC14A.[23]

The Diego system antigenic determinants are carried on the anion exchange multipass membrane glycoprotein band 3. The Diego blood group system comprises 21 antigens, of which 2 antithetical pairs, Di(a/b) and Wr(a/b), are commonly significant.[24] Di(b) and Wr(b) are high-incidence antigens, whereas the other Diego systems antigens are low incidence. The Yt blood group system (sometimes incorrectly referred to as the Cartwright system) consists of 2 antithetical antigens encoded by an SNP that are carried on acetylcholinesterase glycoprotein (ACHE). The Yt(b) antigen has moderately low incidence the United States but is common in the Israeli population. Because ACHE is GPI-linked to the RBC membrane, RBCs of patients with paroxysmal nocturnal hemoglobinemia lack Yt antigens as well as Cromer antigens.[24]

The Dombrock blood group system comprises an antithetical pair, Do(a/b), and the high-incidence antigens Hy and Jo to which antithetical antigens have not been identified. Although anti-Do(a) and anti-Do(b) are uncommon, they may cause hemolytic transfusion reactions. Genotyping is essential to identify compatible blood donors because reliable reagent Dombrock antisera are extremely rare.

The Colton blood group system comprises an antithetical pair, Co(a/b), and a high-incidence antigen Co3, carried on the aquaporin water channel protein AQP1. Absence of Co3 results in the null phenotype, Co(a–b–), which has only been described in rare individuals.

The LW blood group system comprises an antithetical pair, LW(a/b), carried on the intracellular adhesion molecule ICAM-4. Expression of LW antigens is strongly influenced by the presence or absence of Rh proteins, so that anti-Lw(a) may be confused with anti-D. Genotyping can be helpful in making this distinction correctly.

The Cromer blood group system comprises 12 high-incidence and 3 low-incidence antigens that are carried on CD55, the complement regulatory protein decay accelerating factor.[25,26] The Cr(a-) phenotype is found mainly in the African American population, although it is still rare. The antithetical antigens to Cr(a) has not been identified. The rare Cromer null phenotype, also termed Inab, is associated with lack of CD55 on RBCs. In contrast to patients with paroxysmal nocturnal hemoglobinuria, Inab RBCs are resistant to complement-mediated lysis. The molecular basis of the Inab phenotype is an SNP or introduction of an alternate splice site, which results in a premature stop codon.

The Knops blood group system contains 8 antigens that are carried on complement receptor 1.[27] In the white population, McC(b) and Sl(a) are low incidence but in the

African American population they are common. Antibodies to Knops antigens are clinically insignificant but are often encountered in pretransfusion testing as so-called high-titer, low-avidity antibodies, which often demonstrate observable hemagglutination through serial dilutions and can complicate the immunohematology work-up when there is suspicion of an underlying clinically significant antibody. In such cases, genotyping can be a useful adjunct in identification and in excluding clinically significant specificities.

PLATELET ANTIGEN EXPRESSION

Platelets carry antigens of importance to the transfusion medicine, including ABO HLA class I and platelet-specific antigens. The antigens whose expression are restricted to platelets, and as such must be investigated separately from the RBC antigens, are grouped into the human platelet antigen (HPA) nomenclature system (**Table 2**).[28]

Table 2
Genetic basis of human platelet antigens

Antigen	Glycoprotein	HGNC Identifier	Chromosome	Nucleotide Change	Mature Protein
HPA-1a/1b	GPIIIa	ITGB3	17	176T > C	L33P
HPA-2a/2b	GPIba	GP1BA	17	482C > T	T145M
HPA-3a/3b	GPIIb	ITGA2B	17	2621T > G	I843S
HPA-4a/4b	GPIIIa	ITGB3	17	506G > A	R143Q
HPA-5a/5b	GPIa	ITGA2	5	1600G > A	E505K
HPA-6w	GPIIIa	ITGB3	17	1544G > A	R489Q
HPA-7w	GPIIIa	ITGB3	17	1297C > G	P407A
HPA-8w	GPIIIa	ITGB3	17	1984C > T	R636C
HPA-9w	GPIIb	ITGA2B	17	2602G > A	V837M
HPA-10w	GPIIIa	ITGB3	17	263G > A	R62Q
HPA-11w	GPIIIa	ITGB3	17	1976G > A	R633H
HPA-12w	GPIbb	GP1BB	22	119G > A	G15E
HPA-13w	GPIa	ITGA2	5	2483C > T	T799M
HPA-14w	GPIIIa	ITGB3	17	1909_1911delAAG	K611del
HPA-15a/15b	CD109	CD109	6	2108C > A	S682Y
HPA-16w	GPIIIa	ITGB3	17	497C > T	T140I
HPA-17w	GPIIIa	ITGB3	17	662C > T	T195M
HPA-18w	GP1a	ITGA2	5	2235G > T	Q716H
HPA-19w	GPIIIa	ITGB3	17	487A > C	K137Q
HPA-20w	GPIIb	ITGA2B	17	1949C > T	T619M
HPA-21w	GPIIIa	ITGB3	17	1960G > A	E628K
HPA-22bw	GPIIb	ITGA2B	17	584A > C	K164T
HPA-23bw	GPIIIa	ITGB3	17	1942C > T	R622W
HPA-24bw	GPIIb	ITGA2B	17	1508G > A	S472N
HPA-25bw	GPIa	ITGA2	5	3347C > T	T1087M
HPA-26bw	GPIIIa	ITGB3	17	1818G > T	K580N
HPA-27bw	GPIIb	ITGA2B	17	2614C > A	L841M

Abbreviation: HGNC, Human Genome Organisation Gene Nomenclature Committee.
Data from European Molecular Biology Institute–European Bioinformatics Institute. IPD-HPA database. Available at: http://www.ebi.ac.uk/ipd/hpa/. Accessed April 16, 2013.

To date, 33 HPAs have been defined at the molecular level. Six biallelic HPA pairs (HPA-1a/1b, HPA-2a/2b, HPA-3a/3b, HPA-4a/4b, HPA-5a/5b, HPA-15a/15b) have been identified, with the higher frequency allele being designated with a lowercase "a." Antigens for which the corresponding allele has not been defined serologically are designated by "w" (workshop).

Identification of platelet antigens by phenotype is more difficult than RBC phenotyping. The most commonly used method is flow cytometry. This, however, requires specialized instrumentation. In addition, high-quality antisera are difficult to obtain. Most human sera containing platelet antibodies also contain HLA class I antibodies or are multispecific. Antisera for low-frequency antigens are rare. For these reasons, genotyping has largely replaced phenotyping as a means of HPA determination.

A variety of molecular methods can be used for HPA genotyping. Because almost all of HPAs arise from single base substitutions, the most commonly used method for HPA genotyping is PCR DNA amplification using oligonucleotide PCR-SSPs. The amplification conditions must be optimized for each specific primer set. PCR-SSP is commonly used because it is a simple and inexpensive procedure; however, post-PCR processing steps are required. Melting curve analysis is another commonly used method for HPA genotyping. In this technique, PCR amplification of DNA containing the platelet SNP of interest is performed using flanking primers. The product is detected using 2 differently labeled fluorescent oligonucleotide probes that bind to adjacent sequences on a patient's DNA near the SNP. Binding of both probes is detected by fluorescence resonance energy transfer. The instrument takes a series of readings at increasing temperatures that allow the probes to dissociate, or melt off, at different temperatures, generating a melting curve, the shape of which depends on the presence or absence of the SNP of interest. A third method is the 50-nuclease assay, or TaqMan, real-time (RT) PCR assay. This uses 3 sequence-specific, single-stranded DNA probes (TaqMan probes) 5′ labeled with different reporter fluorophores, and a quencher molecule attached to the 3′ ends. The probes are designed to bind to the platelet SNP of interest on the DNA template. When bound in close proximity to the quencher, the fluorescence of the reporter is reduced through fluorescence resonance energy transfer. Practical genotyping for large-scale screening, such as blood donor or fetal and neonatal alloimmune thrombocytopenia (FNAIT) screening, requires high-throughput methods. Several multiplex, PCR-based, high-throughput systems using glass slide microarrays, microplate arrays, and liquid bead arrays have been described.[29-33]

The most common clinical situations in which platelet antigen determination are used are FNAIT and post-transfusion purpura. Less common uses include evaluation of platelet transfusion refractoriness, immune thrombocytopenia (ITP), and drug-induced ITP. In FNAIT, maternal IgG alloantibodies to platelet antigens cross the placenta causing fetal and subsequently neonatal thrombocytopenia. Determination that the mother is negative for the implicated platelet antigen establishes that the pregnancy is at risk; however, it does not necessarily indicate that the pregnancy is affected. Determination that the father is homozygous for the implicated antigen or that the fetus is positive identifies the pregnancy as high risk. Post-transfusion purpura is a rare complication of transfusion in which alloimmunization to a platelet antigen is coincident with a period of severe thrombocytopenia. Determination that a patient is negative for the implicated platelet antigen establishes the diagnosis. For both of these applications, genotyping has distinct advantages compared with phenotyping, because it does not require platelets and may be performed on somatic DNA obtained from peripheral blood, buccal swab, or amniotic fluid. Platelet antigen determination has a limited role in management of the multitransfused platelet refractory patient because antibodies to HPA are rare in this setting and, when they do occur, are usually in conjunction with HLA antibodies.[26] In ITP and drug-induced ITP, antibody identification rarely requires HPA typing.

CELL FREE NUCLEIC ACID TESTING

During the past decade, the discovery of cell-free nucleic acids in serum, plasma, urine, or other body fluids has promoted investigation of genes encoding proteins as a means to detect diseases with potentially greater sensitivity. Normally, DNA is isolated from tissue through standard procedures using phenol chloroform extraction followed by ethanol precipitation. DNA can also be obtained, however, directly from serum, plasma, or other body fluids by centrifugation, separating it from cells and platelets and subsequently interrogated using amplification methods, such as RT-PCR or other detection methods.[34] The use of cell-free nucleic acid interrogation also has application to the discipline of transfusion medicine.[35] Studies on fetal *RHD* typing in maternal plasma samples of pregnant women in different periods of pregnancy have been reported.[36–38] Studies by Brojer and colleagues[36] found that maternal plasma may be confidently used as a sample source for detection of fetal *RHD* genotyping (99.6% predictive value) after 1 set of RT-PCR procedures, with the understanding that implementation of additional polymorphisms can increase the predictive value to 100%. Recent studies on noninvasive genotyping of other blood group alloantigens (D, c, E, and Kell) have also been reported.[39] In the setting of FNAIT, genotyping for fetal platelet antigens can also be performed on cell-free fetal DNA extracted from maternal plasma.[40,41]

Future applications of molecular technology to the field of transfusion medicine will continue to provide additional diagnostic opportunities for increased sensitivities, reduced turnaround times, cost containment, and population informatics for optimal patient care.

REFERENCES

1. Reid ME. Transfusion in the age of molecular diagnostics. Hematology Am Soc Hematol Educ Program 2009;171–7.
2. Fasano RM, Chou ST. Red blood cell antigen genotyping for sickle cell disease, thalassemia, and other transfusion complications. Transfus Med Rev 2016;30(4): 197–201.
3. Singleton BK, Frayne J, Anstee DJ. Blood group phenotypes resulting from mutations in erythroid transcription factors. Curr Opin Hematol 2012;19:486–93.
4. Westhoff CM, Vege S, Nickle P, et al. Nucleotide deletion in RHCE*cE (907delC) is responsible for a D- - haplotype in Hispanics. Transfusion 2011;51:2142–7.
5. Daniels G, van der Schoot CE, Olsson ML. Report of the fourth International Workshop on molecular blood group genotyping. Vox Sang 2011;101:327–32.
6. Monteiro F, Tavares G, Ferreira M, et al. Technologies involved in molecular blood group genotyping. ISBT Sci Ser 2011;6:1–6.
7. Latini FRM, Castilho LM. An overview of the use of SNaPshot for predicting blood group antigens. Immunohematology 2015;31(2):53–7.
8. Veldhuisen B, van der Schoot CE, de Haas M. Multiplex ligation-dependent probe amplification (MLPA) assay for blood group genotyping, copy number quantification, and analysis of RH variants. Immunohematology 2015;31(2):58–61.
9. Denomme GA, Schanen MJ. Mass-scale donor red cell genotyping using real-time array technology. Immunohematology 2015;31(2):69–74.
10. Immucor, Inc. Molecular immunohematology. Available at: http://www.immucor.com/Global/Products/Pages/Molecular.aspx. Accessed April 16, 2013.

11. Paccapelo C, Trugilo F, Villa MA, et al. HEA BeadChip technology in immunohe-matology. Immunohematology 2015;31(2):81–90.
12. Immucor, Inc. LIFECODES. Available at: http://www.immucor.com/en-us/Pages/LIFECODES.aspx. Accessed April 16, 2013.
13. Goldman M, Nogues N, Castilho LM. An overview of the Progenika ID CORE XT: an automated genotyping platform based on a fluidic microarray system. Immu-nohematology 2015;31(2):62–8.
14. Progenika, Inc. BLOODchip reference. Available at: http://www.progenika.com/ eu/index.php?option5com_content&task5view&id5302&Itemid5384. Accessed April 16, 2013.
15. McBean RS, Hyland CA, Flower RL. Blood group genotyping: the power and lim-itations of the Hemo ID Panel and MassARRAY platform. Immunohematology 2015;31(2):75–80.
16. Drago F, Karpasitou K, Poli F. Microarray beads for identifying blood group single nucleotide polymorphisms. Transfus Med Hemother 2009;36:157–60.
17. Lee S. Molecular basis of Kell blood group phenotypes. Vox Sang 1997;73:1–11.
18. Storry JR, Castilho L, Daniels G, et al. International Society of Blood Transfusion Working Party on red cell immunogenetics and blood group terminology: Berlin report. Vox Sang 2011;101:77–82.
19. ABO Blood Group System. Available at: http://www.ncbi.nlm.nih.gov/projects/gv/mhc/xslcgi.cgi?cmd5bgmut/systems_info&system5abo. Accessed April 16, 2013.
20. Reid ME. MNS blood group system: a review. Immunohematology 2009;25:95–101.
21. Shih MC, Yang LH, Wang NM, et al. Genomic typing of human red cell milten-berger glycophorins in a Taiwanese population. Transfusion 2000;40:54–61.
22. Westhoff CM, Reid ME. Review: the Kell, Duffy, and Kidd blood group systems. Immunohematology 2004;20:37–49.
23. Frohlich O, Macey RI, Edwards-Moulds J, et al. Urea transport deficiency in Jk(ab) erythrocytes. Am J Physiol 1991;260:C778–83.
24. Byrne KM, Byrne PC. Review: other blood group systems—Diego, Yt, Xg, Scianna, Dombrock, Colton, Landsteiner-Wiener, and Indian. Immunohematology 2004;20:50–8.
25. Telen MJ. Glycosyl phosphatidylinositol-linked blood group antigens and parox-ysmal nocturnal hemoglobinuria. Transfus Clin Biol 1995;2:277–90.
26. Storry JR, Reid ME, Yazer MH. The Cromer blood group system: a review. Immu-nohematology 2010;26(3):109–18.
27. Moulds JM. The Knops blood-group system: a review. Immunohematology 2010; 26(1):2–7.
28. European Molecular Biology Institute–European Bioinformatics Institute. IPD-HPAdatabase. Available at: http://www.ebi.ac.uk/ipd/hpa/. Accessed April 16, 2013.
29. Beiboer SH, Wieringa-Jelsma T, Maaskant-Van Wijk PA, et al. Rapid genotyping of blood group antigens by multiplex polymerase chain reaction and DNA microar-ray hybridization. Transfusion 2005;45:667–79.
30. Denomme GA, Van Oene M. High-throughput multiplex single-nucleotide poly-morphism analysis for red cell and platelet antigen genotypes. Transfusion 2005;45:660–6.
31. Peterson JA, Gitter ML, Kanack A, et al. New low-frequency platelet glycoprotein polymorphisms associated with neonatal alloimmune thrombocytopenia. Transfusion 2010;50:324–33.
32. Shehata N, Denomme GA, Hannach B, et al. Mass-scale high-throughput multi-plex polymerase chain reaction for human platelet antigen single-nucleotide poly-morphisms screening of apheresis platelet donors. Transfusion 2011;51:2028–33.

33. Vassallo RR. Recognition and management of antibodies to human platelet antigens in platelet transfusion-refractory patients. Immunohematology 2009;25: 119–24.

34. Goldstein H, Hausmann MJ, Douvdevani A. A rapid direct fluorescent assay for cell-free DNA quantification in biological fluids. Ann Clin Biochem 2009;46: 488–94.

35. Chiu RW, Lo YM. Clinical applications of maternal plasma fetal DNA analysis: translating the fruits of 15 years of research. Clin Chem Lab Med 2013;51: 197–204.

36. Brojer E, Zupanska B, Guz K, et al. Noninvasive determination of fetal *RHD* status by examination of cell-free DNA in maternal plasma. Transfusion 2005;45: 1473–80.

37. Van der Schoot CE, Soussan AA, Koelewijn J, et al. Non-invasive antenatal *RHD* typing. Transfus Clin Biol 2006;13:53–7.

38. Cardo L, García BP, Alvarez FV. Non-invasive fetal *RHD* genotyping in the first trimester of pregnancy. Clin Chem Lab Med 2010;48:1121–6.

39. Scheffer PG, van der Schoot CE, Page-Christiaens GC, et al. Noninvasive fetal blood group genotyping of rhesus D, c, E and of K in alloimmunised pregnant women: evaluation of a 7-year clinical experience. BJOG 2011;118:1340–8.

40. Scheffer PG, Ait Soussan A, Verhagen OJ, et al. Noninvasive fetal genotyping of human platelet antigen-1a. BJOG 2011;118:1392–5.

41. Le Toriellec E, Chenet C, Kaplan C. Safe fetal platelet genotyping: new developments. Transfusion 2013;53(8):1755–62.

Molecular Diagnosis of Hematopoietic Neoplasms
2018 Update

Radhakrishnan Ramchandren, MD[a], Tarek Jazaerly, MD[a],
Martin H. Bluth, MD, PhD[b,c], Ali M. Gabali, MD, PhD[a,*]

KEYWORDS

- Hematopoietic neoplasms • Molecular testing • Cytogenetic testing
- Genetic aberrations

KEY POINTS

- Cytogenetic abnormalities are considered common events in hematologic malignancies.
- These abnormalities generally consist of structural chromosomal abnormalities or gene mutations, which often are integral to the pathogenesis and subsequent evolution of an individual malignancy.
- Improvements made in identifying and interpreting these molecular alterations have resulted in advances in the diagnosis, prognosis, monitoring, and therapy for cancer.
- As a consequence of the increasingly important role of molecular testing in hematologic malignancy management, this article presents an update on the importance and use of molecular tests, detailing the advantages and disadvantages of each test when applicable.

INTRODUCTION

Several hematologic malignancies are associated with diverse genetic aberrations that range from single base-pair substitution to complete chromosomal abnormalities. Before the development of the current modern molecular and cytogenetic techniques, distinguishing between specific diseases was often time consuming and difficult. In the molecular era, however, cytogenetic and molecular tests are commonplace and critical to diagnose hematologic malignancies. Moreover, such testing also plays a significant role in determining prognosis, therapy, and disease status (remission or

This article has been updated from a version previously published in *Clinics in Laboratory Medicine*, Volume 33, Issue 4, December 2013.

[a] Wayne State University, School of Medicine, Department of Pathology, Karmanos Cancer Center, Detroit Medical Center, 3990 John R, Detroit, MI 48201, USA; [b] Department of Pathology, Wayne State University, School of Medicine, 540 East Canfield Street, Detroit, MI 48201, USA; [c] Pathology Laboratories, Michigan Surgical Hospital, 21230 Dequindre Road, Warren, MI 48091, USA
* Corresponding author.
E-mail address: agabal@med.wayne.edu

Clin Lab Med 38 (2018) 293–310
https://doi.org/10.1016/j.cll.2018.02.005
0272-2712/18/© 2018 Elsevier Inc. All rights reserved.

labmed.theclinics.com

relapse). The 2016 update of the World Health Organization (WHO) *Classification of Tumours of Haematopoietic and Lymphoid Tissues* integrates new categories of diseases based on molecular signatures as well as established and provisional entities and expands the 2008 edition in this respect.[1–3] These signatures have the potential to improve understanding of the disease process and may lead to diagnostic and therapeutic advances.

MOLECULAR TESTS USED TO IDENTIFY CLONAL T-CELL AND B-CELL POPULATIONS
Immunoglobulin Gene Rearrangement

Immunoglobulins are B-cell receptors (BCRs) found on B lymphocytes and able to bind antigens with high specificity. At the protein level, each immunoglobulin (antibody) is formed of heavy chains and light chains. Based on size and amino acid composition, the heavy chains are divided into 5 isotypes (classes) represented by the Greek letters α, δ, ε, γ, and μ, which are representative of the immunoglobulins class of heavy chains, IgA, IgD, IgE, IgG, and IgM, respectively. The light chain is much smaller than the heavy chain and consists of 1 of 2 possible isotypes, kappa or lambda, represented by the Greek letters κ and λ, respectively. The Ig contains 2 identical heavy chains and 2 identical light chains. Each chain contains 1 constant region that is similar for each isotype and 1 variable region that is different in amino acid sequence for the same isotype. The variable regions of the heavy and light chains undergo gene rearrangement during B-cell development and maturation. An individual B cell, therefore, produces 1 distinct Ig composed of 1 unique variable region for the heavy chain and another unique variable region for the light chain.

Humans inherit many variable region gene segments called germline genes. The immunoglobulin heavy chain gene locus (IGH@) is located on chromosome 14q32.Genes that encode light chains, however, are located on 1 separate chromosomes. Immunoglobulin kappa locus (IGK@) is located on chromosome 2p11.2 and immunoglobulin lambda locus (IGL@) is located on chromosome 22q11.22. The variable region of the IGH@ contains variable numbers of variable (V), diverse (D), and joining (J) gene regions. The light chains also contain a different number of V and J gene regions but lack the D gene region.[4,5] These genes are vital for generating the diverse number of human antibodies required and encode for more than 100 variable regions that encode for the first 90 to 95 amino acid of the variable region. The rest of the variable region, the last 15 to 20 amino acids, are present further along the chromosome in a linked set of DNA. Chronologically, the heavy chain variable region rearrangement precedes that of the light chain. Successful IGH rearrangement triggers the rearrangement of IGK@ and failure to achieve successful IGK rearrangement subsequently triggers the rearrangement of IGL@. In addition, the recombination of an individual variable region also occurs in an ordered sequence. The heavy chain recombination first occurs between 1 randomly selected D and J gene region followed by the joining of 1 V gene region. Then the constant chain gene is added and similarly the rearrangements of IGK@ and IGL@ start by joining the V and J gene regions to give a VJ complex before the addition of the constant chain gene.[4,5]

T-Cell Gene Rearrangement

Each T-cell receptor (TCR) consists of 2 different chains coupled together. TCRa (TCRA) and TCRb (TCRB) chains are present in approximately 95% of the TCR with the rest formed by TCRg (TCRG) and TCRd (TCRD) chains. The genes encoding the TCRd chain are located within the TCRa gene on chromosome 14q11-12, whereas the TCRb and TCRg genes are located on chromosome 7q32-35 and 7p15, respectively. Each chain consists of 1 V and 1 constant (C) region.[6] The variable coding regions of TCRa and TCRg are generated by the recombination of VJ regions (like Ig light chain), whereas those that form TCRb and TCRd are generated by the recombination of VDJ regions (like Ig heavy chain). The TCR contains different numbers of V, D, and J gene regions. The recombination occurs in a similar pattern to that of immunoglobulin heavy and light chains. Because TCRd genes are located within the TCRa genes, the rearrangement of TCRa, which occurs first, causes the deletion of the embedded TCRd gene region.[6]

The basic concept behind testing for immunoglobulin and TCR gene rearrangement is that large numbers of B cells and/or T cells respond to any single antigen encountered and this leads to having many B cells and T cells each with different rearranged non-germline variable regions. Neoplastic T calls and B cells have the same rearranged variable region of the TCR or heavy chain and of the light chain. Most T-cell and B-cell neoplasms have clonal rearrangement of the variable region that can be detected by various methods including the Southern blot hybridization assay and polymerase chain reaction (PCR) assay.

Southern Blot Analysis for Rearrangement of Immunoglobulin and T-Cell Receptors

In the past, Southern blot hybridization assay was considered the gold standard assay for detecting rearrangements of both B-cell and T-cell receptors. Currently, however, this test is rarely used in clinical molecular testing.

Polymerase Chain Reaction Assay for Rearrangement of Immunoglobulin and T-Cell Receptors

The most targeted region for B-cell neoplasm is the immunoglobulin heavy chain gene, and for the T-cell neoplasm, the TCRg gene region. Accurate knowledge of the rearranged gene segments is required to design primers, and this problem is solved by the commercial availability of many tested probes with great specificity. In B-cell neoplasm, most PCR probes target the consensus sequence of the J region and the framework segment of the V region of the heavy chain. For many years the drawback of PCR assay of these regions was the false-negative results, especially in tumors that undergo somatic hypermutation and subsequently change the primer binding site.

Diffuse large B-cell lymphoma (DLBCL), follicular lymphoma, subset of chronic lymphocytic leukemia/small lymphocytic lymphoma, and marginal zone lymphoma tend to undergo somatic hypermutation more than others, and the use of additional primers may decreases the false-negative rate in such lesions.[7] Recently, most diagnostic laboratories are using the newly described BIOMED-2 protocol.[8] The assay targets multiple variable gene segments in rearranged immunoglobulin and TCR genes. The primers are designed to probe 3 VH-JH regions, 2 DH-JH regions, 2 IGK regions, 1 IGL region, 3 TCRb regions, 2 TCRg regions, and 1 TCRd region. This protocol detects almost all clonal B-cell populations, including those with a high rate of somatic hypermutation.

In addition, because TCRg region is rearranged in almost all T-cell neoplasms and many show TCRB gene rearrangements, BIOMED-2 protocol has the ability to detect virtually all clonal T-cell populations.[8,9] Small clonal B-cell and T-cell populations, however, have the potential to be missed. On the other hand, because of the high sensitivity of PCR assay, a small number of polyclonal B cells or T cells could be amplified and cause erroneous interpretation of the presence of a clonal population. Therefore, correlation with the morphologic and immunophenotypic findings is required at all times.

OTHER MOLECULAR TESTS USED IN NON-HODGKIN B-CELL AND T-CELL LYMPHOMAS
B-Cell Leukemia/Lymphoma 2 Translocation Assay

B-cell leukemia/lymphoma (BCL)-2 is located on chromosome 18q21.33 and is normally expressed by mantle zone B cells. Immunohistochemical studies demonstrate that primary follicles composed predominantly of B cells are usually positive for BCL-2.[10] T cells also express BCL-2, in particular interfollicular T cells. Germinal center B cells are negative for BCL-2, and positive results may indicate a lymphoma. Follicular lymphoma is the most common lymphoma to express BCL-2 (approximately 85%–90%), and approximately 20% to 30% of DLBCLs are positive for BCL-2. In lymphomas, BCL-2 protein is abnormal, and results from translocation between chromosomes 14 and 18: t(14;18) (q32;q21). The placement of the antiapoptotic gene BCL-2 in close proximity to the highly active immunoglobulin gene of the heavy chain causes excessive up-regulation of this protein and this potentiates its antiapoptotic activity.

The 2016 update of the WHO *Classification of Tumours of Haematopoietic and Lymphoid Tissues* replaced the provisional category of B-cell neoplasms with features intermediate between DLBCL and Burkitt lymphoma (BL) with 2 categories based on the presence or absence of MYC, BCL-2, and or BCL-6 gene rearrangements. The first category is called high-grade B-cell lymphoma with *MYC, BCL-2,* and/or *BCL-6* translocation (double-hit or triple-hit lymphoma). Cases that are confirmed to be follicular lymphoma by morphology or B-lymphoblastic lymphoma by immunophenotype are excluded. The second category of this high-grade B cell lymphoma is characterized by having the same morphologic and immunophenotypic findings but lacks *MYC* translocation. This entity is called high-grade B-cell lymphoma, not otherwise specified (NOS).

Studies reported that approximately 65% of the breakpoints in BCL-2 gene (18q21.33) are located at the major breakpoint region (MBR) and approximately 9% are located at the minor cluster region. The rest of the breakpoints with documented BCL-2 translocation could not be mapped. Survival studies, however, did not show any correlation between breakpoint location and clinical outcome. The joining (JH6) segment of the immunoglobulin heavy chain was the most frequently involved whatever the breakpoint location. Most primers used in PCR assays target the MBR of BCL-2 and JH6 region of the immunoglobulin heavy chain.

Fluorescence in situ hybridization (FISH) is more sensitive in detecting BCL-2 translocation than PCR assay. This is because PCR assay is limited by the size of the primer needed for the PCR reaction, whereas FISH can use large spanning probes, because all that is needed is hybridization of the probe to its complementary sequence. Studies found that the higher the grade of follicular lymphoma the more likely it is not to show BCL-2 translocation. As with all ancillary tests, correlation with the morphologic findings is required, because low levels of BCL-2 can be detected in the peripheral blood of normal individuals.

Cyclin-D1 Translocation Assay

Cyclin-D 1 (CCND1), also known as BCL-1, is located on chromosome 11q13.3 and is the hallmark of mantle cell lymphoma (MCL). CCND1 is also expressed by a subset of plasma cell myeloma. CCND1-positive myeloma is also positive for t(11;14), and most myeloma cells are CD20 positive with the morphologic appearance of small plasmcytoid lymphocytes. In addition, a small subset of hairy cell leukemia may show weak expression of CCND1 protein and predominantly negative for t(11;14). The t(11;14) places CCND1 gene in juxtaposition to the highly active immunoglobulin gene of the heavy chain causing overexpression of CCND1 protein. CCND1 is a nuclear, cell-cycle control protein and in normal cells is maximally expressed in G1 phase.[11] All normal lymphocytes are negative for CCND1 expression by immunohistochemical studies.

In approximately 50% of MCLs, the breakpoint of the translocation is located at 1 area, termed major translocation cluster. The rest of the breakpoints, however, are not linked to any specific region. Therefore, the PCR assay is not that sensitive for CCND1 translocation. FISH analysis using large, dual-fusion probes is the most sensitive assay. Less than 5% of classic cases of MCLs are CCND1-negative. The diagnosis of such category becomes more difficult because this lymphoma is usually negative for t(11;14). Identification of SOX11 protein in neoplastic cells may be helpful in such a scenario.[12]

Recently, the detection of the mutational status of the IGHV gene in MCL has started to gain ground. MCL that has unmutated IGHV tends to express SOX11 protein expression by immunohistochemistry and show more aggressive clinical course and more nodal involvement. On the other hand, MCL with mutated IGHV has indolent clinical course, is SOX11 negative, shows blood, and has bone marrow involvement pattern.

B-Cell Lymphoma 6 Translocation Assay

B-Cell Lymphoma 6 (BCL-6) is a transcriptional repressor that blocks the maturation of B cells to plasma cells and is essential for the formation of germinal centers.[13] The BCL6 gene is located on chromosome 3q27.3, and the protein is normally expressed in the nuclei of germinal center B cells and T cells. The 3q27 translocation affecting BCL-6 gene has been observed in 20% to 40% of DLBCLs and in 5% to 10% of follicular lymphomas. The partner of a BCL-6 translocated gene can be an Ig or non-Ig partner. In 1 study, a total of 120 BCL-6 breakpoint found that 62 breakpoints (52%) joined to immunoglobulin heavy chain; 12 to immunoglobulin light chains (10%); and 46 to non-Ig partners (38%). Approximately 20 non-Ig partner genes have been identified, including 1p32, 7p11, 7p21, 14q11, and 16p13. Some studies suggest that DLBCL with non-Ig/BCL-6 fusion has a poor prognosis. Breakpoints at 3q27 are predominantly located in the 5^0 untranslated region of BCL6 that has been called the MBR.[14] As with BCL-2, many of the break-points may locate outside the MBR. Thus, the PCR assay using specific probes may not detect BCL-6 rearrangement. Many diagnostic laboratories are using FISH break-apart probes spanning the BCL6 locus and not the dual-fusion IGH@/BCL6-specific probes.

Cellular Myelocytomatosis Translocation Assay

Cellular myelocytomatosis (C-MYC) gene is a transcription factor located on chromosome 8q24. In normally growing cells, C-MYC is produced in small amounts. This production is tightly regulated during cell cycle and it returns back to its basal level in nondividing cells. Abnormally produced C-MYC activates a protective pathway through the induction of p53-dependent cell death pathway, among others, such as p14ARF and BCL-2 like protein 11, which forces such cells to undergo apoptosis. p53 plays an important role in MYC-induced apoptosis, and approximately 30% of endemic BLs harbor a p53 mutation. BL is characterized by having C-MYC translocation with the JH region of immunoglobulin heavy chain (14q32) (80%) and less frequently with the loci of immunoglobulin light chains (kappa or lambda), with slight preference for partnering with kappa (15%) than lambda (5%) gene segments.

C-MYC is detected in virtually all cases of BL and in high numbers of AIDS-related lymphoma, including EBV-positive and EBV-negative cases. In addition to being reported in de novo cases of DLBCL (10%), some cases of Richter transformation of chronic lymphocytic leukemia/small lymphocytic lymphoma have C-MYC translocation.[15] C-MYC is also detected in other lymphomas and plasma cell myeloma with much less frequency.

Based on the chromosomal breakpoints relative to the C-MYC gene, the translocations have been classified into 3 classes. Translocations within the 5^0 first noncoding exon or intron of 5^0 region of C-MYC gene have been designated as class I, those with breakpoints immediately upstream of the gene as class II, and those with breakpoints distant as class III. Studies have found that the breakpoints in BL are different between the sporadic and endemic entities of BL. All cases of BL have C-MYC translocation; however, rearrangement of C-MYC gene, close to the 5^0 first noncoding exon or intron region, is predominantly demonstrated in sporadic BL (class I). C-MYC gene in most cases of endemic BL is translocated as an intact nonrearranged gene. In this case, the breakpoint in chromosome 8 is found outside the C-MYC gene (class III).

Several methods are used to detect C-MYC translocation, including conventional cytogenetics (CCs), Southern blot, and FISH. Among all, FISH detection is the method most used by laboratories. Because C-MYC translocations show no constant clustering of breakpoints, the PCR detection method is not the best test to look for C-MYC translocation. Both fusion and break-apart probes are used. Break-apart probes, designed to span most of the C-MYC region, are usually applied to test for C-MYC rearrangement including those arising from variant translocations. Specific fusion probes are then applied to detect the t(8;14), t(2;8), and t(8;22) abnormalities. Up to 10% of BL cases may lack a demonstrable C-MYC translocation by FISH and southern blot hybridization probes hybridizing to class II and class III region may be helpful to detect translocations in such cases.

The 2016 update of the WHO *Classification of Tumours of Haematopoietic and Lymphoid Tissues* has added the entity of Burkitt-like lymphoma with 11q aberration as a provisional entity to describe a group of lymphomas that has the morphologic features and gene expression profile of BL in the absence of *MYC* rearrangement. The 11q abnormalities that characterize such group of lymphomas include chromosome 11q proximal gain and telomeric gene loss.

Mucosal-Associated Lymphoid Tissue Translocation Assay

The t(11;18) (q21;q21) is the most common translocation in mucosal-associated lymphoid tissue (MALT) lymphomas and is found in approximately 30% to 40% of MALT lymphomas. The next encountered translocation is t(14;18) (q32;q21), which is seen in approximately 10% to 20% of cases.[16,17] The most common sites for the t(11;18) (q21;q21) are stomach and lung, and it involves the gene of API2, member of the apoptosis suppressor family on chromosome 11q21 and MALT1 gene on chromosome 18q21. The t(14;18) involves the immunoglobulin heavy chain locus 14q32 and the MALT gene 18q21 and is detected in MALT lymphoma of the liver, skin, ocular adnexa, and salivary glands but less frequently in MALT lymphoma involving other sites.

Other translocations have been described in MALT lymphoma, including t(1;14)/IGH-BCL10 and t(3;14)/IGH-FOXP1. These two translocations are rare, found in approximately 2% of MALT lymphoma each and they are not confined to any specific site. Continuous activation of nuclear factor kappa B is the main mechanism by which the t(11;18)/API2-MALT1, t(14;18)/IGH-MALT1, and t(1;14)/IGH-BCL10 promote lymphoma. The function of the t(3;14)/IGH-FOXP1 in MALT lymphoma remains unclear.

Gastric lymphomas with t(11;18)/API2-MALT1 respond poorly to treatment directed against *Helicobacter pylori* microorganism. They show less than 10% of durable remission at long-term follow-up, and they may spread to regional lymph nodes or distal sites. Most high-grade transformation of MALT lymphomas, however, is seen in non–translocation-associated lymphoma rather than those with positive translocation. Neoplastic cells of MALT lymphoma associated with either t(11;18) or t(1;14) demonstrate nuclear expression of BCL-10 by immunohistochemistry.

As with other low-grade lymphomas, using CC analysis for detecting MALT translocations is hampered by the low yield and poor quality of metaphase spreads. In addition, cytogenetic analysis cannot differentiate between t(14;18) caused by IGH/BCL-2 and that caused by IGH/MALT1 because the 18q21 region contains the BCL-2 and MALT1 loci. Therefore, interphase FISH is becoming the main test to look for such translocations.

Anaplastic Lymphoma Kinase Translocation Assay

Anaplastic lymphoma kinase (ALK), or CD246, is a type II transmembrane receptor tyrosine kinase and is a member of the insulin receptor superfamily involved in the development of the nervous system. ALK is not expressed in normal and hyperplastic lymphoid tissue. Approximately 85% of pediatric and 35% of adult anaplastic large cell lymphomas (ALCLs) are associated with a recurrent cytogenetic abnormality that involves ALK in locus 2p23.[18] ALK protein is also expressed by a subset of DLBCL. Deregulated ALK fusion protein has been reported in neural origin tumors, such as retinoblastoma and neuroblastoma, and some cases of lung carcinoma and melanoma. In ALCL, ALK expression is associated with better 5-year survival rates compared with ALK-negative ALCL. The most common partner for ALK protein is the nucleophosmin (NPM) gene located at 5q35 and is seen in approximately 80% of the ALK-positive ALCLs. NPM is a nucleolar protein responsible for protein shuttling between the cytoplasm and the nucleus. The t(2;5) results in expression of a novel fusion protein, NPM-ALK (also called p80) that has tyrosine kinase activity and has been shown to induce a lymphoma-like disease in mice. By immunohistochemistry, the NPM-ALK fusion protein can be nuclear or cytoplasmic.

Other partner genes have been described in about 15% to 20% of ALK-positive ALCLs, including TRK fused gene (TFG) at 3q21, TFG-ALK, tropomysin 3 (TPM3) at locus 1q25, topomysin 4 (TPM4) at locus 19p13, and clathrin chain polypeptide-like gene at locus 17q11, among others.[19] No difference in survival is seen between the ALK-NPM translocation and the variant translocations. When ALK partners with other than NPM gene, it produces cytoplasmic or membranous staining patterns by immunohistochemical studies.

NPM-ALK fusion transcripts can be detected by PCR using primers targeting the ALK portion of the transcript. Because low levels of detection can be seen in the peripheral blood and lymph node of healthy individuals, however, only the high-level detection matches with the presence of ALK fusion gene identified by CCs and FISH studies. In most laboratories, the FISH break-apart probes that hybridize to the 2 ends of the ALK gene breakpoint are routinely used to detect the t(2;5) and variant translocations, because documenting ALK translocation is more clinically important than identifying its partner chromosome.

MOLECULAR TESTS USED TO IDENTIFY DEFINING CYTOGENETIC ABNORMALITIES OF THE LEUKEMIAS
Acute Myeloid Leukemia with t(15;17) (q22;q21)/Acute Promyelocytic Leukemia–Retinoic Acid Receptor-Alpha

In acute myeloid leukemia (AML) the identification of t(15;17) (q22;q21) is diagnostic of acute promyelocytic leukemia (APL), representing approximately 10% of AMLs. In addition to having this defining cytogenetic abnormality, APL has its own distinctive morphologic and immunophenotypic characteristics with high prediction of the disease. The urgency of early diagnosis of APL is generally attributed to a tendency to develop disseminated intravascular coagulation and the responsiveness of the disease to all-*trans* retinoic acid (ATRA) and arsenic trioxide therapy. The presence of t(15;17), and t(8;21) and inv(16) as a solo abnormality in AML is associated with a favorable prognosis.

The t(15;17) (q22;q21) involves the promyelocytic leukemia (PML) gene from chromosome 15 and the retinoic acid receptor alpha (RARA) gene from chromosome 17 to produce PML-RARA fusion gene or RARA-PML reciprocal product. In most cases, the breakpoint on chromosome 17 is located in intron 2 of the RARA gene. The PML gene, however, has 3 breakpoint cluster regions (bcr) called bcr1 at intron 6 (long [L-form]), bcr2 at exon 6 (variant [V-form]), and bcr3 at intron 6 (short [S-form]) forms, based on the size of the end products. The L-form and S-form represent approximately 90% of the t(15;17) positive cases.

Generally, the t(15;17) can be detected in 98% of typical APL cases. The rest (2%) of typical APL cases have either a cryptic (submicroscopic) PML breakpoint or RARA translocation with rare variants, including t(11;17) (q23;q21) that forms the PML zinc finger protein RARA fusion (PLZF-RARA), t(5;17) (q35;q21) that forms NPM-RARA fusion, t(11;17) (q13;q21) that generates nuclear mitotic apparatus-RARA transcript (NUMA-RARA), and der(17) that forms the signal transducer and activator of transcription-RARA fusion (STAT5b-RARA).[20,21] Few other variants have been reported to partner with the RARA gene; however, their novelty has to be confirmed. Variants PLZF-RARA and NPM-RARA fusion genes may have reciprocal products. Patients with APL with PLZF-RARA gene fusion may respond to histone deacetylase inhibitors rather than ATRA or arsenic trioxide therapy.

Peripheral blood or bone marrow samples can be used to look for the t(15;17) or other variant translocation abnormalities. CC may detect 75% of the APL associated translocations. The major problem with CC, however, is the increased risk of false-negatives. FISH is considered more sensitive, and it can detect up to 98% of the cases when the correct probes are used. Both dual-color fusion probes and break-apart probes can be used, even though the latter need further work-up. In cases of cryptic PML fusion gene, or when minimal residual disease is to be investigated, FISH analysis on different metaphases and interphases from cytogenetic cultures has been shown useful. Reverse transcriptase (RT)-PCR also can be used in such conditions. The only caveat is that sometimes RT-PCR may produce several bands in patient sample with bcr2 PML breakpoint, and they could be potentially misinterpreted as nonspecific amplification products.

Acute Myeloid Leukemia with t(8;21) (q22;q22)/RUNX1-RUNX1T1

The t(8;21) constitutes approximately 5% to 10% of all cases of AML and it results from the fusion of Runt-related transcription factor 1 (RUNX1) gene on 21q22 and the RUNX1T1 (RUNX1-translocated to 1) gene on 8q22.[22] RUNX1, also known as AML 1 protein (AML1) and core-binding factor subunit alpha-2 (CBFA2), is expressed by all hematopoietic elements. Core binding factor includes the DNA binding unit RUNX1 (in addition to RUNX2 and RUNX3 subunits) and the non-DNA binding CBF subunit-beta (CBFB). All 4 subunits are necessary for the formation of normal hematopoietic stem cells during embryogenesis. RUNX1T1, also known as Eight Twenty One, is a transcription regulatory protein that binds to nuclear histone deacetylases and transcription factors to block differentiation of hematopoietic elements. Some reports indicate that approximately 3% of AMLs associated with t(8;21) have variant translocations for which their significance needs to be clarified. The breakpoint in both genes of RUNX1 and RUNX1T1 are clustered in highly conserved regions, intron 5 to 6 in RUNX1and in intron 1b-2 in RUNX1T1. Therefore, most of the translocations create a fusion transcript made of the 5^0 region of RUNX1 fused to the 3^0 region of RUNX1T1 gene and form the same fusion transcript that can be detected in all patients. The t(8;21) can be detected by CC and FISH analysis using locus-specific probes for AML1–Eight Twenty One fusion. False-negative results in FISH analysis may occur if the malignant cells represent less than 10% of the cells present in the specimen. In such situations, RT-PCR analyses can also be used to detect and confirm the presence of the RUNX1-RUNX1T1 fusion gene.

Acute Myeloid Leukemia with inv(16) (p13.1q22) or t(16;16) (p13.1;q22)/CBFB-MYH11

The inv(16) and t(16;16) occur in approximately 5% of pediatric cases and 7% of adult AML cases. Most cases of AML, however, with abnormal eosinophils (AML-M4Eo) are associated with inv(16) (p13.1q22) or, to a lesser extent, with t(16;16) (p13.1;q22).[23] Both result in the fusion of the CBFB gene at 16q22 to the myosin heavy chain 11 (MYH11) gene at 16p13.1 locus. Even though the CBFB–MYH11 chimeric protein tends to be sequestered in the cytoplasm, it has the ability to interfere with the function, in a dominant-negative manner, of CBF. Such mechanism is postulated to impair cell differentiation and increase predisposion to leukemic cell transformation. The breakpoint in CBFB gene occurs in intron 5, but the breakpoint in MYH11 is variable and includes more than 8 regions on the gene. Therefore, CC analysis may overlook cryptic (submicroscopic) fusion. In such conditions, the use of FISH and RT-PCR methods may be important to detect CBFB/MYH11 fusion gene. Other structural abnormalities are seen in approximately 30% to 40% of cases, including trisomy 22, trisomy 8, and 7q deletion. Because trisomy 22 is rare in other acute leukemias, the presence of trisomy 22 without detectable inv(16) or t(16;16) by CC may suggest the presence of a possible cryptic genetic alteration.

Acute Leukemia with 11q23/Mixed Lineage Leukemia Translocation

Mixed lineage leukemia (MLL) gene is located at 11q23 locus and it functions as a positive regulatory gene in hematopoiesis development during embryogenesis.[24] The presence of rearranged MLL gene is considered an unfavorable prognostic indicator and is observed in approximately 3% to 4% of AMLs and in approximately 3% to 7% of acute lymphoblastic leukemias (ALLs). Translocated MLL gene is seen in AML and ALL affecting adult and infant patients and in most patients with therapy-related acute leukemia caused by previous history of topoisomerase II inhibitor therapy.[24] Breakpoints in the MLL gene are located between exon 5 and exon 11. To date, more than 100 translocations have been reported to partner with the MLL gene and most of them are cloned. Three partners have been identified in approximately 80%, including AF4 (ALL-1 fused gene on chromosome 4) gene to form t(4;11) (q21;q23); MLLT3 (myeloid/lymphoid mixed lineage leukemia translocate 3) gene to create t(9;11) (q21;q23); and MLLT1 gene to form t(11;19) (q23;p13). Rearrangement of 11q23 can be detected by CC, FISH analysis, and other molecular tests, including Southern blot hybridization and RT-PCR. The CC ability to detect such rearrangement is limited by the presence of cryptic fusion, particularly when its partner has a telomeric location. FISH is useful in such circumstances. In addition, FISH can discriminate between true 11q23/MLL and rearrangements clustering within the 11q22 to 25 regions without MLL involvement. RT-PCR is the most sensitive approach for detecting specific subtypes of MLL rearrangements when the partner gene is known, otherwise multiplex RT-PCR approach is used.

ACUTE LEUKEMIA WITH OTHER TRANSLOCATIONS
Acute Myeloid Leukemia with t(6;9) (p23;q34)/DEK-NUP214

This translocation is seen in approximately 1% to 2% of acute leukemias affecting children and adults. The DEK-NUP214 chimeric protein encodes for altered nucleoporin fusion protein with an aberrant transcription factor activity that affects nuclear transport. This translocation is associated with poor prognosis, multilineage dysplasia, basophilia, and higher association with FLT3-ITD mutation. Some reports indicate the presence of terminal deoxynucleotidyl transferase (TdT) in neoplastic cells. The breakpoints in both genes are constant and this allows for the design of specific probe for precise detection by RT-PCR.

Acute Myeloid Leukemia with inv(3) (q21q26.2) or t(3;3) (q21;q26.2)/RPN1-EVI1

This translocation is seen in 1% to 2% of adult AMLs and is associated with poor response to therapy and dismal outcome. It results in the juxtaposition of the ribophorin 1(RPN1) gene with the ecotropic viral integration site-1 (EVI1) gene that causes defective cellular proliferation and differentiation and subsequent leukemic transformation. Inv(3) AML is associated with multilineage dysplasia with atypical megakaryocytes, variable fibrosis, and peripheral thrombocytosis.[25] Secondary cytogenetic abnormalities are seen in approximately 40% of cases, including monosomy 7, 5q del, and complex karyotypes. Rearrangement of EVI1 gene at 3q26 locus with other chromosomes, including t(1;3) (p36.3;q21.1) and t(3;21) (q26.2;q22.1), t(2;3) (p15;q26.2), and t(3;12) (q26.2;p13), are excluded. The former 2 translocations are commonly seen in AML with myelodysplasia-related changes. The chromosomal breakpoints at 3q26 in the translocation are in the 5^0 of the EVI1 gene, whereas the breakpoints in the inversion cases are at the 3^0 of the gene. The fusion transcript can be detected by RT-PCR and FISH analysis using dual-color probes, now commercially available.

Acute Myeloid Leukemia (Megakaryoblastic) with t(1;22) (p13;q13)/RBM15-MKL1

This translocation is restricted to patients younger than 3 years old and constitutes approximately 1% of AMLs. Morphologically, it is linked to acute megakaryoblastic leukemia and commonly associated with variable amounts of bone marrow fibrosis, hepatosplenomegaly, and poor outcome. The translocation results in the fusion of RNA-binding motif protein 15 (RBM15) and megakaryocyte leukemia 1 genes (MKL1). It has been postulated that the fusion protein causes impairment of megakaryoblastic proliferation and differentiation.

The t(1;22) can be detected by CC or FISH analysis. Some laboratories are using RT-PCR to identify the chimeric mRNA.

ACUTE LEUKEMIA WITH GENE MUTATIONS

NPM1-mutated AML NPM1 mutations occur in approximately 50% of normal karyotypes of AML and approximately 35% of AML associated with chromosomal aberration.[26,27] Physiologically, NPM1 is a nucleolar protein that mediates the transport of ribosomal proteins through the nuclear membrane. Aberration affecting NPM1 causes its sequestration in the cytoplasm, thus preventing its function as a transport protein. Deregulated NPM1 gene (5q35) may result from balanced translocation (t(2;5) (p23;q35)/ALK-NPM1, t(5;17) (q35;q21)/NPM-RARA, and t(3;5) (q25.1;q34)/MLF1-NPM1) or mutation.

The most common mutation is an insertion of 4 base pairs, in exon 12, resulting in a frame-shift and replacement of the 7 C-terminal amino acids of the NPM1 protein by

11 different residues that cause the disruption of the nucleolar localization signal. Some studies indicated that mutated NPM1 inhibits the tumor-suppressor gene p14-ARF. NPM1 mutations often coincide with mutations in FLT3 and such association may decrease its favorable outcome. NPM1 mutation is analyzed by PCR amplification followed by fragment analysis by capillary electrophoresis to detect small insertional mutations.

CCAAT Enhancer Binding Protein Alpha–Mutated Acute Myeloid Leukemia

CCAAT enhancer binding protein alpha is a transcription factor that is involved in myeloid cell differentiation. Mutated CCAAT enhancer binding protein alpha is found in approximately 10% of AMLs and is associated with good prognosis. Mutations may involve both alleles with 1 allele having mutation in C-terminus and the other allele in N-terminus.[26,27] Less frequently, 1 allele with both C-terminus and N-terminus mutations may present. Mutations are detected by PCR amplification followed by sequencing.

Fms-Related Tyrosine Kinase 3 Gene–Mutated Acute Myeloid Leukemia

Fms-related tyrosine kinase 3 gene (FLT3) is a tyrosine kinase receptor that is involved in cell maturation and inhibition of apoptosis. Mutated FLT3 is found in approximately 30% of AMLs and is associated with poor outcome.[26,27] FLT3 may undergo point mutation of the aspartic acid residue 835 (D835) on exon 20 or internal tandem duplication (ITD) of the juxtamembrane domain on exon 14/15. FLT3 mutations are detected by multiplex PCR amplification followed by capillary electrophoresis for length mutations (FLT3-ITD) and resistance to EcoRV digestion (D835). Studies have found that high mutant/wild-type ratio is associated with worse prognosis.

KIT-Mutated Leukemia

cKIT (CD117) is the cellular homolog of the feline sarcoma viral oncogene v-kit. It is a class III receptor tyrosine kinase that is involved in stem cell homing to their microenvironment, and the gene is located at 4q11-q12.[26,27] cKIT mutations are gain of function mutations, and they result from an ITD of exon 11 or insertion/deletion of exon 8 at the tyrosine kinase domain. The presence of cKIT mutation, particularly in the setting of core binding leukemia (t[8;21] and inv[16]), is associated with poor outcome. cKIT mutations are detected by using allele-specific PCR and sequencing.

Wilms Tumor Gene–Mutated Leukemia

Wilms tumor gene (WT1) is a transcription factor that has tumor suppressor and, paradoxically, oncogenic functions. The gene is located at 11p13 and most mutations are present on exons 7 and 9.[26,27] It is seen in approximately 10% to 14% of AMLs and its expression is associated with poor prognosis. WT1 mutations are detected by using allele-specific PCR followed by amplicon sequencing and computer analysis for the presence of mutation.

Leukemia Associated with Isocitrate Dehydrogenase 1 and 2 or Brain and Acute Leukemia, Cytoplasmic

Some proteins have been reported to be overexpressed in AML, particularly in AML with normal karyotype, and they may act as adverse prognostic factors.[26,27] Mutations involving isocitrate dehydrogenase 1 (IDH1, IDH1^{R132}) and 2 (IDH2, IDH2^{R172}) and the brain and acute leukemia, cytoplasmic genes are among this group. Basically, they are detected by PCR amplification and mutational analysis by sequencing and comparison with the published unmutated sequence.

Acute Lymphoblastic Leukemia with t(9;22) (q34;q11)/BCR-ABL

The t(9;22) is seen in 25% and 5% of adult B-ALLs and pediatric B-ALLs, respectively. All cases of conventional chronic myelogenous leukemia (CML) have t(9;22). The translocation involves the fusion of Abelson murine leukemia viral oncogene homolog 1 (ABL) gene at 9q34 with breakpoint cluster region (BCR) gene at 22q11. Philadelphia (Ph) chromosome is the derivative chromosome 22 and is associated with poor outcome in B-ALL. In CML and ALL, the cluster region in ABL gene is somewhat constant but variable for BCR gene. Depending on the site of BCR within chromosome 22 (major-BCR [M-BCR], minor-BCR [m-BCR], and micro-BCR [mu-BCR]), three fusion transcripts with high tyrosine activities are produced. Breakpoints in the cluster regions M-BCR, m-BCR, and mu-BCR translate into producing p210, p190, and p230 proteins, respectively. M-BCR is the most common breakpoint in CML (95%) and almost all cases of B-ALL have a breakpoint in the m-BCR region. The t(9;22) can be detected by several methods including CC, Southern blotting, FISH, and RT-PCR. The RT-PCR method is the most commonly used test when looking for minimal residual disease.

BCR-ABL1–Like B Lymphoblastic Leukemia

This new entity is added to the 2016 update of the WHO classification to describe a group of B-ALL with translocations involving tyrosine kinases or cytokine receptors. This entity is characterized by having poor prognosis, potential response to TKI treatment and gene expression profiles similar to those seen in cases of BCR-ABL1 positive lymphoblastic leukemia. More than 30 genes are identified, including ABL1, EBF1, ABL2, PDGFRB, NTRK3, TYK2, CSF1R, CRLF2, EPOR, TSLPR, and JAK2. Next-generation sequencing is the gold standard method to detect this group of leukemia; however, specific testing for some of the involved genes by FISH is done in same laboratory.[28,29]

Acute Lymphoblastic Leukemia with t(12;21) (p13;q22)/TEL/RUNX1

This translocation is found in approximately 20% to 30% and 3% of pediatric and adult B-ALLs, respectively, and most of the time in cryptic form. B-ALL with t(12;21) demonstrates favorable prognosis but this observation is hindered by late relapse. The translocation involves fusion of intron 5 of TEL gene at 12p13 locus with intron 1 of RUNX1 gene at 21q22. The mechanism by which this fusion protein works is not completely revealed; however, it seems to interfere with RUNX1-dependent gene regulation. Because of the cryptic nature of this translocation CC analysis is not the preferred test. Both FISH and RT-PCR are used to detect t(12;21).

Acute Lymphoblastic Leukemia with t(1;19) (q23;p13)/TCF3-PBX1

This translocation is seen in approximately 5% of pediatric B-ALLs and is associated with poor prognosis. It results from the fusion of T-cell factor 3 (TCF3) gene at 19p13 and the pre–B-cell leukemia transcription factor 1 (PBX1) at 1q23. The chimeric protein causes impairment of B-cell maturation and proliferation. In approximately 25% of cases, the translocation is cryptic, thus precluding its detection by CCs. FISH and RT-PCR can be also used to detect t(1;19).

Acute Lymphoblastic Leukemia with t(4;11) (q11;q23)/AF4-MLL

This translocation is seen in approximately 10% of adult and pediatric B-ALLs and in approximately 80% of infantile B-ALLs. B-ALL associated with this translocation has poor prognosis in all age groups. It results from the fusion of MLL gene at 11q23 with AF4 gene at 4q11. FISH and RT-PCR can be used to detect this translocation.

Chronic Myelogenous Leukemia with t(9;22) (q34;q11)/BCR-ABL1

The discovery of Ph chromosome in 1960 provided the first evidence of a genetic association to cancer. The translocation involves the fusion of ABL gene at 9q34 with the BCR gene at 22q11.[30,31] Ph chromosome is the shortened chromosome number 22 because of this translocation. Ph chromosome harbors the gene that encodes for the chimeric protein BCR-ABL1 that exhibits high kinase activity and results in phosphorylation and recruitment of several cellular substrates. BCR-ABL1 fusion protein induces myeloid proliferation through many pathways, including P13K/AKT, JAK/STAT, RAS/RAF, and JUN.[31] Studies show that the reciprocal ABL/BCR on chromosome 9 encodes p96 and p40 fusion proteins. Their leukemogenic potential is under investigation.

Almost all cases of typical CML are positive for t(9;22). The CML cases of negative Ph chromosome by cytogenetic and molecular studies are in the category of myelodysplastic/myeloproliferative neoplasm (MDS/MPN) in the 2016 update of the WHO classification. Further description of the BCR-ABL1 fusion protein is described previously. Imatinib mesylate (Gleevec, NOVARTIS, Switzerland) has an inhibitory effect on the continuously activated ABL1 domain of the BCR-ABL1 chimeric protein. In addition to imatinib, the new-generation drugs dasatinib and nilotinib have improved the outcome of CML. New BCR-ABL1 mutations, however, have been implicated in some resistant cases of CML. Approximately 85% of all resistance-associated mutations are caused by a single amino acid substitution, including T315I, F359V, Y253F/H, M244V, G250E, E255K/V, and M351T. The new-generation drugs can be used in cases with resistance-associated mutations.

Conventional karyotype can detect the t(9;22), except the cryptic forms (approximately 5%), where FISH analysis can be used. The advantage of CC over FISH is that it also can reveal additional chromosomal abnormalities that are harbingers of accelerated phase or blast crisis. Most laboratories are using quantitative RT-PCR to measure BCR-ABL1 p210, P230, and p190 transcripts. The quantitative RT-PCR results are normalized to the international standard (IS) and presented in IS % ratio units. For example, a sensitivity of 0.001 IS % ratio indicates the detection of 1 translocation positive cell per 100,000 cells.[32]

MUTATIONS ASSOCIATED MYELOPROLIFERATIVE NEOPLASMS

Myeloproliferative neoplasms (MPNs) are a heterogeneous group of clonal diseases associated with excessive production of mature hematopoietic elements, including BCR-ABL1–positive CML, polycythemia vera (PV), primary myelofibrosis (PMF) essential thrombocythemia (ET), chronic neutrophilic leukemia, chronic eosinophilic leukemia (CEN) NOS, and MPN, NOS. Mutations involving Janus kinase 2 (JAK2V617F), myeloproliferative leukemia (MPL) protein, and JAK2 exon 12 cause constitutive activation of cytokine-regulated intracellular signaling pathways, which are considered the major driving mechanism of BCR-ABL1–negative MPN. The 2016 update of the WHO incorporates JAK2 mutations (V617F and exon 12) in the diagnostic criteria for the diagnosis of PV, PMF, and ET. In JAK2 mutation–negative cases of MPN, the finding of MPL mutation addresses the WHO criteria.

The JAK2 mutations are the most common mutations in MPN, where they are identified in most patients with PV (95%), in approximately half of the patients with PMF or ET, and rarely with other MPNs, myelodysplastic syndrome (MDS), and MPN/MDS. JAK2 is a downstream tyrosine kinase involved in the phosphorylation and activation of different cellular proteins, which mediate different cellular functions, including cell growth and differentiation. The gene encoding JAK2 is located at 9p24 locus. The first identified JAK2 mutation involves a change of valine to phenylalanine at the 617 position in exon 14 (JAK2V617F). Other mutations have been found to occur in the 3^0 terminus of exon 12 of JAK2 gene (JAK2 exon 12 mutation) in patients with JAK2V617F-negative MPN (1%–5%). JAK2 mutations are gain-of-function mutations causing constitutive activa-tion of tyrosine kinase and subsequent activation of cytokine-regulated intracellular signaling pathways. MPL is another protein that was found to play a role in the pathogenesis of MPN with negative JAK2 mutations. MPL mutations are caused by a substitution of leucine, lysine, or alanine for tryptophan at codon 515 (W515L, W515K, and S505N), and these mutations have been reported in approximately 5% and 1% of PMF and ET cases, respectively. The presence of MPL mutations is associated with severe anemia and thrombocytosis. JAK2 and MPL mutations are detected by using allele-specific PCR amplification followed by amplicon sequencing for mutation detection. The tests are resulted as positive or negative. The sensitivity of the test is limited by the presence of mutant allele (1%–10%) in the background of wild-type allele. In JAK2V617F-positive cases evaluating melting curve differentiates wild-type (GG) from homozygous (GT) and heterozygous (TT) mutants.

In addition to JAK2 (exon12 and exon14) mutations, the 2016 update of the WHO also incorporated two additional mutations in the BCR-ABL1 negative MPN categories. These mutations are CALR (calreticulin, exon 9) and MPL, (exon10)mutations and they appear in different frequencies in BCR-ABL1 negative MPN. The occurrence of JAK2, CALR, and MPL mutations is found mutually exclusive in ET and PMF. Approximately 90% of PV cases show JAK2 (5% for exon 12) and be negative for MPL and CALR. The rest of PV cases (5%–10%) are triple negative for JAK2, CALR and MPL gene mutations. Approximately 10% to 25% of ET and PMF cases show MPL and CALR mutations, respectively. The significance of these mutations in the clinical course of ET and PMF is still under investigation. Some studies suggest that CALR mutation may be associated lower white blood cell count in peripheral blood but more disease progression to acute leukemia.

The 2016 update of the WHO classification did not change the category that is initially incorporated in the 2008 WHO edition, including myeloid and lymphoid neoplasms associated with eosinophilia and abnormalities of platelet-derived growth factor (PDGF) receptor alpha (PDGFRA) at 4q12 locus, PDGF receptor beta (PDGFRB) at 5q33 locus, or epidermal growth factor receptor 1 at 8p11.2 locus. These genes encode cell surface tyrosine kinase receptors that regulate embryonic development and cell proliferation and differentiation. Cases associated with rearrangement of PDGFRA and FGFR1 tend to have a lymphoid component and may present initially as T or B-lymphoblastic leukemia/lymphoma with eosinophilia, whereas cases associated with PDGFRB tend to present as chronic myelomonocytic leukemia with eosinophilia or as CEL. Myeloid neoplasms associated with PDGFRA or PDGFRB rearrangements are sensitive to imatinib (Gleevec) therapy. Rearrangement of PDGFRB and FGFR1 can be detected by CC and by FISH and PCR amplification and sequencing. Because of the cryptic nature of PDGFRA rearrangement, however, molecular testing through PCR amplification and sequencing PCR is usually necessary.

CYTOGENETIC ABNORMALITIES ASSOCIATED WITH MYELODYSPLASTIC SYNDROME

MDS is a group of diseases associated with ineffective hematopoiesis, dysplastic changes in bone marrow elements, and peripheral cytopenia. The 2016 update of the WHO classification of MDS includes MDS with single-lineage dysplasia

(MDS-SLD); MDS with multilineage dysplasia (MDS-MLD); MDS with ring sideroblasts (MDS-RS); MDS with excess blasts (MDS-EB); myelodysplastic syndrome with isolated del(5q); MDS-unclassifiable; and MDS of childhood (refractory cytopenia of childhood). The MDS-RS category is further subtyped into MDS-RS-SLD and MDS-RS-MLD. Most cytogenetic abnormalities are either numerical (loss/gain) or, less commonly, unbalanced/balanced chromosomal abnormalities. They are seen in approximately 80% of secondary MDS cases after chemotherapy or radiotherapy and in approximately 50% of de novo cases. The most common abnormalities observed in MDS include monosomy 5 (5−) or deletions in the long arm of chromosome 7 (7q−), 7− or 7q−, 13− or 13q−, trisomy 8 (8†), and 20q−.[33] The balanced translocation that may be seen include t(11;16) (q23;p13.3), t(3;21) (q26.2;q22.1), t(1;3) (p36.3;q21.1), t(2;11) (p21;q23), inv(3) (q21q26.2), and t(6;9) (p23;q34). Approximately 33% and 40% of MDS cases show a single abnormality or are part of a monosomal karyotype, respectively. Complex karyotypes are seen in approximately 11% of MDS cases. Conventional karyotypes detect most of the chromosomal abnormalities associated with MDS. FISH analysis and spectral karyotyping also can be used; however, they do not show increased sensitivity over CC.

THE IMPORTANCE OF CHROMOSOMAL ABERRATIONS IN HEMATOPOIETIC MALIGNANCIES

It is not surprising that an accurate diagnosis is important in the management of hematopoietic neoplasms. Given the ever-expanding list of diagnostic disorders, an increasing understanding of the molecular biology of cancer, the proliferation of sensitive testing methods, and novel targeted therapies designed to capitalize on these findings, it is also clear this process has never been more difficult or critical for appropriate patient care. When coupled with the appropriate clinical scenario, molecular markers have proved beneficial and often vital to the diagnosis, prognosis, and therapy for hematologic malignancies.

A prime example of this is detailed in the story of CML. The identification of the t(9;22) translocation resulting in the fusion of BCR and ABL results in constitutively active fusion tyrosine kinase. The identification of this abnormality by cytogenetics, FISH, or PCR is necessary for the diagnosis of CML. The phenotypic and clinical conditions that mimic CML, such as other myeloproliferative syndromes, leukemoid reactions, and chronic myelomonocytic leukemia, fail to possess this crucial translocation. This critical discrepancy allows physicians to more accurately diagnose CML in the molecular era. More importantly, scientists have developed several tyrosine kinase inhibitors to inhibit the hyperactive fusion protein coded by the (9;22) translocation. These tyrosine kinase inhibitors have transformed a universally fatal illness to one with an excellent prognosis.

Other such examples of molecularly targeted therapies are noted in other hematologic disorders. For instance, the use of ATRA in APL has capitalized on the improved understanding of disease pathophysiology. In APL a translocation of the retinoic acid receptor on chromosome 17 occurs (most commonly with the PML gene on chromosome 15) and the resultant fusion protein inhibits myeloid differentiation. The use of ATRA overcomes this phenomenon and has been used extensively in the treatment of APL.

Other chromosomal abnormalities in AML engender a favorable, intermediate, or unfavorable prognosis and are used in combination with other factors to help determine when allogeneic transplants are considered. In this way the prognostic implications of molecular testing may also result in alteration of management.

Molecular findings also provide potential insights into the underlying pathophysiology of malignancy and help clinicians understand why in some instances treatment is unsuccessful. For instance, the inv(16) chromosomal abnormality in AML is generally associated with a good prognosis with conventional chemotherapy. Studies suggest high rates of complete remission and 10-year survival rates of more than 50% in this population with conventional therapy. Several patients with this cytogenetic abnormality fail to remain in remission, however, and studies have suggested that at least a proportion of these failures may be related to mutations in c-kit. In 1 study, approximately 30% of inv(16) patients harbored a c-kit mutation and had higher incidences of relapse and a lower overall survival rate compared with their wild-type c-kit counterparts. Consequently, because of interactions between individual molecular abnormalities, favorable prognosis leukemia may be altered negatively. Similarly in lymphoma, overexpression of C-MYC and BCL-2 translocations, so called double-hit lymphomas, have been shown to confer a poorer prognosis to conventional therapy. Neither C-MYC overexpression, however, nor presences of the BCL-2 translocation have been shown to result in poorer outcomes, which raises the possibility of important interactions between individual abnormalities.

Lastly, the ability to identify these signatures of malignancy allows for sensitive monitoring of response or relapse. The (9;22) translocation in CML is assessed by PCR to determine the depth of response. This translocation is also commonly seen in ALL and is a sensitive predictor of relapse on completion of therapy.

SUMMARY

The progress made by advances in molecular medicine has had far-reaching effects in all aspects of clinical treatment of hematologic malignancies. These findings, and numerous others, have provided a doorway into understanding the molecular drivers of disease but have also yielded excellent targets for therapy, thereby saving numerous lives.

REFERENCES

1. Arber DA, Orazi A, Hasserjian R, et al. The 2016 revision to the World Health Organization classification of myeloid neoplasms and acute leukemia. Blood 2016; 127:2391–405.
2. Swerdlow SH, Campo E, Pileri SA, et al. The 2016 revision of the World Health Organization classification of lymphoid neoplasms. Blood 2016;127:2375–90.
3. Vardiman JW, Thiele J, Arber DA, et al. The 2008 revision of the World Health Organization (WHO) classification of myeloid neoplasms and acute leukemia: rationale and important changes. Blood 2009;114:937–51.
4. Alt FW, Yancopoulos GD, Blackwell TK, et al. Ordered rearrangement of immunoglobulin heavy chain variable region segments. EMBO J 1984;3:1209–19.
5. Tonegawa S. Somatic generation of antibody diversity. Nature 1983;302:575–81.
6. Davis MM, Bjorkman PJ. T-cell antigen receptor genes and T-cell recognition. Nature 1988;334:395–402.
7. Tobin G, Rosenquist R. Prognostic usage of V(H) gene mutation status and its surrogate markers and the role of antigen selection in chronic lymphocytic leukemia. Med Oncol 2005;22:217–28.
8. van Dongen JJ, Langerak AW, Brüggemann M, et al. Design and standardization of PCR primers and protocols for detection of clonal immunoglobulin and T-cell receptor gene recombinations in suspect lymphoproliferations: report of the BIOMED-2 concerted action BMH4-CT98-3936. Leukemia 2003;17:2257–317.

9. Bruggemann M, White H, Gaulard P, et al. Powerful strategy for polymerase chain reaction-based clonality assessment in T-cell malignancies. Report of the BIOMED-2 Concerted Action BHM4 CT98-3936. Leukemia 2007;21:215–21.

10. Aster JC, Longtine JA. Detection of BCL2 rearrangements in follicular lymphoma. Am J Pathol 2002;160:759–63.

11. Sherr CJ. Mammalian G1 cyclins. Cell 1993;73:1059–65.

12. Mozos A, Royo C, Hartmann E, et al. SOX11 expression is highly specific for mantle cell lymphoma and identifies the cyclin D1-negative subtype. Haematologica 2009;94:1555–62.

13. Albagli-Curiel O. Ambivalent role of BCL6 in cell survival and transformation. Oncogene 2003;22:507–16.

14. Basso K, Dalla-Favera R. BCL6: master regulator of the germinal center reaction and key oncogene in B cell lymphomagenesis. Adv Immunol 2010;105:193–210.

15. Nakamura N, Nakamine H, Tamaru J, et al. The distinction between Burkitt lymphoma and diffuse large B-Cell lymphoma with c-myc rearrangement. Mod Pathol 2002;15:771–6.

16. Kalla J, Stilgenbauer S, Schaffner C, et al. Heterogeneity of the API2-MALT1 gene rearrangement in MALT-type lymphoma. Leukemia 2000;14:1967–74.

17. Dierlamm J. Genetic abnormalities in marginal zone B-cell lymphoma. Haematologica 2003;88:8–12.

18. Morris SW, Kirstein MN, Valentine MB, et al. Fusion of a kinase gene, ALK, to a nucleolar protein gene, NPM, in non-Hodgkin's lymphoma. Science 1995;267:316–7.

19. Hernandez L, Pinyol M, Hernandez S, et al. TRK-fused gene (TFG) is a new partner of ALK in anaplastic large cell lymphoma producing two structurally different TFG-ALK translocations. Blood 1999;94:3265–8.

20. Breen KA, Grimwade D, Hunt BJ. The pathogenesis and management of the coagulopathy of acute promyelocytic leukaemia. Br J Haematol 2012;156:24–36.

21. De Botton S, Chevret S, Sanz M, et al. Additional chromosomal abnormalities in patients with acute promyelocytic leukaemia (APL) do not confer poor prognosis: results of APL 93 trial. Br J Haematol 2000;111:801–6.

22. Nucifora G, Birn DJ, Erickson P, et al. Detection of DNA rearrangements in the AML1 and ETO loci and of an AML1/ETO fusion mRNA in patients with t(8;21) acute myeloid leukemia. Blood 1993;81:883–8.

23. Le Beau MM, Larson RA, Bitter MA, et al. Association of an inversion of chromosome 16 with abnormal marrow eosinophils in acute myelomonocytic leukemia. A unique cytogenetic-clinicopathological association. N Engl J Med 1983;309:630–6.

24. Kaneko Y, Maseki N, Takasaki N, et al. Clinical and hematologic characteristics in acute leukemia with 11q23 translocations. Blood 1986;67:484–91.

25. Lugthart S, Groschel S, Beverloo HB, et al. Clinical, molecular, and prognostic significance of WHO type inv(3)(q21q26.2)/t(3;3)(q21;q26.2) and various other 3q abnormalities in acute myeloid leukemia. J Clin Oncol 2010;28:3890–8.

26. Grimwade D, Hills RK, Moorman AV, et al. Refinement of cytogenetic classification in acute myeloid leukemia: determination of prognostic significance of rare recurring chromosomal abnormalities among 5876 younger adult patients treated in the United Kingdom Medical Research Council trials. Blood 2010;116:354–65.

27. Marcucci G, Mrozek K, Bloomfield CD. Molecular heterogeneity and prognostic biomarkers in adults with acute myeloid leukemia and normal cytogenetics. Curr Opin Hematol 2005;12:68–75.

28. Thorsten Klampfl T, Gisslinger H, Harutyunyan, et al. Somatic mutations of calreticulin in myeloproliferative neoplasms. N Engl J Med 2013;369:2379–90.
29. Roberts KG, Li Y, Payne-Turner D, et al. Argetable kinase-activating lesions in Ph-like acute lymphoblastic leukemia. N Engl J Med 2014;371:1005–15.
30. Faderl S, Talpaz M, Estrov Z, et al. The biology of chronic myeloid leukemia. N Engl J Med 1999;341:164–72.
31. Verfaillie CM. Biology of chronic myelogenous leukemia. Hematol Oncol Clin North Am 1998;12:1–29.
32. Gabert J, Beillard E, van der Velden VH, et al. Standardization and quality control studies of 'real-time' quantitative reverse transcriptase polymerase chain reaction of fusion gene transcripts for residual disease detection in leukemia: a Europe against cancer program. Leukemia 2003;17:2318–57.
33. Pozdnyakova O, Miron PM, Tang G, et al. Cytogenetic abnormalities in a series of 1,029 patients with primary myelodysplastic syndromes: a report from the US with a focus on some undefined single chromosomal abnormalities. Cancer 2008;113: 3331–40.

Molecular Diagnostics in Colorectal Carcinoma

Advances and Applications for 2018

Amarpreet Bhalla, MBBS, MD[a],*, Muhammad Zulfiqar, MD[b],
Martin H. Bluth, MD, PhD[c,d]

KEYWORDS

- Colorectal carcinoma • Serrated polyp pathway • KRAS • BRAF
- CpG island methylator phenotype

KEY POINTS

- The molecular pathogenesis and classification of colorectal carcinoma are based on the traditional adenoma–carcinoma sequence in the Vogelstein model, serrated polyp pathway, and MSI.
- The genetic basis for hereditary nonpolyposis colorectal cancer is based on detection of mutations in the MLH1, MSH2, MSH6, PMS2, and EPCAM genes.
- Genetic testing for the Lynch syndrome includes MSI testing, methylator phenotype testing, BRAF mutation testing, and molecular testing for germline mutations in mismatch repair genes.
- Molecular makers with predictive and prognostic implications include quantitative multi-gene reverse transcriptase polymerase chain reaction assay and KRAS and BRAF mutation analysis.
- Mismatch repair-deficient tumors have higher rates of programmed death-ligand 1 expression.

INTRODUCTION

The pathogenesis of colorectal carcinoma is heterogeneous and involves complex multistep molecular pathways initiated by genetic and epigenetic events. The molecular classification of colorectal carcinoma provides the basis for evaluation of prognostic, predictive, and theranostic markers. The goal is precise, efficient, and accurate application of molecular tests for patient management.[1–3]

This article has been updated from a version previously published in Clinics in Laboratory Medicine, Volume 33, Issue 4, December 2013.

[a] Department of Pathology and Anatomical Sciences, Jacobs School of Buffalo, Buffalo, NY 14203, USA; [b] SEPA Labs, Brunswick, GA, USA; [c] Department of Pathology, Wayne State University School of Medicine, 540 East Canfield Street, Detroit, MI 48201, USA; [d] Pathology Laboratories, Michigan Surgical Hospital, 21230 Dequindre Road, Warren, MI 48091, USA
* Corresponding author.
E-mail addresses: ABhalla@KaleidaHealth.org; bhallapreet7@gmail.com

EPIDEMIOLOGY

Constitutional (endogenous) as well as environmental (exogenous) factors are associated with the development of colorectal carcinoma. Multiple risk factors have been linked to colorectal carcinoma. Colorectal carcinoma is more common in late-middle-aged and elderly individuals. Men are at a higher risk for developing this malignancy. There is a strong association with a Western type of diet consisting of high-calorie food, rich in animal fat.[4]

Clinical Features

Clinical presentation includes change in bowel habit, constipation, abdominal distension, hematochezia, tenesmus, weight loss, malaise, fever, and anemia. Regarding screening, the American Gastroenterological Association, American Medical Association, and American Cancer Society recommend endoscopy with biopsy as the standard screening approach. Radiologic evaluation by computed tomography scan and MRI are used to assess locoregional spread and distant metastases.[4–9]

PATHOPHYSIOLOGY AND MOLECULAR GENETICS

The various molecular alterations described in colorectal carcinoma are enlisted in **Box 1**.[10] The diagrams depict the adenoma–carcinoma sequence and serrated polyp pathway arising from a complex interplay of genetic alterations (**Figs. 1–4**).[1]

TRADITIONAL VOGELSTEIN MODEL AND APC GENE PATHWAY

The traditional model of Vogelstein describes the classic adenoma–carcinoma sequence and accounts for approximately 80% of sporadic colon tumors. The pathogenesis involves mutation of the APC gene early in the neoplastic process.[2]

APC Gene

A tumor suppressor gene located on the long (q) arm of chromosome 5 between positions 21 and 22 plays a key role in regulating cell division cycle and regulates the WNT/β-catenin signaling pathway. With loss of APC function, β-catenin accumulates and activates the transcription of MYC and cyclin D1 genes, resulting in enhanced proliferation of cells. More than 700 mutations in the APC gene have been identified in familial adenomatous polyposis (FAP), both classic and attenuated types. In this regard,

---

Box 1
Common genetic and epigenetic alterations in colorectal cancer

Tumor Suppressor Genes	Proto-Oncogenes	Other Molecular Alterations
• APC	• BRAF	• Chromosome instability
• ARID1A	• ERBB2	• CpG island methylator phenotype
• CTNNB1	• GNAS	• Microsatellite instability
• DCC	• IGF2	• Mismatch-repair genes
• FAM123B	• KRAS	• SEPT9
• FBXW7	• MYC	• VIM, NDRG4, BMP3
• PTEN	• NRAS	• POLE/POLD1
• RET	• PIK3CA	
• SMAD4	• RSPO2/RSPO3	
• TGFBR2	• SOX9	
• TP53	• TCF7L2	

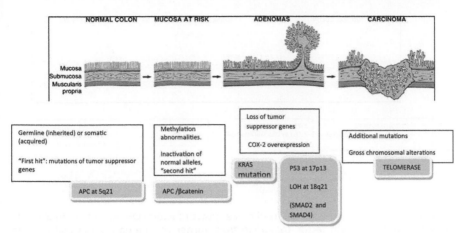

Fig. 1. Adenoma-carcinoma sequence. COX-2, cyclooxygenase-2; LOH, loss of heterozygosity. (*Modified from* Turner JR. The gastrointestinal tract. In: Kumar V, Abbas AK, Fausto N, et al, editors. Robbins and Cotran pathologic basis of disease. 8th edition. Philadelphia: Elsevier; 2010. p. 823; with permission.)

FAP is a syndrome with an inherited truncating APC mutation, leading to the production of an abnormally short, nonfunctional version of the protein that cannot suppress the cellular overgrowth and leads to the formation of polyps and subsequent progression to carcinoma. Both copies of the APC gene must be functionally inactivated, either by mutation or by the epigenetic events for development of adenomas; the second allele in adenomas harbors a loss or similar mutation, whereas homozygous deletions of APC are rare or absent. In sporadic colorectal tumors, the mutation may be in a mutation cluster region in the APC gene with allelic loss, or mutations may be outside this region with a tendency to harbor truncating mutations (**Fig. 5**).[2,3,11]

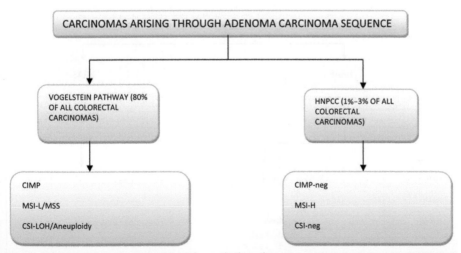

Fig. 2. Subtypes of carcinoma arising through the adenoma-carcinoma sequence. CIMP, CpG island methylator phenotype; LOH, loss of heterozygosity; MSI, microsatellite instability; MSS, microsatellite stable.

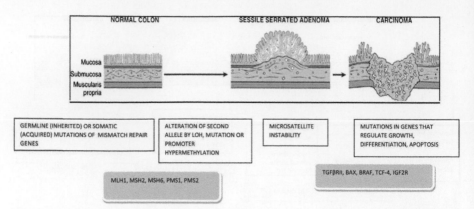

Fig. 3. Serrated polyp pathway. IGF, insulin-like growth factor; LOH, loss of heterozygosity; TGF, transforming growth factor. (*Modified from* Turner JR. The gastrointestinal tract. In: Kumar V, Abbas AK, Fausto N, et al, editors. Robbins and Cotran pathologic basis of disease. 8th edition. Philadelphia: Elsevier; 2010. p. 824; with permission.)

Neoplastic progression is associated with additional mutations and chromosomal instability, with involvement of the following.

- KRAS, an oncogene that enhances growth and prevents apoptosis;
- SMAD2 and SMAD4 (DPC4), tumor suppressor genes that are effectors of transforming growth factor-β signaling and allows unrestrained cell growth;
- DCC, a tumor suppressor gene located at 18q2.3;
- p53, which are tumor suppressor genes and are mutated in 70% to 80% of colon cancers; and
- Telomerase, which increases as lesions become more advanced.

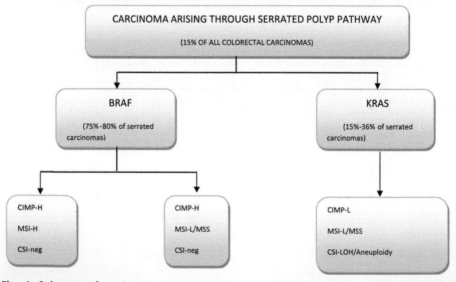

Fig. 4. Subtypes of carcinoma arising through serrated polyp pathway. CIMP, CpG island methylator phenotype; LOH, loss of heterozygosity; MSI, microsatellite instability; MSS, microsatellite stable.

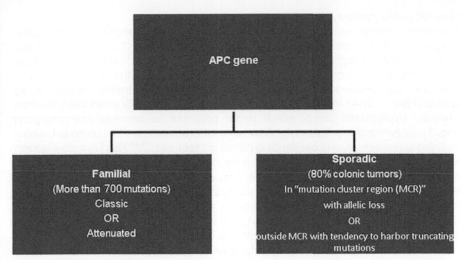

Fig. 5. APC gene mutations.

Other causes of chromosomal instability may be heterogeneous and include mutations in genes encoding mitosis checkpoint proteins such as BUB1 and BUB1B, abnormal centrosome number, amplification of aurora kinase A (AURKA, STK 15/BTAK), mutations of FBXW7, CHFR.1,2,11 Alternatively, tumor suppressor genes may also be silenced by methylation of a CpG-rich zone or CpG island (**Fig. 6**).[8] GNAS mutations have been reported in villous adenomas.[12]

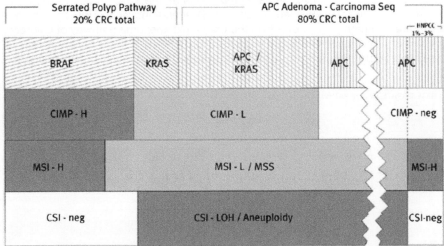

Fig. 6. Molecular genetic profiles of colorectal carcinoma. CIMP, CpG island methylator phenotype; CRC, colorectal cancer; HPNCC, hereditary nonpolyposis colorectal cancer; LOH, loss of heterozygosity; MSI, microsatellite instability; MSI-H, high-frequency microsatellite instability; MSS, microsatellite stable. (*Modified from* O'Brien MJ, Yang S, Huang CS, et al. The serrated polyp pathway to colorectal carcinoma. Mini-symposium: pathology of the large bowel. Diagn Histopathol 2008;14(2):90; with permission.)

Serrated polyp pathway

The serrated polyp pathway comprises a group of colorectal neoplasms with distinct morphologic and molecular characteristics. There are 20% to 30% of colorectal carcinomas that are thought to develop from serrated precursors.[13] Aberrant crypt focus and hyperplastic polyps comprise the earliest lesions. The other serrated polypoid lesions include sessile serrated adenoma/polyp (SSA/P), and traditional serrated adenoma (TSA).[14] BRAF mutation has been described as an early event seen in microvesicular hyperplastic polyp, which might progress to serrated adenoma/polyp (**Fig. 7**). SSA/P and hyperplastic polyps have different cancer risks, different recommended surveillances, and overlapping histologic features.[13,15] Hes1 is a downstream target of Notch signaling pathway and is found to be ubiquitously expressed in the nuclei of normal colonic epithelial cells. The complete loss or weak expression of Hes1 is observed in majority of SSA/P compared with normal expression of Hes1 in hyperplastic polyps. The dysplastic areas in sessile serrated adenomas, however, reveal the cytoplasmic staining of Hes1. Tubular adenoma and TSA show variable mixed positive and negative staining patterns.[16]

TSA are a heterogenous group of polyps with mutually exclusive KRAS and BRAF mutations. Molecular analysis of TSAs shows highly variable frequencies of KRAS, BRAF, and GNAS mutations in 10% to 46%, 29% to 90%, and 8% of tumors, respectively. Unlike SSA/P, TSA rarely reveal diffuse expression of ANXA10. BRAF-mutated TSA reveal more widespread methylation of a 5 marker CpG island panel compared with KRAS-mutated polyps.[12] In general, TSA may be CpG island methylator phenotype (CIMP) high, CIMP low, or CIMP negative. The CIMP-high tumors exclusively reveal methylation of RUNX3 and SOCS1, and are associated with BRAF mutations. The CIMP-low tumors are associated with KRAS mutations. They reveal restricted methylation pattern confined to NEUROG1. A strong association between KRAS mutations and high-grade dysplasia has been reported in a patient cohort from Korea.[17] Contiguous serrated lesions resembling SSA/P or hyperplastic polyps, when present, share the same mutations as the TSA. Tumors arising from TSA are predominantly left sided. Wnt/CTNNB1 alterations, and KRAS and p53 mutations are common genetic events in the traditional adenoma pathway of colorectal carcinoma. The characteristic genetic alteration PTPRK-RSPO3 fusion is also reported in a study. The TSA with the aforementioned fusion reveal distal localization,

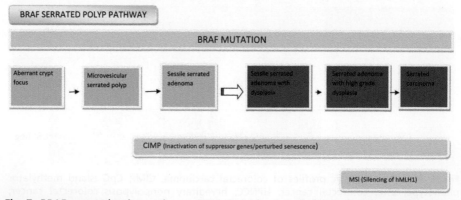

Fig. 7. BRAF serrated polyp pathway. CIMP, CpG island methylator phenotype; MSI, microsatellite instability. (*Modified from* O'Brien MJ, Yang S, Huang CS, et al. The serrated polyp pathway to colorectal carcinoma. Mini-symposium: pathology of the large bowel. Diagn Histopathol 2008;14(2):79; with permission.)

larger size, prominent ectopic crypt foci, association with high-grade component, progression to carcinoma, and the presence of KRAS mutations. Slitlike serrations are less prominent and associations with hyperplastic polyps and SSA/P are rare. RSPO overexpression is mutually exclusive with Wnt pathway gene mutation, but is involved in its activation[18] ANXA10 protein is highly expressed in the majority of SSA/P, but not in the TSA or contiguous precursor polyps associated with them.[19] The progress of nondysplastic serrated polyps to more advanced neoplasms is associated with increasing levels of CpG island methylation, leading to inactivation of tumor suppressor genes.

Carcinomas arising in the serrated pathway The carcinomas of this pathway frequently show MSI as a result of epigenetic silencing of hMLH 1.[14] Some studies have shown that transition to high-grade dysplasia and carcinoma is facilitated by methylation-induced silencing of p16 and escape from activation-induced senescence (**Fig. 8**).[20] The other major pathway of pathogenesis of serrated carcinomas arises after KRAS mutations. The carcinomas are microsatellite stable (MSS) and CIMP low, but show chromosomal instability and loss of heterozygosity of tumor suppressor genes. It is one of the earliest genetic mutations in colon carcinogenesis, detected in approximately 40% of the tumors. Along with BRAF mutations, it has been found in the earliest detectable lesions with a serrated morphology. They have been reported in 18% of aberrant crypt foci, 4% to 37% of hyperplastic polyps, 60% of admixed polyps, 80% of TSAs, and up to 10% of sessile serrated adenomas. KRAS mutation has been observed to be associated with a right-sided tumor location. The mutation has significant association with usual tumor histology (vs mucinous, signet ring, medullary), extramural tumor extension, peritumoral lymphocytic host response, presence of distant metastases, and absence of lymphovascular invasion at the time of diagnosis.[21–28] SSA/P with dysplasia are frequently associated with loss of MLH1 expression, which is critical to progression. The patterns of dysplasia have been classified in a recent study as minimal deviation, serrated, adenomatous, and not otherwise specified. The loss of immunostaining may help in supporting

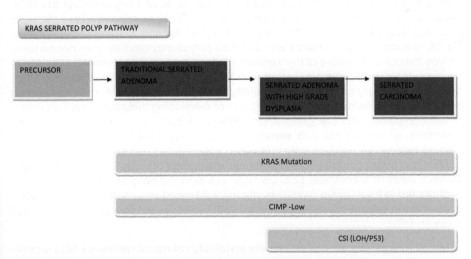

Fig. 8. KRAS serrated polyp pathway. CIMP, CpG island methylator phenotype; LOH, loss of heterozygosity. (*Modified from* O'Brien MJ, Yang S, Huang CS, et al. The serrated polyp pathway to colorectal carcinoma. Mini-symposium: pathology of the large bowel. Diagn Histopathol 2008;14(2):79; with permission.)

minimal deviation pattern of dysplasia, resolving the equivocal nature of atypical lesions, and differentiating sporadic adenomas from fragments of dysplasia associated with SSA/P. Tumors arising from SSA/P are predominantly right sided, microsatellite unstable, BRAF mutated, and hypermethylated at CpG islands (CIMP high).[19] They commonly present as interval colorectal carcinomas, because of missed precursor lesions, incomplete resection and rapid progression.[28]

Serrated polyposis Serrated polyposis is a clinically defined syndrome characterized by occurrence of multiple serrated polyps in the large intestine. A significant number of patients may have synchronous or metachronous tumors. Small numbers of conventional adenomas may also be present. Individuals with serrated polyps and their relatives are at increased risk of colorectal carcinoma. Mutations in BRAF along with CpG island mutator phenotype is the molecular marker for serrated neoplasia, with serrated polyps being precursor lesions.[29] The reported incidences of colorectal cancer (CRC) in serrated polyposis patients vary from 14% to 54%. They have diverse molecular alterations encompassing features of at least of the serrated neoplasia pathway and traditional adenoma pathway. The concomitant presence of conventional adenomas also increases the risk of development of carcinoma. However, the carcinomas contiguous to conventional adenoma are not associated with BRAF mutation.[29] Colorectal carcinoma with adjacent TSA or sessile serrated adenoma demonstrate more frequent mucinous differentiation, BRAF mutation, and mismatch repair (MMR) deficiency. Serrated colorectal carcinomas in distal colon are usually BRAF/KRAS wild type and MMR proficient. Activation of β-catenin was found in CRC with or without BRAF mutation. A large proportion of CRC from patients with serrated polyps do not develop CRC through the serrated neoplasia pathway and show various molecular phenotypes, including the traditional adenoma pathway. A few tumors show KRAS mutation along with low levels of CIMP, MSI, downregulation of MGMT by methylation, and frequent KRAS mutation. Atypical conventional adenomas in individuals who have at least 1 sessile serrated adenoma share some morphologic characteristics with serrated polyps and are all BRAF/KRAS wild type. This polyp may possibly be a precursor lesion of a large number of CRCs. Up to 95% of sessile serrated adenomas harbor a BRAF mutation and are the likely precursor lesions of CRC. Tumors with residual contiguous serrated polyps harbor V600E mutation. CRC in patients with serrated polyps may develop from nonserrated polyps through a derivative of the traditional adenoma pathway. Serrated polyps may be considered a disorder associated with hypermature mucosa secondary to alteration in DNA methylation with a propensity to develop early onset multiple serrated polyps. These patients are at increased risk of developing metachronous carcinoma when compared with the general population. In patients with a high-risk CRC syndrome, when patients with serrated polyps present with CRC more extensive colonic resection should be considered for both subsequent risk of metachronous cancer and future control of polyps. A high proportion of interval CRCs, diagnosed within 5 years of a complete colonoscopy, are serrated neoplasia pathway CRC. It is attributed to lower polyp detection rate for right-sided polyps or rapid progression of serrated lesions to dysplasia and carcinoma even for polyps less than 1 cm.[13,19,29–31]

Sporadic high-frequency microsatellite instability colorectal carcinoma MSI is prevalent in 10% to 15% of all sporadic colorectal carcinomas. Biallelic transcriptional silencing of MLH1 gene secondary to promoter hypermethylation leads to loss of normal MMR function in sporadic CRCs. The malignancy develops through the serrated pathway, with sessile serrated adenoma as the precursor lesion. The molecular abnormality includes methylation of multiple regions of C-G dinucleotide or CpG islands within the promoter region of genes and subsequent downregulation of these genes. It is known as CIMP and is associated with BRAF mutation in 40% to 50% cases.[32] Genetic instability may operate at the chromosomal level (chromosomal instability), affecting the whole chromosome or parts of chromosomes or at a more subtle level affecting DNA sequences resulting from replication errors (high-frequency MSI). These forms of instability are mutually exclusive, so that CRCs with chromosomal instability are MSS (Table 1).[33–37] Appropriate caution must be exercised when correlating single molecular events with patient outcomes. The molecule examined might be associated with global genomic or epigenetic aberrations, and improved or adverse outcomes might be associated with alterations in other molecules. A positive correlation has been reported between BRAF mutated colorectal carcinoma, female sex, proximal tumor location, mucinous or serrated adenocarcinoma histologic type, and the presence of tumor infiltrating lymphocytes (Tables 2 and 3).[29] Metaanalyses of MSI status and survival of patients with colorectal carcinoma showed that high-frequency MSI tumors were associated with a better prognosis compared with MSS tumors. High-frequency MSI tumors show no benefit from adjuvant 5-fluorouracil. Patients with CIMP-positive tumors experience a significant survival benefit from chemotherapy in contrast with those with CIMP-negative tumors. CIMP in non–high-frequency MSI tumors predicts worse survival.[20]

Hereditary nonpolyposis colon cancer/the Lynch syndrome The Lynch syndrome is a hereditary autosomal-dominant syndrome with high penetrance. Its associated tumors show MSI owing to mutations in MMR proteins. The 4 DNA MMR genes are involved in the repair of mismatches resulting from misincorporation, or slippage events, during replication. Hereditary defects in 1 of the 4 MMR genes accounts for 80% to 90% of cases of hereditary nonpolyposis colon cancer (HNPCC).[38–41] Clinically, the Lynch syndrome is defined by applying either the Amsterdam I or Amsterdam II criteria and represents about 2% to 3% of all CRCs. An additional 2% to 3% of patients with CRC harbor similar MMR gene defects, but do not fulfill the criteria. Contrarily, some patients with attenuated FAP-associated and MUTYH- associated polyposis might fulfill Amsterdam criteria for having HNPCC. Revised Bethesda criteria show a higher sensitivity in the detection of new patients with the Lynch syndrome.[42–46] The subset of HNPCC cases caused by MMR gene defects is referred to as hereditary MMR-deficiency syndrome. The MMR-deficient cancers arise after loss of DNA MMR in tumor cells, leading to an increase in the rate of frameshift mutations in microsatellites. The frequency of mutations in short repetitive sequences located in coding regions of genes, such as transforming growth factor-BR2, is also increased. Germline mutations in 4 MMR proteins (MLH1, MSH2, MSH6, and PMS2) account for majority of the cases. Of the cases reported, 80% are attributed to mutations in MLH1 and MSH2.[19] Most of the genetic defects are a result of point mutations, insertions, and deletions.[47] Deletion in the EPCAM gene may cause epigenetic inactivation of MSH2. There are 20% to 25% of the cases that are suspected of having a mutation in MSH2, but without germline mutations, may be accounted for by germline deletions in EPCAM/TACSTD1. They account for about 1% of patients with the Lynch syndrome.

EPCAM is a calcium-independent cell adhesion membrane protein and is not involved in the physiologic functions of MMR. The EPCAM gene is located on the short (p) arm of chromosome 2 at position 21. Large germline deletions and rearrangement

Table 1
Molecular pathologic classification of colorectal cancer

Group Number	CIMP Status	MLH1 Status	MSI Status	Chromosomal Status	Precursor	Proportion (%)
1	CIMP high	Full methylation	MSI-H	Stable (diploid)	Serrated polyp	12
2	CIMP high	Partial methylation	MSS/MSI-L Associated with BRAF mutation	Stable (diploid)	Serrated polyp	8
3	CIMP low	No methylation	MSS/MSI-L Associated with KRAS mutation	Unstable (aneuploid)	Adenoma/serrated polyp	20
4	CIMP negative	No methylation	MSS Associated with KRAS mutation	Unstable (aneuploid)	Adenoma	57
5	CIMP negative	Germline MLH1 or other mutation	MSI-H	Stable (diploid)	Adenoma	3

Abbreviations: CIMP, CpG island methylator phenotype; MSI-L, low-frequency microsatellite instability; MSS, microsatellite stable.

Modified from Jass JR. Classification of colorectal cancer based on correlation of clinical, morphological and molecular features. Histopathology 2007;50:119, with permission; and *Adapted from* Redston M. Epithelial neoplasms of the large intestine. In: Odze RD, Goldblum JR, editors. Surgical pathology of the GI tract, liver, biliary tract and pancreas. 2nd edition. Philadelphia: Elsevier; 2009. p. 597–637, with permission.

Table 2
Clinical presentation of microsatellite instability and BRAF mutation in colorectal carcinoma

BRAF v600E	MMR/MSI	CIMP	Clinical Presentation	%
−	Unstable/high	Low/negative	Lynch syndrome/other	2–3
−	Unstable/high	High	Sporadic	35–55
+	Unstable/high	High	Sporadic	...
+	Stable/negative	Low/negative	Aggressive phenotype/serrated carcinoma	Rare

Abbreviations: CIMP, CpG island methylator phenotype; MMR, mismatch repair; MSI, microsatellite instability.

encompassing EPCAM-*MSH2* have been characterized from the 30 end region of EPCAM to the 50 initial sequences of the MSH (**Tables 4** and **5**).[39–41,47] The tumors do not, however, reveal expression of annexin 10.[19] A few unclassified variants inclusive of mutations and missense-type nucleotide substitutions have been reported in literature and have unknown clinical significance. Many variants are associated with defects in RNA splicing. The prevalence of variants has been reported to be up to 34% among the HNPCC cohorts.[47] The Lynch syndrome type I is confined to patients presenting only with CRC. The Lynch syndrome type II is associated with additional extracolonic cancers. The DNA MMR system is closely associated with tumor response to radiation. It has a critical role in the repair process of DNA structural damage caused by radiation. The MSI attributes to altered radiosensitivity.[48] Patients with the Lynch syndrome/HNPCC harbor a similar number of adenomatous polyps to the

Table 3
Site-specific variation in molecular phenotypes of colorectal carcinoma

	Predominant Tumor Type		Other Common Tumors	
Cecum	BRAF mutated MMR deficient	BRAF/KRAS wild type, MMR deficient		
Ascending colon	BRAF mutated MMR deficient	BRAF/KRAS wild type, MMR deficient	BRAF/KRAS wild type, MMR proficient	BRAF mutated MMR proficient
Transverse colon	BRAF mutated MMR deficient	BRAF mutated MMR proficient	BRAF/KRAS wild type, MMR deficient	KRAS mutated MMR proficient
Descending colon	BRAF/KRAS wild type MMR proficient			
Sigmoid colon	BRAF/KRAS wild type MMR proficient	BRAF mutated MMR deficient		
Rectum	BRAF/KRAS wild type MMR proficient	KRAS mutated MMR proficient		

Abbreviation: MMR, mismatch repair.
    Data from Rosty C, Walsh MD, Walters RJ, et al. Multiplicity and molecular heterogeneity of colorectal carcinoma in individuals with serrated polyposis. Am J Surg Pathol 2013;37:434–42.

Table 4
Molecular testing for Lynch syndrome

Serial Number	Tests
1	Evaluation of tumor tissue for MSI: immunohistochemistry for 4 MMR proteins followed by MMR gene mutation testing by PCR
2	Molecular testing of the tumor for methylation abnormalities to rule out sporadic cases
3	Molecular testing of the tumor for BRAF mutations to rule out sporadic cases
4	Molecular genetic testing of the MMR genes to identify germline mutations when findings are consistent with Lynch syndrome

Abbreviations: MMR, mismatch repair; MSI, microsatellite instability; PCR, polymerase chain reaction.
Data from Redston M. Epithelial neoplasms of the large intestine. In: Odze RD, Goldblum JR, editors. Surgical pathology of the GI tract, liver, biliary tract and pancreas. 2nd edition. Philadelphia: Elsevier; 2009.

general population. The polyps are indistinguishable from conventional adenomas. Therefore, the detection of index cases is challenging and requires the use of specific testing (**Table 6**).[42–46]

KRAS serrated pathway

KRAS-mutated TSA progresses to a mixed tubulovillous adenomatous phenotype and acquires high-grade dysplasia. The interface of high-grade dysplasia and infiltrating carcinoma is associated with a p53 mutation.[1,14] TSA associated with high-grade dysplasia or malignancy is associated with high rates of MLH1 methylation. CIMP high and CIMP low tumors are reported with variable frequency (**Fig. 9**). An unequivocal diagnosis of serrated carcinoma is made when 6 of the 7 histologic criteria listed in **Box 2** are fulfilled.

Limitations of molecular classification and correlates
- Lack of gold standard and uniform methods, definition, and criteria.
- False-positive and false-negative results.
- Sampling bias.
- Markers used for studies on MSI are not uniform.
- Nonuniform methods of detection of methylation markers.
- Lack of standardized definition of chromosomal instability.[3]

Table 5
Genetic basis of HNPCC

High-Frequency MSI (%)	Gene Mutation (%)
Yes (80–90)	MLH1 (39)
	MSH2 (38)
	MSH6 (11)
	PMS2 (7)
	EPCAM (1)
	Unknown (5)
No (10)	Yes (as above; 10)
	Unknown (90)

Abbreviations: HNPCC, hereditary nonpolyposis colon cancer; MSI, microsatellite instability.
Data from Refs.[4,9,15]

Table 6
Differences in molecular phenotype of sporadic colorectal carcinoma and the Lynch syndrome

	Sporadic	Lynch Syndrome
MMR	MLH1 loss	Loss of any MMR protein
MSI high	+ (approximately 75%)	+
MLH1 promoter methylation	+	Majority negative; rare cases with germline defects
Mutations in MMR	−	+
BRAF	±	−
Annexin 10 IHC	Focal ±	Majority negative Rare cases with germline defects
Precursor lesions	SSA/P	Tubular and tubulovillous adenomas

Abbreviations: IHC, immunohistochemistry; MSI, microsatellite instability; SSA/P, sessile serrated adenoma/polyp.

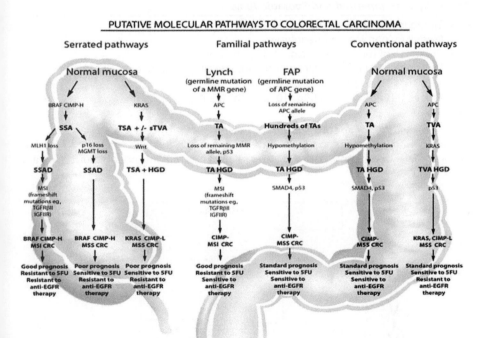

Fig. 9. Molecular pathogenesis of colorectal carcinoma (CRC). CIMP, CpG island methylator phenotype; EGFR, epidermal growth factor receptor; FAP, familial adenomatous polyposis; 5-FU, 5-fluoricail; HGD, high-grade dysplasia; MMR, mismatch repair; MSI, microsatellite instability; MSS, microsatellite stable; SSA, sessile serrated adenoma; SSAD, sessile serrated adenoma with dysplasia; TGF, transforming growth factor; TSA, traditional serrated adenoma. (*Adapted from* Bettington M, Walker N, Clouston A, et al. The serrated pathway to colorectal carcinoma: current concepts and challenges. Histopathology 2013;62:380; with permission.)

Box 2
Histomorphologic features of serrated carcinomas

Epithelial serrations

Eosinophilic or clear cytoplasm

Abundant cytoplasm

Vesicular nuclei with peripheral chromatin condensation and a single prominent nucleolus

Distinct nucleoli

Absence of necrosis (or <10% necrosis)

Intracellular and extracellular mucin

Cell balls and papillary rods

Adapted from Bettington M, Walker N, Clouston A, et al. The serrated pathway to colorectal carcinoma: current concepts and challenges. Histopathology 2013;62:382; with permission.

PATHOLOGIC FEATURES OF COLORECTAL CARCINOMA WITH HIGH-FREQUENCY MICROSATELLITE INSTABILITY
Shared by Both Inherited and Sporadic Tumors

- Tendency to occur on right side of colon.
- Medullary carcinoma phenotype.
- Presence of mucinous or signet ring component.
- Presence of tumor infiltrating and peritumoral lymphocytes.
- Crohnlike inflammatory response.
- Pushing tumor borders (**Fig. 10**; see **Tables 4** and **5**).[32]

Clinical correlation of specific subtypes of colorectal carcinoma
Medullary carcinoma Tumors with " medullary-type" are high-frequency MSI and generally have better prognosis and lower rates of locoregional nodal involvement and

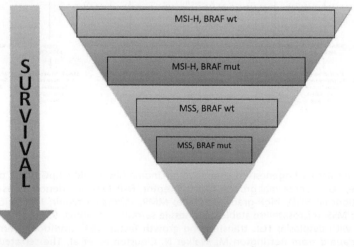

Fig. 10. Effect of microsatellite instability (MSI) and BRAF mutation on survival in colorectal carcinoma. mut, mutation; wt, wild type.

distant metastasis. On comparison of medullary carcinoma with MSS and MSI tumors, significant upregulation of several immunoregulatory genes induced by Interferon gamma including are identified. The specific genes include IDO-1, WARS (tRNA(trp)), GBP1, GBP4, GBP5, PD-1, and programmed death ligand 1 (PD-L1). The tumor reveals higher mean CD8$^+$ and PD-L1 tumor infiltrating lymphocytes compared with other tumors. The CD8 T lymphocytes are presumed to be activated upon presentation of neo-antigens from the tumor cells. The lymphocytes promote a strong interferon response.[49]

Early onset colorectal carcinoma These tumors manifest in patients less than 40 years of age without underlying HNPCC, adenomatous polyposis, or inflammatory bowel disease. The tumor shows pathologic features associated with aggressive behavior. The adenomas and carcinomas reveal increased expression of AMACAR. miR-21, miR-20a, miR-106a, miR-181b, and miR-203 are increased compared with normal tissues. miR-21 was associated with poor clinical outcome.[50]

Adenoma-like adenocarcinoma Adenoma-like adenocarcinoma is an uncommon variant of CRC with a low rate of metastasis and good prognosis. The predominant mutation reported is KRAS in codons 12 or 13. Other mutations included PIK3CA and BRAF V600E.[51]

Micropapillary colorectal carcinoma CRC with micropapillary features have a high likelihood of locoregional and distant metastases. They show significant increase in tp53 mutation and frequent mutations in KRAS and BRAF. Increased expression of stem cell markers SOX2 and NOTCH3 has also been reported.[52,53]

Mucinous tumors Mucinous CRC, which are MMR deficient have similar outcomes as low-grade nonmucinous tumors on survival analysis. Mucinous MMR-proficient CRCs behave slightly better than nonmucinous high-grade tumors but worse than mucinous low-grade nonmucinous tumors.[54]

Sporadic microsatellite unstable colorectal carcinoma The underlying pathogenesis of sporadic microsatellite unstable colorectal carcinoma is attributed to MLH1 promoter hypermethylation, subsequently leading to silencing of gene transcription. A BRAF V600E mutation is highly specific for these tumors, but not sensitive. Focal annexin A10 expression has been reported in both BRAF mutated and wild-type subcategories.[19]

Braf-mutated microsatellite stable adenocarcinoma of the proximal colon Tumors demonstrate adverse histologic features inclusive of lymphatic invasion, lymph node metastasis, perineural invasion, perineural invasion, tumor budding, and mucinous and signet ring histology. It is associated with significantly poor overall and disease-free survivals.[19]

Undifferentiated/rhabdoid carcinomas of the gastrointestinal tract The switch sucrose nonfermenting chromatin remodeling complex components have been reported to reveal loss of expression in the undifferentiated tumors with variable rhabdoid features, pleomorphic giant cells, and spindle cells. The most common components showing loss include SMARCB1(INI1), SMARCA2, SMARCA4, and ARID1A. Concurrent loss of MMR proteins (MLH1/PMS2) has also been reported. Some tumors belong to well-defined molecular subtypes and sustain additional loss of the remodeling complex components.[55]

Synchronous and metachronous cancers Similar genetic changes have been reported in sporadic contiguous tumors. In tumors separated by 1 or more segments, there was less consistency in genetic changes. Metachronous tumors did show variation, which was decreased when the subsequent tumor was located near the first tumor.[56]

Molecular biomarkers for the evaluation of colorectal cancer Guideline statements were established by the American Society for Clinical Pathology, the College of American Pathologists and Laboratory Quality Center, the Association for Molecular Pathology, and the American Society of Clinical Oncology to create standard molecular biomarker testing and guide therapies for patients with colorectal carcinoma. The guidelines follow well-established methods used in their development as well as for regular updates, so that new advances can be integrated in a timely manner in future. The biomarker guideline expert panel strongly recommends that laboratories must incorporate colorectal carcinoma molecular biomarker testing methods into their overall laboratory quality improvement program, establishing appropriate quality improvement monitors as needed to ensure consistent performance in all steps of the testing and reporting process. Laboratories performing the biomarker testing must participate in proficiency testing programs or alternative proficiency assurance activity. Anti-epidermal growth factor receptor (EGFR) monoclonal antibodies have been the main targeted therapies for CRC and require knowledge of mutational status of genes in the pathway as predictive biomarkers of response to therapies. The monoclonal antibodies target the EGFR extracellular domain and block the pathway.[55] Polymerase chain reaction (PCR)–based techniques and Sanger sequencing are mostly used for diagnosis; however, other sequencing techniques, including deep sequencing and hybridization-induced bead aggregation technology, are under evaluation.[57]

KRAS Patients carrying activating mutations of KRAS affecting exon 2 codons 12 and 13 do not benefit from anti-EGFR therapy, such as cetuximab and panitumumab. The expert panel on colorectal biomarker guideline recommends patients with colorectal carcinoma being considered for anti-EGFR therapy must undergo RAS mutational testing. Mutational analysis should include KRAS and NRAS codons 12 and 13 of exons 2, 59, and 61 of exon 3, and codons 117 and 146 of exon 4 ("expanded" or "extended" RAS).[57]

BRAF The expert panel on colorectal biomarker guideline recommends patients with colorectal carcinoma should receive BRAF p. V600 [BRAF c. 1799 (p. V600)] mutational analysis for prognostic stratification. In addition, BRAF p. V600 mutational analysis should be performed in deficient MMR tumors with loss of MLH1 to evaluate for risk of the Lynch syndrome. The presence of BRAF mutation strongly favors a sporadic pathogenesis.[31] Mutations in BRAF and KRAS are mutually exclusive. BRAF mutated stages III and IV CRCs are associated with worse prognosis, including survival after tumor recurrence. BRAF V600E mutation blocks the effect of anti-EGFR antibodies on disease progression in stage IV colorectal carcinoma. The effect of MSI and BRAF mutations on survival in colorectal carcinoma is shown in **Fig. 10**.[19,29–31,57]

Prognostic biomarkers for management of patients with colorectal carcinoma
POLE mutations Colorectal carcinoma with POLE (exonuclease domain of polymerase epsilon) proofreading domain mutations are more immunogenic and portend a better prognosis in stages II and III CRC. The presence of POLE mutations results in better recurrence-free survival and disease-free survival relative to MSI-proficient tumors.[58]

MASPIN MASPIN has been reported to be negative in normal colonic mucosa. Cytoplasmic and nuclear positivity in superficial and deep parts of the tumor have been noted. The staining correlated positively with a right-sided location and a high tumor grade. Increased nuclear grade correlated with more than 4 positive lymph nodes. The tumors belonging to both conventional pathway and MSI pathway reveal MAPSIN expression.[59]

SATB1 SATB1 shows nuclear positivity in normal colonic mucosa and colorectal carcinoma. It has been reported that approximately 22% CRC show loss of expression, which is associated with worse overall survival predominantly in right-sided colon cancers. The loss is associated with younger age, mucinous or signet ring histology, poor differentiation, and less favorable response to chemotherapy. It correlates with CIMP-high phenotype.[60]

Histone deacetylases Global nuclear expression of histone modifications and histone deacetylases correlates with clinical outcomes in CRC. The deacetylases cause epigenetic changes and have been reported to have clinical prognostic value as individual markers and in combination when used for multimarker analysis. The specific deacetylases significantly reported to be dysregulated in CRC include SIRT1 (decreased nuclear expression), HDAC2 (increased nuclear expression), and H4K16Ac (decreased nuclear expression). It may correlate with long interspersed nuclear element-1 hypomethylation.[61]

RSPO fusions CRCs with RSPO fusions are sensitive to repression of WNT pathway signaling with anti-RSPO antibody and PORCN inhibitors.[16]

Phospholipase The expression of PLA2G2A, a phospholipase, is associated with an aggressive phenotype, low survival, and poor therapeutic response in patients receiving concurrent chemoradiotherapy.[62]

Exosomes ALG-2 interacting protein X, an exosome involved in transporting bioactive molecules, potentially mediates epithelial stromal interactions and reveals reduced expression in adenoma and colorectal carcinoma.[63,64]

Mismatch Repair Testing

Scientific rationale
The MMR gene MSH2 binds with MSH3 and MSH6, forming a functional molecular complex that facilitates the recognition of the DNA mismatch. Subsequently, the complex recruits MLH1, its binding partner PMS2, and other enzymes, leading to excision, repolymerization, and ligation of the repaired strand of DNA. Patients with HNPCC and 15% of sporadic tumors have defective DNA MMR and are high-frequency MSI.

Clinical rationale
Molecular testing is recommended in patients with CRC to evaluate for possible Lynch syndrome. It is used in patients less than 70 years of age, with high-grade right-sided colon cancer, mucinous histology, and Crohn's disease–like peritumoral lymphoid infiltrate. Lynch syndrome–associated colorectal adenomas have also been reported to have abnormal MSI or immunohistochemical (IHC) testing results. Initial screening is accomplished by MSI testing using PCR or immunohistochemistry for MMR proteins.[34] Definitive diagnosis of the disorder and presymptomatic detection of carriers in at-risk individuals is possible by follow-up germline testing, with the potential for a reduction in morbidity and mortality. MSI is also a good prognostic marker for patients without lymph node metastases after undergoing neoadjuvant radiotherapy. Guidelines for reporting MMR as a predictive biomarker of response to PD-L1 therapy are

in the pipeline. The information is used for the selection of patients for immunotherapy.[34,48,65–68]

Best method

MSI testing is generally performed with at least 5 microsatellite markers, generally mononucleotide or dinucleotide repeat markers. In 1998, a National Institutes of Health consensus panel proposed that laboratories use a 5-marker panel comprising 3 dinucleotide and 3 mononucleotide repeats for MSI testing. Because mononucleotide markers have a higher sensitivity and specificity, many commercially available kits use 5 mononucleotide markers.

QUALITY ASSURANCE

The detection of MSI in a tumor by microsatellite analysis requires that the DNA used for the analysis be extracted from a portion of the tumor that contains approximately 40% or more tumor cells. Thus, pathologists should help to identify areas of the tumor for DNA isolation that have at least this minimum content of tumor cells. MSI testing is frequently performed in conjunction with IHC testing for MMR protein expression (ie, MLH1, MSH2, MSH6, and PMS expression). If the results of MMR IHC and MSI testing are discordant (eg, high-frequency MSI phenotype with normal IHC or abnormal IHC with MSS phenotype), then the laboratory should ensure that the same sample was used for MSI and IHC testing and that there was no sample mix up. External proficiency testing surveys are available through the College of American Pathologists Molecular Oncology resource committee and other organizations. These surveys are invaluable tools to ensure that the laboratory assays are working as expected.

PITFALLS

- During IHC evaluation of MSI proteins, an intact expression of all 4 proteins indicates that the tested MMR enzymes are intact.
- It is common for intact staining to be patchy.
- Positive IHC reaction for all 4 proteins does not exclude the Lynch syndrome, because approximately 5% of families may have a missense mutation (especially in MLH1), which can lead to a nonfunctional protein with retained antigenicity.
- Defects in lesser known MMR enzymes may also lead to a similar result, but this situation is rare.
- Loss of expression of MLH1 may be caused by the Lynch syndrome or methylation of the promoter region (as occurs in sporadic MSI colorectal carcinoma). BRAF mutation testing can help in differentiating the cases, although definitive interpretation is possible by genetic testing.[65–68]

Recommendations

The National Comprehensive Cancer Network guidelines recommend MMR protein testing to be performed for all patients younger than 50 years of age with colon cancer based on an increased likelihood of the Lynch syndrome in the US population. The testing should also be considered for all patients with stage II disease, because patients with stage II high-frequency MSI may have a good prognosis and do not benefit from 5-fluorouracil adjuvant therapy.

Mismatch repair immunohistochemistry

The DNA MMR proteins are ubiquitously expressed in normal human tissues. HNPCC or the Lynch syndrome results in instability of the truncated messenger RNA transcript and the protein product and results in complete loss of ICH-detectable MMR protein in tumors. Mutation of MLH1 results in its loss from the DNA MMR complex, subsequently leading to loss of PMS2 from the repair protein complex. Therefore, mutation and loss of the MLH1 protein is also usually accompanied by loss of PMS2 expression. The same mechanism holds true for MSH2 and its binding partner, MSH6. These IHC results are summarized in **Table 7**. The specificity of loss of protein expression for an underlying MMR defect is virtually 100%, although up to 10% of these tumors are MSS on MSI testing. The staining pattern of the tumor tissue is compared with the normal-appearing control tissue of the same patient to prevent misinterpretation caused by polymorphisms.[21–25]

Reporting guidelines (College of American Pathologists)

- The results of DNA MMR IHC and MSI testing should be incorporated into the surgical pathology report for the CRC case and an interpretation of the clinical significance of these findings provided.
- If DNA MMR IHC has not been performed, this testing should be recommended for any cases that show a high-frequency MSI phenotype, because this information helps to identify the gene that is most likely to have a germline mutation.
- Examination of expression of MLH1, MSH2, MSH6, and PMS2 is the most common IHC testing method used for suspected high-frequency MSI cases; antibodies to these MMR proteins are available commercially.
- Any positive reaction in the nuclei of tumor cells is considered as intact expression (normal).
- Loss of MSH2 expression essentially always implies the Lynch syndrome.[65–68]

MICROSATELLITE INSTABILITY TESTING

Frameshift mutations in microsatellites are identified by the amplification of selected microsatellites by PCR and analysis of fragment size by gel electrophoresis or an automated sequencer after extraction of DNA from both normal and tumor tissue (usually formalin-fixed, paraffin-embedded tissue). The sensitivity of the revised panel of MSI testing is at least 90% **(Table 8)**.[4–7]

Various fluorescent multiplex PCR-based panels (eg, Promega panel) are used for detection of MSI loci. The prototype Promega panel uses fluorescently labeled primers

Table 7
Interpretation of DNA MMR IHC

MLH1	PMS2	MSH2	MSH6	Interpretation
1	1	1	1	Intact DNA MMR; or rare germline point mutation with intact IHC; or other gene
—	—	1	1	MLH1 methylation silencing or MLH1 germline mutation (HNPCC)
1	1	—	—	MSH2 germline mutation (HNPCC)
1	—	1	1	PMS2 germline mutation (HNPCC); rare MLH1 mutation may also have this pattern
1	1	1	—	MSH6 germline mutation (HNPCC)

Abbreviations: HNPCC, hereditary nonpolyposis colon cancer; IHC, immunohistochemistry; MMR, mismatch repair.

Adapted from Redston M. Epithelial neoplasms of the large intestine. In: Odze RD, Goldblum JR, editors. Surgical pathology of the GI tract, liver, biliary tract and pancreas. 2nd edition. Philadelphia: Elsevier; 2009. p. 631; with permission.

Table 8 Bethesda criteria for MSI	
Loci with MSI (%)	Classification
40	MSI-H
10–30	MSI-L
0	MSS

Abbreviations: MSI, microsatellite instability; MSI-H, high-frequency microsatellite instability; MSI-L, low-frequency microsatellite instability; MSS, microsatellite stable.

Adapted from Redston M. Epithelial neoplasms of the large intestine. In: Odze RD, Goldblum JR, editors. Surgical pathology of the GI tract, liver, biliary tract and pancreas. 2nd edition. Philadelphia: Elsevier; 2009. p. 629; with permission.

for the coamplification of 7 markers for analysis of the high-frequency MSI phenotype, including 5 nearly monomorphic mononucleotide repeat markers (BAT-25, BAT-26, MONO-27, NR-21, and NR-24) and 2 highly polymorphic pentanucleotide repeat markers (Penta C and Penta D). Amplified fragments are detected using special spectral genetic analyzers.[20,21,36,37]

BRAF Mutation Testing

BRAF mutations in colorectal carcinoma neoplasms are activating point mutation at V600E, which may be detected in 6% to 10% of CRCs. This mutation constitutively stimulates other enzymes to promote continuous cell growth. This stimulation abrogates the ability of EGFR inhibitors to block cell proliferation and growth and confers resistance to anti-EGFR antibodies. The test is performed on formalin-fixed paraffin-embedded tumor tissue by sequencing-based technologies or allele-specific PCR. In addition, laboratory developed tests that involve standard genotyping or next-generation sequencing may be used to measure the level of this mutation. BRAF mutation testing is performed for prognostic stratification. It confers a worse clinical outcome and need for adjuvant therapy. Mutations are associated with reduced overall survival, and shorter progression-free survival. The poor prognosis is attributed to the genetic pathway in which it occurs. The adverse effects are negated in CIMP-positive tumors; it is also performed in MMR-deficient tumors to evaluate for the Lynch syndrome. There are insufficient data to guide the use of anti-EGFR therapy in the first-line setting with active chemotherapy based on BRAF V600E mutation status. IHC for mutated BRAFV600 E is not recommended for use in colorectal carcinoma because it is not as sensitive and concordant with genomic sequencing. However, it may be used for screening for the Lynch syndrome in conjunction with molecular genetic testing. Testing should be performed only in laboratories that are certified under the Clinical Laboratory Improvement Amendments of 1988 as qualified to perform high-complexity clinical laboratory (molecular pathology) testing.[19,30,69–72]

CpG Island Methylation Analysis Testing

A subset of CRCs (about 25%) have widespread aberrations in DNA methylation, including promoter silencing of genes. Referred to as CIMP, this subset includes most sporadic high-frequency MSI cancers with methylation silencing of MLH1. CIMP testing is a method to detect abnormal DNA methylation by using a panel of markers/loci and has been used in some studies to differentiate sporadic from hereditary MLH1-deficient cancers. Although there has not yet been an international consensus on the correct choice of markers for CIMP testing, several loci have begun to emerge as the most sensitive and specific for this type of application. The CIMP genes commonly analyzed include CACNA1G, SOCS1, NEUROG1, RUNX3, and IGF2. COL2A repeats serves as normalization control. Methylation-specific PCR is widely used for analysis, although there is lack of standardization. Some high-frequency MSI tumors are CIMP high, but negative for BRAF mutations. Therefore, CIMP testing is not a surrogate for BRAF mutation testing and has additional significance. Sporadic MSI-high colon cancers rarely reveal IHC evidence of Wnt signaling activation.[73] Based on conventional pathway DNA methylation, MSS and CIMP-negative colorectal carcinomas comprise 47% to 55% of CRC, are mostly located in distal colon, and are presumed to arise from conventional adenomas. Distinct methylation patterns involving genes not included in the traditional CIMP assessment panels have been reported in the conventional pathway of CRC. The reported clusters included 30 CpG loci associated with homeobox genes, intestinal transcription factor CDX-2, and the prostate cancer susceptibility genes PRAC1 and PRAC2.[68–72,74]

KRAS MUTATION TESTING

Mutations in codons 12 and 13 in exon 2 of the coding region of the KRAS gene predict a lack of response to therapy with antibodies targeted to EGFR. The presence of the KRAS gene mutation has been shown to be associated with a lack of a clinical response to therapies targeted at EGFR, such as cetuximab and panitumumab. Although clinical guidelines for KRAS mutational analysis are evolving, provisional recommendations from the American Society for Clinical Oncology are that all patients with stage IV colorectal carcinoma who are candidates for anti-EGFR antibody therapy should have their tumor tested for KRAS mutations (available from: http://www.asco.org/CRC-markers-guideline, updated 2017). Testing for mutations in codons 12 and 13 should be performed only in laboratories that are certified under the Clinical Laboratory Improvement Amendments of 1988 as qualified to perform high-complexity clinical laboratory (molecular pathology) testing. The testing can be performed on formalin-fixed paraffin-embedded tissue, on primary or metastatic cancer. Sequencing (Sanger/pyrosequencing) and PCR-based technologies are commonly used. Hybridization-induced aggregation technology and deep sequencing techniques are in the pipeline.[14,75–79]

GERMLINE TESTING
Hereditary Nonpolyposis Colon Cancer

The goal of a genetic workup of families with HNPCC is to identify the underlying germline mutation. Confirmation of the germline mutation allows for the most accurate treatment and follow-up recommendations for the patient, and allows predictive testing to be undertaken in interested family members. The initial approach by most laboratories is to analyze the complete coding sequence of the relevant gene or genes (depending on IHC results), as well as a portion of the intronic regions important to exon splicing. Some laboratories use a variety of rapid screening approaches to find mutations, whereas others undertake a complete sequence analysis.[7,33]

APC Gene

Ninety-eight percent of alterations in FAP include frameshift, nonsense, splice site mutations, large deletions, and duplications of the APC gene. Testing is performed by mutation screening (Sanger sequencing, conformation sensitive gel electrophoresis, and protein truncation testing) with reflex conformation sequencing. Gene deletion or duplication analysis may be performed by multiplex ligation-dependent probe amplification. False-negative results can occur because of deep intronic mutations, allele dropout, somatic mosaicism, and locus heterogeneity for the phenotype. Negative results may be followed by MUTYH targeted mutation testing.[22]

ALGORITHMIC STRATEGIES FOR MANAGEMENT OF MISMATCH REPAIR COLORECTAL CARCINOMA

There is no definitive standardized practice for the triage of colorectal carcinoma for molecular testing. Almost all microsatellite-instable colorectal carcinomas are detected by a combination of MSI and IHC testing. In the presence of deficient MMR, additional loss of protein expression of MSH2/MSH6, MSH6 alone, or PMS2 increases likelihood of the Lynch syndrome. Concomitant incidence of defective MMR, CIMP high, and MLH1 supports the diagnosis of sporadic defective MMR CRC. Detection of a BRAF c.1799T>A mutation serves to exclude diagnosis of the Lynch syndrome. Funkhauser and colleagues have critically analyzed the various recommendations and have advocated a screening algorithm to include MSI testing, BRAF c. 1799T>A mutation, and IHC for the 4 MMR proteins. **Fig. 11** shows MMR subgroup assignment for approximately 94% of colorectal carcinoma cases. Only the high-frequency MSI, MLH1 lost, and BRAF wild-type cases remain unassigned. The

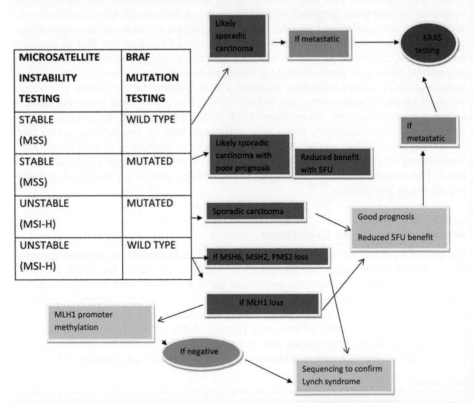

Fig. 11. Algorithmic strategies for prognosis and prediction of therapeutic response. 5-FU, 5-fluoracil; MSI-H, high-frequency microsatellite instability. (*Modified from* Funkhouser WK Jr, Lubin IM, Monzon FA, et al. Relevance, pathogenesis, and testing algorithm for mismatch repair–defective colorectal carcinomas. A report of the Association for Molecular Pathology. J Mol Diagn 2012;14(2):97; with permission.)

group recommends triage of unassigned 6% cases to referral laboratories performing high volumes of hypermethylation, sequencing, and deletion testing for resolution of subgroup assignment. An additional subgroup, comprising 1.7% of the cases (those assigned to the Lynch syndrome subgroup), would also be referred to define the germline mutation/deletion involved. The recommendation is based on the expectation that cost of testing is less than the cost of delayed diagnosis and absent surveillance of Lynch carriers.[32] The National Comprehensive Cancer Network (available from: www.nccn.org) recommends the use of the Amsterdam or revised Bethesda criteria as the initial screening step. This approach would miss the diagnosis of 5% to 58% of new cases of the Lynch syndrome, as well as most sporadic defective MMR CRC cases.

The Evaluation of Genomic Applications in Practice and Prevention model estimated detection rates and costs of testing using 4 different testing strategies:

a. MMR gene sequencing/deletion testing on all probands;
b. MSI testing, followed by MMR gene sequencing/deletion testing on all high-frequency MSI cases;
c. IHC testing, with protein loss guiding targeted MMR gene sequencing/deletion testing; and
d. IHC, with BRAF c.1799T>A testing of cases with MLH1 protein loss. Each of these would fail to detect all defective MMR CRC.

A similar comparison of 4 strategies, each starting with a single test, was recently published by the US Centers for Disease Control and Prevention, with similar limitations to the Evaluation of Genomic Applications in Practice and Prevention model. The IHC sequencing strategy and IHC_/_ BRAF c.1799T>A sequencing strategy were more cost effective for the diagnosis of Lynch syndrome probands and carriers. However, 11% to 12% of cases of the Lynch syndrome would not be diagnosed because of the absence of MSI testing to identify high-frequency MSI tumors with normal IHC in patients with the Lynch syndrome. Published recommendations by other investigators and clinical groups also exist. The aim of molecular subgrouping is improved diagnostic accuracy and appropriate therapy, genetic counseling for patients with germline MMR mutations, and appropriate counseling and screening of unaffected family members of patients with the Lynch syndrome.[32,33]

MOLECULAR INVESTIGATION OF LYMPH NODES IN PATIENTS WITH COLON CANCER USING ONE-STEP NUCLEIC ACID AMPLIFICATION

A diagnostic system called one-step nucleic acid amplification, has recently been designed to detect cytokeratin 19 messenger RNA as a surrogate for lymph node metastases. In a study by Güler and colleagues,[28] analysis of lymph nodes reported negative after standard examination with hematoxylin and eosin resulted in upstaging 2 of 13 patients (15.3%). Compared with histopathology, one-step nucleic acid amplification had a 94.5% sensitivity, 97.6% specificity, and a concordance rate of 97.1%. However, insufficient data are available for routine use in standard clinical practice.[80,81]

MOLECULAR STAGING INDIVIDUALIZING CANCER MANAGEMENT

GUCY2C is a member of a family of enzyme receptors synthesizing guanosine 3'5' cyclic monophosphate from guanosine-5'-triphosphate, which is expressed on intestinal epithelial cells but not in extraintestinal tissues. The expression is amplified in colorectal carcinoma compared with normal intestinal tissues. It is identified in all colorectal human tumors independent of anatomic location or grade, but not in extra-gastrointestinal malignancies. Therefore, it has a potential application in identifying occult metastases in the lymph nodes of patients undergoing staging for CRC. However, there are insufficient data to support its use in standard clinical practice.[82]

NOVEL MOLECULAR SCREENING APPROACHES IN COLORECTAL CANCER

Stool DNA potentially offers improved sensitivity, specificity, and cancer prevention by the detection of adenomas. The basis for stool DNA screening is the identification of genetic alterations in the initiation of a sequenced progression from adenoma to carcinoma, such as mutations in APC, KRAS, DCC, and p53. Key genetic alterations seen in many hereditary forms of CRC correspond with genetic alterations in sporadic CRC, indicating that the somatic occurrence of these genetic alterations leads to the initiation and progression of CRC and supports the targeting of these genes for generalized population screening. DNA methylation of CpG islands of known CRC markers has been shown in DNA samples from serum and stool samples of patients with CRC. SFRP2 methylation in fecal DNA was evaluated for detection of hyperplastic and adenomatous colorectal polyps. SFRP methylation was not found in healthy controls.[83]

PREDICTIVE AND PROGNOSTIC MARKERS
Quantitative Multigene Reverse Transcriptase Polymerase Chain Reaction Assay

Quantitative gene expression assays to assess recurrence risk and benefits from chemotherapy in patients with stages II and III colon cancer have been evaluated and are commercially available. The test provides information on the likelihood of disease recurrence in colon cancer (prognosis) and the likelihood of tumor response to standard chemotherapy regimens (prediction). The Oncotype D_x colon cancer assay evaluates a 12-gene panel consisting of 7 cancer genes and 5 reference genes to determine the recurrence score. This score was validated in the QUASAR (Quick and Simple and Reliable) study. The score improves the ability to discriminate high-risk from low-risk patients who have stage II colon cancer beyond known prognostic factors even in the cohort of apparently low-risk patients. Similar proportional reductions in recurrence risks with 5-fluorouracil/leucovorin chemotherapy were observed across the range of recurrence scores. Another Oncotype D_x score was validated in the National Surgical Adjuvant Breast and Bowel Project C-07 study, which differentiated risk of recurrence for patients with stage III disease and in the context of oxaliplatin-containing adjuvant therapy.[25,65,83–85]

Future trends
Other gene mutations associated with resistance to anti-EGFR therapy
- KRAS mutations at codons 61 and 146,
- PIK3CA exon 20 mutation, and
- PTEN protein inactivation.[33]

MicroRNAs Upregulated microRNAs in colorectal carcinoma include miR-96 oncogenic microRNAs involved in key signaling pathways. miR-96, miR-21, miR-135, and miR17 to 92 potentially target CHES1 (transcription factor involved in apoptosis inhibition). miR-21 correlates with the downregulation of tumor suppressor protein PDCD4. It may target PTEN, a tumor suppressor gene. miR-135a and miR135b correlate with reduced expression of the APC gene. Overexpression of miR17-92 results in the suppression of the antiangiogenic factors Tsp1 and connective tissue growth factor. It also mediates myc-dependent tumor growth promoting.

Downregulated microRNAs The downregulated microRNAs include 143 and 145, 31, 96, 133b, 145, and 183. microRNA-133 targets kras, which is known to be involved in signaling pathway for cell proliferation. Expression level of microRNA-31 correlates with development and stage of colorectal carcinoma. Experimentally mediated over-expression of microRNA-34a subsequent effects associated with actions of p53, such as cell cycle arrest and apoptosis, could be phenocopied. There is potential for early detection and staging. It detects precancerous adenomas. It relies on real-time qual-itative PCR, which yields results within a 24- to 48-hour period.[85] hsa-miR-663b, hsa-miR-4539, hsa-miR-17-5p, hsa-miR-20a-5p, hsa-miR-21-5p, hsa-miR-4506, hsa-miR-92a-3p, hsa-miR-93-5p, hsa-miR-145-5p, hsa-miR-3651, hsa-miR-378a-3p, and hsa-miR-378 have been reported to be differentially expressed in colorectal carcinoma versus normal colonic mucosa. On comparison of MSI and MSS tumors, the majority of differentially expressed microRNAs were downregulated. The micro-RNAs most significantly associated with survival include miR-196b-5p, miR-31-5p, miR-99b-5p, miR-636, and miR-192-3p. Higher levels of expression increase the risk of dying from colon cancer, but improve survival if diagnosed in rectal cancer. miR-196a-5p and miR-196b-5p were downregulated in both CIMP-high and BRAF-mutated tumors. Tp53 mutated tumors revealed significant difference in expression of miR-224, miR-17, miR-1226, miR-532-5p, miR-17, miR-574-5p, miR-424, and miR-16. KRAS-mutated tumors revealed significant downregulation in expression of microRNA-204-3p, upregulation in miR-4255, and miR-518e-5p.[85–88]

EPIGENETIC INACTIVATION OF ENDOTHELIN 2 AND ENDOTHELIN 3 IN COLON CANCER

Therapeutic strategies target overexpressed members of the endothelin axis via small molecule inhibitors and receptor antagonists, but this work supports a complementary approach based on the reexpression of endothelin 2 and endothelin 3 as natural an-tagonists of endothelin 1 in colon cancer.[89]

Role of Programmed Death Ligand 1 Expression in Colorectal Carcinoma

At the time of detection of a tumor, the balance of power between the immune system and the cancer has shifted in favor of the growing tumor, and a state of immune toler-ance has been established. The goal of cancer immunotherapy is to reestablish a tar-geted antitumor immune response. Blockade of inhibitory immune check point molecules enhances immune response to tumors. Immune checkpoint blockade tar-geting the programmed death-1 (PD-1) pathway has shown efficacy in several types of cancers, including MMR-deficient colorectal carcinoma. PD-L1 expression detected by immunohistochemistry has shown usefulness as a predictive marker for response to anti–PD-1 therapies. Most colorectal carcinomas with significantly increased lym-phocytes fall into the MMR-deficient subset. The tumors also possess clinicopatho-logic parameters associated with MMR deficiency. The features included medullary morphology, a right side location, younger age, higher tumor infiltrating lymphocyte score, and peritumoral lymphocyte aggregates. In a study characterizing PD-L1–pos-itive colorectal tumors, the significant features included poor differentiation, MMR deficiency, "stemlike" immunophenotype defined by loss or weak expression of CDX-2, and stem cell marker ALCAM positivity. Eighty-eight percent of the tumors also revealed the BRAF V 600E mutation. These features are associated with tumors arising via the serrated neoplasia pathway. In 1 study, it was found that 5% of colo-rectal carcinomas exhibited high tumor PD-L1 expression and 19% had increased PD-1–positive tumor-infiltrating lymphocytes. MMR-deficient tumors had significantly higher rates of PD-1 and PD-L1 expression and a stronger intensity of staining when compared with MMR-proficient tumors. Tumors with proficient MMR function (96%) are less likely to respond to anti-PD1 therapy. Further, PD-1/PD-L1 expression stratified recurrence-free survival in an interdependent manner. Patients whose tumors had both PD-1–positive tumor infiltrating lymphocytes and high PD-L1 expression had a significantly worse recurrence-free survival rate. Tumors with high PD-1–positive tumor-infiltrating lymphocytes and low-level PD-L1 expression revealed improved recurrence-free survival rates.[90,91]

Cell-free nucleic acid analysis

Although solid tissue based analysis has been the mainstay of CRC diagnosis, interrogation of cell-free DNA (cfDNA) in fluids including serum, plasma, urine, spinal fluid has proven beneficial for diagnosis and prognosis of these disease states.[92–97] Studies by Pereira and colleagues[94] showed that in 78% of the samples tested (100/128), there were detectable somatic genomic alteration in studies comparing formalin-fixed, paraffin-embedded tissue from prior resections or biopsies with cfDNA obtained from peripheral blood samples in certain cases. In addition, 50% of cfDNA cases had potentially actionable alterations, and physicians reported that the cfDNA testing improved the quality of care they could provide in 73% of the cases. Furthermore, 89% of patients reported greater satisfaction with the efforts to personalize experimental therapeutic agents. Studies by Zhuang and colleagues[95] showed in a meta analysis that KRAS mutation in cfDNA obtained from plasma or serum was associated with a poorer survival in patients with cancer for overall survival in patients with CRC and that ethnicity did not seem to influence the prognostic value of this mutation. Similarly, other metaanalyses[97] have suggested that the cfDNA of both KRAS and BRAF mutations can serve as poor prognostic biomarkers associated with worse survival outcomes in patients undergoing hepatic resection as a result of CRC-related liver metastasis. Hypomethylation of long interspersed nuclear element-1 in plasma cf DNA obtained from patients with CRC with large tumors ($\geq$6.0 cm), advanced N stage ($\geq$2), and distant metastasis (M1) had statistically significantly higher cfDNA long interspersed nuclear element-1 hypomethylation index than other patients with CRC.[96] Furthermore, patients with early stages I and II CRC as well as patients with advanced stages III and IV CRC had significantly higher cfDNA long interspersed nuclear element-1 hypomethylation index than healthy donors, suggesting cfDNA long interspersed nuclear element-1 hypomethylation index as a disease progression biomarker for CRC.[96] cfDNA analysis in CRC may provide timely information on potentially actionable mutations and amplifications, thereby facilitating clinical trial enrollment, personalized treatment and improving the overall quality of care.

REFERENCES

1. O'Brien MJ, Yang S, Huang CS, et al. The serrated polyp pathway to colorectal carcinoma. Mini-symposium: pathology of the large bowel. Diagn Histopathol 2008;14(2).

2. Vogelstein B, Fearon ER, Stanley SR, et al. Genetic alterations during colorectal tumor development. N Engl J Med 1988;319:525–32.

3. Ogino S, Goel A. Molecular classification and correlates in colorectal cancer. J Mol Diagn 2008;10(1):13–27.

4. Redston M. Epithelial neoplasms of the large intestine. In: Odze RD, Goldblum JR, editors. Surgical pathology of the GI tract, liver, biliary tract and pancreas. 2nd edition. Philadelphia: Elsevier; 2009.

5. Omundsen M, Lam FF. The other colonic polyposis syndromes. ANZ J Surg 2012; 82:675–81.
6. Lynch HT, Lynch JF. What the physician needs to know about Lynch syndrome: an update. Oncology 2005;19:455–63.
7. Abdel-Rahman WM, Mecklin JP, Peltomaki P. The genetics of HNPCC: application to diagnosis and screening. Crit Rev Oncol Hematol 2006;58:208–20.
8. Gruber SB. New developments in Lynch syndrome (hereditary nonpolyposis colorectal cancer) and mismatch repair gene testing. Gastroenterology 2006; 130:577–87.
9. Woods MO, Williams P, Careen A, et al. A new variant database for mismatch repair genes associated with Lynch syndrome. Hum Mutat 2007;28:669–73.
10. Kuipers EJ, Grady WM, Lieberman D, et al. Colorectal cancer. Nat Rev Dis Primers 2015;1:1–25. Article number 15065.
11. Rowan AJ, Lamlum H, Ilyas M, et al. APC mutations in sporadic colorectal tumors: a mutational "hotspot" and interdependence of the "two hits". Proc Natl Acad Sci U S A 2000;97(7):3352–7.
12. Wiland HO, Shadrach B, Allende D, et al. Morphologic and molecular characterization of traditional serrated adenomas of the distal colon and rectum. Am J Surg Pathol 2014;38:1290–7.
13. Mesteri I, Bayer G, Meyer J, et al. Improved molecular classification of serrated lesions of the colon by immunohistochemical detection of BRAF V600E. Mod Pathol 2014;27:135–44.
14. O'Brien MJ. Hyperplastic and serrated polyps of the colorectum. Gastroenterol Clin North Am 2007;36:947–68.
15. Rex DK, Ahnen DJ, Baron JA, et al. Serrated lesions of the colorectum: review and recommendations from an expert panel. Am J Gastroenterol 2012;107: 1315–29.
16. Cui M, Awadallah A, Liu W, et al. Loss of Hes1 differentiates sessile serrated adenoma/polyp from hyperplastic polyp. Am J Surg Pathol 2016;40:113–9.
17. Kim K-M, Lee EJ, Kim Y-H, et al. KRAS mutations in traditional serrated adenomas from Korea herald an aggressive phenotype. Am J Surg Pathol 2010;34:667–75.
18. Sekine S, Ogawa R, Hashimoto T, et al. Comprehensive characterization of RSPO fusions in colorectal traditional serrated adenomas. Histopathology 2017;71: 601–9.
19. Pai RK, Shadrach BL, Carver P, et al. Immunohistochemistry for annexin A10 can distinguish sporadic from lynch syndrome associated microsatellite unstable colorectal carcinoma. Am J Surg Pathol 2014;38:518–25.
20. Bettington M, Walker N, Clouston A, et al. The serrated pathway to colorectal carcinoma: current concepts and challenges. Histopathology 2013;62:367–86.
21. Rajagopalan H, Bardelli A, Lengauer C, et al. Tumorigenesis: RAF/RAS oncogenes and mismatch-repair status. Nature 2002;418:934.
22. Kerr SE, Thomas CB, Thibodeau SN, et al. APC germline mutations in individuals being evaluated for familial adenomatous polyposis. A review of the Mayo Clinic experience with 1591 consecutive tests. J Mol Diagn 2013;15(1):31–43.
23. Smyrk TC, Watson P, Kaul K, et al. Tumor-infiltrating lymphocytes are a marker for microsatellite instability in colorectal carcinoma. Cancer 2001;91:2417–22.
24. Güller U, Zettl A, Worni M, et al. Molecular investigation of lymph nodes in colon cancer patients using one-step nucleic acid amplification (OSNA). Cancer 2012; 118:6039–45.
25. Kuebler JP, Wieand HS, O'Connell MJ, et al. Oxaliplatin combined with weekly bolus fluorouracil and leucovorin as surgical adjuvant chemotherapy for stage

II and III colon cancer: results from NSABP C-07. J Clin Oncol 2007;25(16): 2198–204.

26. Toyota M, Ahuja N, Ohe-Toyota M, et al. CpG island methylator phenotype in colorectal cancer. Proc Natl Acad Sci U S A 1999;96:8681–6.

27. Weisenberger DJ, Siegmund KD, Campan M, et al. CpG island methylator phenotype underlies sporadic microsatellite instability and is tightly associated with BRAF mutation in colorectal cancer. Nat Genet 2006;38:787–93.

28. Liu C, Walker N, Leggett BA, et al. Sessile serrated adenomas with dysplasia: morphologic patterns and correlations with MLH1 immunohistochemistry. Mod Pathol 2017;30:1728–38.

29. Rosty C, Walsh MD, Walters RJ, et al. Multiplicity and molecular heterogeneity of colorectal carcinoma in individuals with serrated polyposis. Am J Surg Pathol 2013;37:434–42.

30. Lasota J, Kowalik A, Wasag B, et al. Detection of BRAF V600E mutation in colon carcinoma. Critical evaluation of the immunohistochemical approach. Am J Surg Pathol 2014;38:1235–41.

31. Adackpara CA, Sholl LM, Barletta JA, et al. Immunohistochemistry using the BRAF V600 E mutation-specific monoclonal antibody VE1 is not a useful surrogate for genotyping in colorectal adenocarcinoma. Histopathology 2013;63: 187–93.

32. Funkhouser WK Jr, Lubin IM, Monzon FA, et al. Relevance, pathogenesis, and testing algorithm for mismatch repair-defective colorectal carcinomas. A report of the association for molecular pathology. J Mol Diagn 2012;14(2):91–103.

33. Umar A, Boland CR, Terdiman JP, et al. Revised Bethesda guidelines for hereditary nonpolyposis colorectal cancer (Lynch syndrome) and microsatellite instability. J Natl Cancer Inst 2004;96:261–8.

34. National Comprehensive Cancer Network (NCCN). NCCN clinical practice guidelines in oncology (NCCN guidelines). Colon cancer. Version 3. 2013. Available at: nccn.org/professionals/physician_gls/pdf/colon.pdf. Accessed May 2, 2013.

35. Gray R, Barnwell J, McConkey C, et al. Adjuvant chemotherapy versus observation in patients with colorectal cancer: a randomised study. Lancet 2007; 370(9604):2020–9.

36. Bedeir A, Krasinskas AM. Molecular diagnostics of colorectal cancer. Arch Pathol Lab Med 2011;135(5):578–87.

37. Boland CR, Thibodeau SN, Hamilton SR, et al. A National Cancer Institute workshop on microsatellite instability for cancer detection and familial predisposition: development of international criteria for the determination of microsatellite instability in colorectal cancer. Cancer Res 1998;58:5248–57.

38. Pérez-Cabornero L, Infante Sanz M, Velasco Sampedro E, et al. Frequency of rearrangements in Lynch syndrome cases associated with MSH2: characterization of a new deletion involving both EPCAM and the 5' part of MSH2. Cancer Prev Res (Phila) 2011;4:1556–62.

39. Jass JR. Classification of colorectal cancer based on correlation of clinical, morphological and molecular features. Histopathology 2007;50:113–30.

40. Thibodeau SN, Bren G, Schaid D. Microsatellite instability in cancer of the proximal colon. Science 1993;260:816–9.

41. Goel A, Arnold CN, Boland CR. Multistep progression of colorectal cancer in the setting of microsatellite instability: new details and novel insights. Gastroenterology 2001;121:1497–502.

42. Marcus VA, Madlensky L, Gryfe R, et al. Immunohistochemistry for hMLH1 and hMSH2: a practical test for DNA mismatch repair-deficient tumors. Am J Surg Pathol 1999;23:1248–55.

43. Ribic CM, Sargent DJ, Moore MJ, et al. Tumor microsatellite-instability status as a predictor of benefit from fluorouracil-based adjuvant chemotherapy for colon cancer. N Engl J Med 2003;249(3):247–57.

44. Umar A, Boland CR, Redston M. Carcinogenesis in the GI tract: from morphology to genetics and back again. Mod Pathol 2001;14:236–45.

45. Popovici V, Budinska E, Tejpar S, et al. Identification of a poor-prognosis BRAFmutant–like population of patients with colon cancer. J Clin Oncol 2012; 20:1288–95.

46. Markowitz S, Wang J, Myeroff L, et al. Inactivation of the type II TGF-beta receptor in colon cancer cells with microsatellite instability. Science 1995;268:1336–8.

47. Perez-Cabornero L, Infante M, Velasco E, et al. Evaluating the effect of unclassified variants identified in MMR genes using phenotypic features, bioinformatics prediction and RNA assays. J Mol Diagn 2013;15:380–90.

48. Du C, Zhao J, Xue W, et al. Prognostic value of microsatellite instability in sporadic locally advanced rectal cancer following neoadjuvant therapy. Histopathology 2013;62:723–30.

49. Friedman K, Brodsky AS, Lu S, et al. Medullary carcinoma of the colon: a distinct morphology reveals a distinctive immunoregulatory microenvironment. Mod Pathol 2016;29:528–41.

50. Yantiss RK, Goodarzi M, Zhou XK, et al. Clinical, pathologic and molecular features of early-onset colorectal carcinoma. Am J Surg Pathol 2009;33:572–82.

51. Gonzalez RS, Cates JM, Washington MK, et al. Adenoma-like adenocarcinoma: a subtype of colorectal carcinoma with good prognosis, deceptive appearance on biopsy and frequent KRAS mutation. Histopathology 2016;68:183–90.

52. Gonzalez RS, Huh WJ, Cates JM, et al. Micropapillary colorectal carcinoma : clinical pathological and molecular properties, including evidence of epithelial-mesenchymal transition. Histopathology 2017;70:223–31.

53. Lee HJ, Eom DW, Kang GH, et al. Colorectal micropapillary carcinomas are associated with poor prognosis and enriched in markers of stem cells. Mod Pathol 2013;26:1123–31.

54. Liddell C, Droy-Dupre L, Metairie S, et al. Mapping clinic-pathologic entities within colorectal mucinous adenocarcinomas: hierarchical clustering approach. Mod Pathol 2017;30:1177–89.

55. Agaimy A, Daum O, Mark B, et al. SWI/SNF complex-deficient undifferentiated/rhabdoid carcinomas of the gastrointestinal tract. A series of 13 cases highlighting mutually exclusive loss of SMARCA4 and SMARCA2 and frequent co-inactivation of SMARCB1 and SMARCA2. Am J Surg Pathol 2016;40:544–53.

56. Zauber P, Huang J, Sabbath-Solitare M, et al. Similarities of Molecular Genetic changes in synchronous and metachronous colorectal cancers are limited and related to the cancers' proximities to each other. J Mol Diagn 2013;15:652–9.

57. Sepulveda AR, Hamilton SR, Allegra CJ, et al. Special article: molecular biomarkers for the evaluation of colorectal cancer. guideline from the American society for clinical pathology, college of American pathologists, association for molecular pathology, and American society of clinical oncology. J Mol Diagn 2017;19(2):187–223.

58. Guerra J, Pinto C, Pinto D, et al. POLE somatic mutations in advanced colorectal cancer. Cancer Med 2017;6(12):2966–71.

59. Fung CLS, Chan C, Jankova L, et al. Clinicopathological correlates and prognostic significance of maspin expression in 450 patients after potentially curative resection of node-positive colonic cancer. Histopathology 2010;56:319–30.

60. Al-Sohaily S, Henderson C, Selinger C, et al. Loss of special AT-rich sequence –binding protein 1 (SATB1) predicts poor survival in patients with colorectal cancer. Histopathology 2014;65:155–63.

61. Benard A, Goossens-Beumer IJ, van Hoesel AQ, et al. Nuclear expression of histone deacetylases and their histone modifications predicts clinical outcome in colon cancer. Histopathology 2015;66:270–82.

62. He HL, Lee YE, Shiue YL, et al. PLA2G2A overexpression is associated with poor therapeutic response and inferior outcome in rectal cancer patients receiving neoadjuvant concurrent chemotherapy. Histopathology 2015;66:991–1002.

63. Valcz G, Galamb O, Krenacs T, et al. Exosomes in colorectal carcinoma formation: ALIX under the magnifying glass. Mod Pathol 2016;29:928–38.

64. Pino MS, Mino-Kenudson M, Wildemore BM, et al. Deficient DNA mismatch repair is common in lynch syndrome-associated adenomas. J Mol Diagn 2009;11:237–47.

65. QUASAR: a randomized study of adjuvant chemotherapy (CT) vs observation including 3238 colorectal cancer patients. J Clin Oncol 2004;22(14S):3501, 2004 ASCO Annual Meeting Proceedings (Post-Meeting Edition).

66. Sargent DJ, Marsoni S, Monges G, et al. Defective mismatch repair as a predictive marker for lack of efficacy of fluorouracil-based adjuvant therapy in colon cancer. J Clin Oncol 2010;28(20):3219–26.

67. Stack E, Dubois RN. Role of cyclooxygenase inhibitors for the prevention of colorectal cancer. Gastroenterol Clin North Am 2001;30:1001–10.

68. Thibodeau SN, French AJ, Roche PC, et al. Altered expression of hMSH2 and hMLH1 in tumors with microsatellite instability and genetic alterations in mismatch repair genes. Cancer Res 1996;56:4836–40.

69. Shen L, Toyota M, Kondo Y, et al. Integrated genetic and epigenetic analysis identifies three different subclasses of colon cancer. Proc Natl Acad Sci U S A 2007;104:18654–9.

70. Loupakis F, Ruzzo A, Cremolini C, et al. KRAS codon 61, 146 and BRAF mutations predict resistance to cetuximab plus irinotecan in kras codon 12 and 13 wild-type metastatic colon cancer. Br J Cancer 2009;101:715–21.

71. Spring KJ, Zhao ZZ, Karamatic RR. High prevalence of sessile serrated adenomas with BRAF mutations: a prospective study of patients undergoing colonoscopy. Gastroenterology 2006;131(5):1400–7.

72. Adar T, Rodgers LH, Shannon KM, et al. A tailored approach to BRAF and MLH1 methylation testing in a universal screening program for Lynch syndrome. Mod Pathol 2017;30:440–7.

73. Panarelli NC, Vaughn CP, Samowitz WS, et al. Sporadic microsatellite instability-high colon cancers rarely display immunohistochemical evidence of Wnt signaling activation. Am J Surg Pathol 2015;39:313–7.

74. Koestler DC, Li J, Baron JA, et al. Distinct patterns of DNA methylation in conventional adenomas involving the right and left colon. Mod Pathol 2014;27:145–55.

75. Amado RG, Wolf M, Peeters M, et al. Wild-type KRAS is required for panitumumab efficacy in patients with metastatic colorectal cancer. J Clin Oncol 2008;26:1626–34.

76. Lievre A, Bachet JB, Boige V, et al. KRAS mutations as an independent prognostic factor in patients with advanced colorectal cancer treated with cetuximab. J Clin Oncol 2008;26:374–9.

77. Wijesuriya RE, Deen KI, Hewavisenthi J, et al. Neoadjuvant therapy for rectal cancer down-stages the tumor but reduces lymph node harvest significantly. Surg Today 2005;35(6):442–5.
78. Rechsteiner M, von Teichman A, Ruschoff JH, et al. KRAS, BRAF and tp53 deep sequencing for colorectal carcinoma patient diagnostics. J Mol Diagn 2013;5: 299–311.
79. Sloane HS, Landers JP, Kelly KA. Hybridization-Induced aggregation technology for practical clinical testing. KRAS mutation detection in lung and colorectal tumors. J Mol Diagn 2016;18:546–53.
80. Lindor NM, Burgart LJ, Leontovich O, et al. Immunohistochemistry versus microsatellite instability testing in phenotyping colorectal tumors. J Clin Oncol 2002;20: 1043–8.
81. Lagerstedt Robinson K, Liu T, Vandrovcova J, et al. Lynch syndrome (hereditary nonpolyposis colorectal cancer) diagnostics. J Natl Cancer Inst 2007;99:291–9.
82. Mejia A, Schulz S, Hyslop T, et al. Molecular staging individualizing cancer management. J Surg Oncol 2012;105:468–74.
83. Miller S, Steele S. Novel molecular screening approaches in colorectal cancer. J Surg Oncol 2012;105:459–67.
84. O'Connell MJ, Laurie JA, Kahn M, et al. Prospectively randomized trial of postoperative adjuvant chemotherapy in patients with high risk colon cancer. J Clin Oncol 1998;16:295–300.
85. Menéndez P, Villarejo P, Padilla D, et al. Diagnostic and prognostic significance of serum MicroRNAs in colorectal cancer. J Surg Oncol 2013;107:217–20.
86. Pellatt DF, Stevens JR, Wolff RK, et al. Expression profiles of miRNA subsets distinguish human colorectal carcinoma and normal colonic mucosa. Clin Transl Gastroenterol 2016;7:e152.
87. Paul S, Lakatos P, Hart Mann A, et al. Identification of miRNA-mRNA modules in colorectal cancer using rough hypercuboid based supervised clustering. Sci Rep 2017;7:42809.
88. Slattery ML, Lee FY, Pellatt AJ, et al. Infrequently expressed miRNAs in colorectal cancer tissue and tumor molecular phenotype. Mod Pathol 2017;30:1152–69.
89. Wang R, Löhr CV, Fischer K, et al. Epigenetic inactivation of endothelin-2 and endothelin-3 in colon cancer. Int J Cancer 2012;132:1004–12.
90. Lee LH, Cavalcanti MS, Seigal NH, et al. Patterns and prognostic relevance of PD-1 and PD-L1 expression in colorectal carcinoma. Mod Pathol 2016;29: 1433–42.
91. Inaguma S, Lasota J, Wang Z, et al. Clinicopathologic profile, immunophenotype, and genotype of CD274 (PD-L1)- positive colorectal carcinomas. Mod Pathol 2017;30:278–85.
92. Agah S, Akbari A, Talebi A, et al. Quantification of plasma cell-free circulating DNA at different stages of colorectal cancer. Cancer Invest 2017;35:625–32.
93. Vietsch EE, Graham GT, McCutcheon JN, et al. Circulating cell-free DNA mutation patterns in early and late stage colon and pancreatic cancer. Cancer Genet 2017; 218-219:39–50.
94. Pereira AAL, Morelli MP, Overman M, et al. Clinical utility of circulating cell-free DNA in advanced colorectal cancer. PLoS One 2017;12:e0183949.
95. Zhuang R, Li S, Li Q, et al. The prognostic value of KRAS mutation by cell-free DNA in cancer patients: a systematic review and meta-analysis. PLoS One 2017;12:e0182562.

96. Nagai Y, Sunami E, Yamamoto Y, et al. LINE-1 hypomethylation status of circulating cell-free DNA in plasma as a biomarker for colorectal cancer. Oncotarget 2017;8:11906–16.
97. Passiglia F, Bronte G, Bazan V, et al. Can KRAS and BRAF mutations limit the benefit of liver resection in metastatic colorectal cancer patients? A systematic review and meta-analysis. Crit Rev Oncol Hematol 2016;99:150–7.

Molecular Diagnostics in the Neoplasms of Small Intestine and Appendix

2018 Update

Yingtao Zhang, MD, PhD[a], Muhammad Zulfiqar, MD[b],
Martin H. Bluth, MD, PhD[c,d], Amarpreet Bhalla, MBBS, MD[a,*],
Rafic Beydoun, MD[e]

KEYWORDS

- Microsatellite instability • Small intestine • GNAS • Appendix
- Pseudomyxoma peritonei • Goblet cell carcinoid • Serrated appendiceal lesions

KEY POINTS

- Small intestinal adenocarcinomas are frequent in Lynch syndrome.
- KRAS mutations are found in small intestinal adenomas and adenocarcinoma and imply poor prognosis.
- P53 mutation is a late event in adenoma carcinoma sequence.
- Crohn disease–associated adenocarcinoma reveals p53 mutation as an early event.
- Celiac disease–associated adenocarcinomas have high level of CpG island methylation.
- Microsatellite instability and loss of MMR is extremely rare in pseudomyxoma peritonei.

INTRODUCTION

Neoplasms of the small intestine are rare in comparison with colorectal tumors. The most common tumor types arising in the small intestine are adenocarcinomas

Disclosure: The authors have nothing to disclose.
This article has been updated from a version previously published in *Clinics in Laboratory Medicine*, Volume 33, Issue 4, December 2013.
[a] PGY-3 Department of Pathology and Anatomical Sciences, Jacobs School of Medicine and Biomedical Sciences, University at Buffalo, Buffalo General Hospital, A-701, 100 High Street, Buffalo, NY 14203, USA; [b] Southeastern Pathology Associates (SEPA Labs), 203 Indigo Drive, Brunswick, GA 31525, USA; [c] Department of Pathology, Wayne State University, School of Medicine, 540 East Canfield Street, Detroit, MI 48201, USA; [d] Pathology Laboratories, Michigan Surgical Hospital, 21230 Dequindre Road, Warren, MI 48091, USA; [e] Department of Pathology, Harper University Hospital, Detroit Medical Center, 3990 John R Street, Detroit, MI 48201, USA
* Corresponding author.
E-mail address: ABhalla@KaleidaHealth.org

Clin Lab Med 38 (2018) 343–355
https://doi.org/10.1016/j.cll.2018.03.002
0272-2712/18/© 2018 Elsevier Inc. All rights reserved.

(24%–44%), well-differentiated neuroendocrine tumors (20%–42%), gastrointestinal stromal tumors (7%–9%), and lymphoma (12%–27%).[1,2]

Small-intestinal adenocarcinomas (SIAs) are uncommon malignancies, occurring 50-fold to 100-fold less often than cancers of the large intestine. SIAs are commonly seen between 60 and 70 years of age with slight male predominance. Adenocarcinoma originates in the duodenum in 52.0% (usually in the vicinity of the ampulla of Vater), jejunum in 18.7%, ileum in 17.2%, and unspecified sites in 12.0% of patients.[3] Some diseases can lead to small intestinal adenomas or/and carcinomas, such as familial adenomatous polyposis, celiac disease (CD), Crohn disease, Peutz-Jeghers syndrome, juvenile polyposis syndrome, and Lynch syndrome.[4] Most small-intestinal and ampullary adenocarcinomas are believed to arise from an adenoma-carcinoma sequence (APC, KRAS, TP53, SMAD4, EGFR), such as CD-associated adenocarcinoma. However, adenocarcinomas arising in the background of inflammatory bowel disease (Crohn disease) develop through the dysplasia-carcinoma sequence and it is more common in the ileum (70%).[4] SIAs share many common molecular alterations with colorectal adenocarcinomas, but significant differences exist.

MUTATIONS IN ADENOCARCINOMA
KRAS Mutations

The KRAS gene codes for a GTPase involved in the signaling pathways of several tyrosine kinase receptors. A KRAS mutation has been described in around 40% of colorectal carcinomas (CRCs) and it is predictive of the lack of efficacy of anti-EGFR antibody in treatment of metastatic CRC.[5] Frequent KRAS mutations (43%–57%) have been reported in SIA, with higher frequency in duodenal adenocarcinomas than in other SIAs.[6–8] KRAS mutation (G > A transitions and G12D mutations) is a poor prognostic predictor for patients.[7] KRAS mutations have also been detected in 50% to 62% of small-intestinal adenomas.[9]

TP53 Mutations

TP53 is a nuclear oncosuppressor protein that is involved in the maintenance of genomic integrity. Mutations in the TP53 gene occur commonly in a wide range of cancers and result in overexpression of inactive p53 protein in the nuclei. TP53 mutations are a late event in the adenoma-carcinoma sequence and are identified in 20% to 52% of SIAs cases.[8,10–12]

APC and β-Catenin Mutations

APC mutation leads to an accumulation of β-catenin in the nuclei, which is a key component of the Wnt signaling pathway to increased proliferation of epithelial cells and is considered an early event in most colorectal carcinogenesis.[13,14] The accumulation of β-catenin could occur either in the case of APC gene mutation preventing β-catenin degradation or by gain-of-function mutations. APC mutations have been reported in 0% to 26.8% of SIAs cases.[8,10,11] Abnormal expression of β-catenin was observed in 7.4% to 48% of SIAs[11,15,16] and it is much less frequent than in CRCs, which is seen in around 80% of tumor,[17] suggesting the Wnt pathway has a much less important role in SIAs than in colorectal carcinogenesis.

Mismatch Repair Genes and Microsatellite Instability

Inactivation of the DNA mismatch repair MMR is characterized by tumor microsatellite instability (MSI) and was detected in 15% of CRC. A deficient MMR is caused either by a germline mutation of one of the four MMR genes (usually MSH2 or MLH1, and more rarely MSH6 or PMS2) in the case of Lynch syndrome, or by hypermethylation of the MLH1 promoter in sporadic tumors.[18] Patients with Lynch syndrome have a predisposition to SIAs. In SIAs, the frequency of the deficient MMR phenotype is variable, ranging from 5% to 35% of the cases.[11,19,20]

Epigenetic Alterations

The CpG island methylation phenotype (CIMP) is an epigenetic phenomenon found in a variety of cancers.[21] In colorectal and gastric cancers, CIMP frequently associates with *MLH1* methylation, loss of *MLH1* transcription, and MSI-H.[21] High-level DNA methylation was found in 16% of chromosomal instable tumors and in 44% of microsatellite instable and microsatellite/chromosomally stable carcinomas.[22]

SMAD4/DPC4 Mutations

SMAD4/DPC4 (deleted in pancreatic cancer, locus 4, DPC4) is a mediator of growth suppression through transforming growth factor (TGF)-β signaling, located at 18q21. SMAD4/DPC4 is known to be mutated in several tumor types, most frequently in pancreatic carcinoma.[23] SMAD4/DPC4 mutation has been reported in 17% to 24% of small intestinal nonampullary adenocarcinomas[7,23,24] and in 34% of the ampullary adenocarcinomas.[25]

EGFR Mutations

A recent report showed that a high percentage of tumors express EGFR (71%) and VEGF-A (96%) in young populations, suggesting a potential benefit from anti-EGFR therapy, especially in those patients harboring a wild-type KRAS status.[26–28] However, another study revealed that mutations and amplification in EGFR genes are minor events, and most SIAs may be unsuitable to EGFR-TKIs treatment.[29] Further prospective studies are needed to determine the role of anti-EGFR therapy in SIAs.

ERBB2/HER2 Alterations

HER2 is one of a family of human epidermal growth factor receptors (HERs). Gene amplification and overexpression of HER2/neu have been reported in around 15% of gastric cancers.[30] ERBB2/HER2 mutation has been reported in 1.7% to 8.2% of SIA cases.[7,15,20] ERBB2 alterations are present in 12% through mutations (8.4%) or amplifications (3.6%) and ERBB2 mutations were significantly associated with duodenal tumor location.[24] This may suggest that more than 10% of the patients with SIAs could be treated using an anti-ERBB2-targeted agent.[24]

Programmed Death 1/Programmed Death 1 Ligand 1

Programmed death 1 or programmed death 1 ligand 1 (PD-1/PD-L1) are known as immune checkpoints and have been recently rapidly developing as oncotherapy for various carcinomas. PD-1 and PD-L1 are highly expressed by most SIAs.[31] PD-1 was expressed by intratumoral and peritumoral lymphocytes in 83% of SIA cases. PD-L1 expression on tumor cells and immune cells was observed in 17% and 43% cases, respectively. PD-L1 was mainly expressed by histiocytes capping cancerous glands/nests at the invasive front or by most tumor cells in medullary carcinomas. All the PD-L1-positive tumors also expressed PD-1. The tumors expressing PD-L1 contained more CD3$^+$, CD4$^+$, and CD8$^+$ T cells, but showed a lower CD4$^+$/CD8$^+$ ratio than those without expression of PD-L1. Blockage of the PD-1 pathway should be evaluated in the treatment of SIA.

BRAF Mutations

Infrequently BRAF mutations were observed in a subset of SIA, ranging from 1% to 14%.[7,15,24] Also BRAF mutations were associated with higher pT classification and more frequent pancreatic invasion.[7] BRAF V600E mutations were much less common in SIAs, representing only 10.3% of BRAF-mutated cases.[7] Anti-EGFR targeted therapy could be applied to patients if wild-type KRAS and BRAF exist, similar to patients with colorectal cancer.[7]

CELIAC DISEASE–ASSOCIATED ADENOCARCINOMA

CD is associated with a significantly increased risk (as much as 80-fold compared with the general population) of small bowel adenocarcinoma following the adenoma-carcinoma sequence.[4,32] Adenocarcinoma of the duodenum and proximal jejunum is the most common location. The high-level CpG island methylation/MSI pathway is typical of CD-associated small bowel carcinomas indicating that small bowel adenocarcinomas in CD follow the CpG island methylation-MSI pathway and aberrant CpG island methylation links CD and carcinogenesis.[33] Medullary carcinoma of the small bowel is characteristic for CD and showed loss of MutL homologue 1 (MLH1) expression, consistent with high-level MSI.[34]

CROHN DISEASE–ASSOCIATED ADENOCARCINOMA

Crohn disease is associated with an increased risk of carcinoma of the colon and small intestine. The incidence of SIA in Crohn disease is 40- to 86-fold greater than that observed in the general population following the inflammation-dysplasia-carcinoma sequence.[4] In CRCs, TP53 mutations occur early in this pathway, associated with the development of low-grade dysplasia. In addition, hypermethylation of CpG islands leads to promoter silencing, among others of p16 and p27. Accumulation of such events drives progression toward high-grade dysplasia. Additional events, such as KRAS mutations and activation of the Wnt pathway (APC mutation/β-catenin), are involved in the progression toward invasive carcinoma.[35] Crohn disease–associated SIAs showed similar carcinogenesis to those observed in chronic colitis-related CRCs including mutations in KRAS, BRAF, TP53, and MSI. Nuclear localization of β-catenin and p16 positivity were more frequently observed in SIAs than in small bowel dysplasia, suggesting an accumulation of genetic abnormalities during carcinogenesis.[36]

SERRATED ADENOMA

The serrated pathway in colorectal cancer occurs because of the epigenetic silencing of MLH1 by hypermethylation resulting sporadic MSI-high CRCs, and BRAF mutations are also frequently (up to 70%) identified. KRAS and TP53 are not typically mutated in serrated pathway. Serrated polyps are uncommon in small intestine, but they do occur. A study showed abnormal β-catenin expression in 23% of the small-intestinal serrated adenomas, abnormal p53 expression in 31%, KRAS mutation in 38%, and CIMP in 50% of the cases.[9] However, no BRAF V600E mutations were observed, suggesting that the serrated adenomas in the small intestine may undergo a distinct pathway that is different from those in the colon. More sample size of studies is needed to clarify this phenomenon.[9]

AMPULLARY ADENOCARCINOMA

Ampullary adenocarcinomas are subdivided into intestinal or pancreatobiliary subtype cancers. More frequent KRAS alterations in pancreatobiliary-type ampullary carcinoma (61 vs 29%) and more frequent mutations in APC in intestinal-type ampullary carcinoma (43 vs 17%) were observed.[37] Gain of 13q and 3q, and deletions of 5q, were found specific to the intestinal subtype.[38] KRAS mutation, which occurs in most pancreatic cancers, is found to occur less frequently in ampullary adenocarcinomas (approximately one-third).[39] A whole-genome sequence analysis has identified deletions of KRAS, SMAD4, and PTEN, suggesting a distinct oncogenesis of the ampullary cancers.[40] Studies investigating microRNA expression profiles confirm ampullary cancers are distinct compared with pancreatic adenocarcinoma.[41] PD-L1 is overexpressed in ampulla of Vater carcinoma and most of the PD-L1-positive tumors (70%) were intestinal-type and poorly differentiated (G3), suggesting a role of the PD-1/PD-L1 axis in ampullary adenocarcinomas, and a potential immunotherapy for these tumors.[42]

SMALL-INTESTINE NEUROENDOCRINE TUMOR

Small-intestinal neuroendocrine tumor (SINET) is a common malignancy of the small intestine. The incidence of SINET is increasing and accounts for 25% of all NETs.[43] The most frequent genomic event identified in SINETs is loss of heterozygosity at chromosome 18, occurring in 70% of tumors.[44] Chromosome losses were also frequently found of chromosomes 11 (23%), 16 (20%), and 9 (20%).[44] Recurrent mutations in the cell cycle regulator CDKN1B (cyclin-dependent kinase inhibitor 1B) have been identified in approximately 8% of tumors in large-scale sequencing studies.[45] Mutations occurring in CDKN1B are loss-of-function truncating mutations that occur throughout the gene. Mutational status does not seem to correlate with expression of p27 (the protein product of CDKN1B) and has no detectable association with clinical characteristics or survival.[45] In addition to CDKN1B, other somatic mutations in MEN1 and other genes involved in the PI3K/AKT/mTOR signaling pathway have been identified,[46] suggesting a potential benefit from targeting the mTOR signaling therapy.[47] SINETs are highly epigenetically dysregulated and characterized a panel of 21 genes including CDX1, CELSR3, FBP1, and GIPR, which are epigenetically altered in 70% to 80% of cases, highlighting epigenetic mechanisms as potential drivers of tumorigenesis.[48] MSI, a common feature of SIA,[19,22] is uncommon in SINET,[49] suggesting that SINETs evolve differently than epithelial neoplasia in this organ. The latter exhibited high frequencies of activating BRAF/KRAS mutations, which are typically absent in SINET. PD-1/PD-L1 expression is a frequent occurrence in poorly differentiated neuroendocrine carcinomas of the digestive system including SINET.[50] PD-L1 expression was significantly associated with a high-grade World Health Organization (WHO) classification (G3) but not with gender, primary site, or lymph node status, suggesting that PD-L1 expression is a poor prognostic indicator.[51] Checkpoint blockade targeting the PD-1/PD-L1 pathway may have a potential role in treating patients with this disease.

APPENDICEAL NEOPLASMS
Introduction

Primary appendiceal neoplasms are rare and found in less than 2% of appendectomy specimens with an incidence of approximately 1.2 cases per 100,000 people per year in the United States.[52,53] WHO (2010) diagnostic terminology for primary appendiceal neoplasms includes precursor lesions (conventional adenoma, (SSA/P), (TSA), (HP)), adenocarcinomas, mucinous adenocarcinoma, signet ring cell carcinoma, low-grade appendiceal mucinous neoplasm (LAMN), goblet cell carcinoids (GCC), and neuroendocrine carcinoma.[54] High-grade appendiceal mucinous neoplasm is a new diagnostic category and is included in the Americal Joint Committee on Cancer (AJCC) AJCC 8th edition. High-grade appendiceal mucinous neoplasms are rare tumors that resemble LAMN in lacking destructive invasion but show high-grade cytologic features. This term is not part of the current WHO terminology, but has been recommended in a recent consensus publication and has been included in the AJCC 8th edition.[55,56] Pseudomyxoma peritonei (PMP) results from peritoneal dissemination of mucinous appendiceal neoplasms.[57] Primary appendiceal adenocarcinomas (AA) are the most common subtype of appendiceal tumors and constitute 50% to 70% of all appendiceal neoplasms and 0.5% of all neoplasms of gastrointestinal origin.[52] The most frequent histology was a mucinous adenocarcinoma followed by nonmucinous adenocarcinoma. Carcinoids represent 11% of the appendiceal neoplasms and neuroendocrine carcinoma is extremely rare.[52] GCC tumor is a rare neuroendocrine tumor, comprising approximately 6% of appendiceal carcinoids.[54]

Appendiceal (Nonmucinous) Adenocarcinoma

Despite their anatomic contiguity, AA and CRC are two molecularly distinct tumor types.[6] A large cohort of patients revel significant differences as assessed by the Cancer Genomic Atlas data.[57] KRAS mutations are seen at a high rate in AA,[57–59] and are strongly associated with moderately differentiated histology compared with poorly differentiated tumors.[58,60] BRAF, EGFR, and c-KIT mutations are less frequent in AA. The prevalence of MSI is low in comparison to colon adenocarcinomas.[59,61] The presence of chromosome 18q loss and DPC4 mutations in AA suggests involvement of DPC4 and nearby genes on chromosome 18q (DCC and/or JV-18) in the pathogenesis of AA.[62] Next-generation sequencing revealed mutations in 50.4% KRAS, 21.9% TP53, 17.6% GNAS, 16.5% SMAD4, 10% APC, 7.5% ATM, 5.5% PIK3CA, 5.0% FBXW7, and 1.8% BRAF.[63] GNAS encodes the α subunit of the stimulatory G protein (Gs-alpha), a guanine-nucleotide binding protein (G protein) involved in hormonal regulation of adenylate cyclase. Overall, appendiceal cancers have similar patterns in their molecular profile to pancreatic cancers and have differential expression from colorectal cancers.[63]

Mucinous Appendiceal Neoplasm

Appendiceal mucinous neoplasms are characterized by KRAS mutations most cases that may drive the progression of PMP.[64–66] GNAS mutations are also frequently observed in low-grade appendiceal mucinous tumors and may play a crucial role in mucin production in patients with PMP,[67,68] but do not affect survival.[67,69] GNAS codon 201 is mutated with high frequency in PMP.[70] Alterations in APC, ATM, PIK3CA, SMAD4, NRAS, TP53, and the TGF-β pathway, particularly in adenocarcinomas, are also present.[71–76]

Low-grade appendiceal mucinous neoplasm/high-grade appendiceal mucinous neoplasm

A total of 100% of LAMN had a KRAS mutation either in codon 12 or 13, with G12D and G12V being the most common.[60] GNAS alterations have been reported to occur in 50% of LAMN cases.[16] MSI and BRAF mutations have not been demonstrated.[60]

Pseudomyxoma peritonei

PMP is a subtype of mucinous adenocarcinoma mainly restricted to the peritoneal cavity and most commonly originating from the appendix. KRAS and/or GNAS mutations are common genetic features of PMP. A study identified 58% of PMP are positive for KRAS mutation, and 89% of the mutations were in codon 12 and 11% in codon 13.[58] Codon 12 mutations may be associated with mucin production. Mutations in TP53 and/or genes related to the PI3K-AKT pathway may render malignant properties to PMP.[71] Aberrantly expressed p53 is associated with high-grade histology and reduced survival.[71] GNAS mutation or an alternative mutation in the PKA pathway was identified in most of PMP patients, so inhibition of the PKA pathway might reduce mucin production in most of the PMP patients and potentially suppress disease progression. TGF-β pathway is dysregulated in PMP, and SMAD4, SMAD2, SMAD3, TGFBR1, and TGFBR2 mutations have been the most often detected ones.[77] BRAF V600E, PIK3CA, and APC mutations are rare. All the studied tumors expressed MMR proteins MLH1, MSH2, and MSH6. No MSI and BRAF mutations are present.[69] The presence of an LKB1 mutation possibly linked to activation of mTOR pathway.[68] Also, the involvement of SMAD4 was already described.[68,70] New mutations in angiogenic tyrosine kinase receptors, such as FGFR3 or PDGFRA, are discovered, which may be targeted by specific inhibitors.[25]

Neuroendocrine Neoplasm

Appendiceal neuroendocrine neoplasms comprise the largest subgroup of appendiceal neoplasms with at least 30% of all appendiceal neoplasms.[78] Neuroendocrine neoplasms of the appendix include well-differentiated neuroendocrine tumor (carcinoid tumor), poorly differentiated neuroendocrine carcinoma (including small cell and large cell neuroendocrine carcinomas), mixed adenoneuroendocrine tumors, and GCC.[54]

Appendiceal carcinoid tumor

Allelic loss of chromosome 11q25 was not found in any of the seven classical appendiceal carcinoids compared with 40% of ileal carcinoids.[79] Allelic loss of chromosomes 16q and 18q was less frequent in nonileal carcinoid tumors, such as appendiceal carcinoid tumor, than in GCC.[80] No K-ras and p53 mutations were detected. It suggests that ras oncogenes are probably not involved in the pathogenesis of appendiceal carcinoids.[81]

Goblet cell carcinoid

GCC is a distinctive group of heterogeneous appendiceal neoplasm having glandular and neuroendocrine morphology.[52] Most molecular studies have indicated the similarity between ileal carcinoids and GCC. Stancu and colleagues[80] found infrequent allelic loss of chromosome 11q (25%) but frequent allelic loss of chromosomes 16q (38%) and 18q (56%) in GCC, which is similar to ileal carcinoids (14%, 29%, and 86%). No mutations were shown in K-ras, DPC-4 (Smad4), or β-catenin genes, which are usually present in colonic adenocarcinoma. They show negative staining for nuclear β-catenin and for p53. Ramnani and colleagues[82] also similarly reported the lack of mutation of K-ras in GCC; however, p53 mutations in 25% of GCCs and 44% of classical appendiceal carcinoids suggest that this is a possible pathway for molecular pathogenesis of GCCs. Dimmler and colleagues[83] reported that EGFR, BRAF-mutations, and MSI are absent in GCC of the appendix. Modlin and colleagues[84] showed elevated expression of CgA, NAPIL1, MAGE-D2, and MTA1, along with decreased expression of NALP1 in GCC, compared with normal mucosa, and similar to malignant or small intestinal carcinoid.[85] A recent study from Jesinghaus and colleagues[86] revealed that mutations in colorectal cancer–related genes (eg, TP53, KRAS, APC) were rare to absent in GCC and adenocarcinomas ex-goblet cell carcinoid, but frequent in primary colorectal–type adenocarcinomas of the appendix. Mutations in Wnt-signaling-associated genes (USP9X, NOTCH1, CTNNA1, CTNNB1, TRRAP) were also present in GCC, which may act as potential drivers of these neoplasms.[86] These data suggest that appendiceal GCC and adenocarcinomas ex-goblet cell carcinoid are genetically distinct from primary colorectal-type

Table 1
Appendicular neoplasms with their key genetic alterations

	Major Genetic Alterations
Nonmucinous adenocarcinoma	KRAS, TP53, GNAS, SMAD4, APC, ATM, PIK3CA; BRAF rare
Mucinous adenocarcinoma	KRAS, GRAS, APC, ATM, PIK3CA, SMAD4, TP53
LAMN/HAMN	KRAS, GNAS, APC, MET
PMP	KRAS, GNAS, TP53
Goblet cell carcinoid	Loss of heterozygosity of chromosome 11q, 16q, and 18q; no KRAS, SMAD4, and BRAF mutations
Precursor lesions (conventional adenoma, SSA/P, TSA, HP)	KRAS, not BRAF

Abbreviations: HAMN, high-grade appendiceal mucinous neoplasm; HP, Hyperplastic polyp; SSA/P, Sessile serrated polyp/adenoma; TSA, Traditional serrated adenoma.

adenocarcinoma of the appendix and its colorectal counterparts. Further molecular studies are warranted to understand their molecular mechanisms.[87]

Precursor Lesions (Conventional Adenoma, SSA/P, TSA, HP)

Appendiceal cancers can develop through the serrated pathway of carcinogenesis, indicating that serrated lesions are neoplastic. A large study of serrated polyps from Yantiss and coworkers[88] in 2007 demonstrated that MSI is extremely rare even though the MLH1 and MGMT expressions were reduced. KRAS mutations were present, especially in dysplastic polyps. BRAF mutations were also present but they were less common in dysplastic serrated polyps and in invasive carcinomas arising in serrated polyps suggesting that the biologic potential of BRAF in the appendix is limited. No abnormal nuclear localization of β-catenin in serrated lesions of the appendix is identified so far.[89] Pai and colleagues[90] have demonstrated that serrated lesions of the appendix frequently harbor KRAS mutations but not BRAF mutations. They identified KRAS mutations in 52% of the appendiceal serrated lesions, and BRAF V600E mutations in only 4% of the patients, indicating that serrated pathway in the appendix is likely different than in the colon and rectum (**Table 1**).

REFERENCES

1. Zeh HJ, Federle M. Cancer of the small intestine. In: DeVita VT, Hellman S, Rosenberg SA, editors. Cancer: principles and practice of oncology. 8th edition. Philadelphia: Lippincott Williams & Wilkins; 2008. p. 1186–204.

2. Bosman FT, Carneiro F, Hruban RH, et al. In: WHO classification of tumours of the digestive system. Geneva (Switzerland): WHO Press; 2010. p. 95–118.

3. Verma D, Stroehlein JR. Adenocarcinoma of the small bowel: a 60-yr perspective derived from M. D. Anderson Cancer Center Tumor Registry. Am J Gastroenterol 2006;101:1647–54.

4. Noffsinger A. Epithelial neoplasms of the small intestine [Chapter 26]. In: Odze RD, Goldblum JR, editors. Odze and Goldblum surgical pathology of the GI tract, liver, biliary tract and pancreas. 3rd edition. Philadelphia: Saunders Elsevier; 2015. p. 722–36.

5. Lièvre A, Bachet JB, Boige V, et al. KRAS mutations as an independent prognostic factor in patients with advanced colorectal cancer treated with cetuximab. J Clin Oncol 2008;26(3):374–9.

6. Younes N, Fulton N, Tanaka R, et al. The presence of K-12 ras mutations in duodenal adenocarcinomas and the absence of ras mutations in other small bowel adenocarcinomas and carcinoid tumors. Cancer 1997;79:1804–8.

7. Jun SY, Kim M, Jin Gu M, et al. Clinicopathologic and prognostic associations of KRAS and BRAF mutations in small intestinal adenocarcinoma. Mod Pathol 2016; 29:402–15.

8. Schrock AB, Devoe CE, McWilliams R, et al. Genomic profiling of small-bowel adenocarcinoma. JAMA Oncol 2017;3:1546–53.

9. Rosty C, Campbell C, Clendenning M, et al. Do serrated neoplasms of the small intestine represent a distinct entity? Pathological findings and molecular alterations in a series of 13 cases. Histopathology 2015;66:333–42.

10. Arai M, Shimizu S, Imai Y, et al. Mutations of the Ki-ras, p53 and APC genes in adenocarcinomas of the human small intestine. Int J Cancer 1997;70:390–5.

11. Wheeler JM, Warren BF, Mortensen NJ, et al. An insight into the genetic pathway of adenocarcinoma of the small intestine. Gut 2002;50:218–23.

12. Svrcek M, Jourdan F, Sebbagh N, et al. Immunohistochemical analysis of adenocarcinoma of the small intestine: a tissue microarray study. J Clin Pathol 2003;56: 898–903.

13. Behrens J. The role of the Wnt signalling pathway in colorectal tumorigenesis. Biochem Soc Trans 2005;33:672–5.

14. Zhan T, Rindtorff N, Boutros M. Wnt signaling in cancer. Oncogene 2017;36: 1461–73.

15. Aparicio T, Svrcek M, Zaanan A, et al. Small bowel adenocarcinoma phenotyping, a clinicobiological prognostic study. Br J Cancer 2013;109:3057–66.

16. Lee HJ, Lee OJ, Jang KT, et al. Combined loss of E-cadherin and aberrant beta-catenin protein expression correlates with a poor prognosis for small intestinal adenocarcinomas. Am J Clin Pathol 2013;139:167–76.

17. Hao X, Tomlinson I, Ilyas M, et al. Reciprocity between membranous and nuclear expression of beta-catenin in colorectal tumours. Virchows Arch 1997;431: 167–72.

18. Zaanan A, Meunier K, Sangar F, et al. Microsatellite instability in colorectal cancer: from molecular oncogenic mechanisms to clinical implications. Cell Oncol (Dordr) 2011;34:155–76.

19. Planck M, Ericson K, Piotrowska Z, et al. Microsatellite instability and expression of MLH1 and MSH2 in carcinomas of the small intestine. Cancer 2003;97:1551–7.

20. Overman MJ, Pozadzides J, Kopetz S, et al. Immunophenotype and molecular characterisation of adenocarcinoma of the small intestine. Br J Cancer 2010; 102:144–50.

21. Bariol C, Suter C, Cheong K, et al. The relationship between hypomethylation and CpG island methylation in colorectal neoplasia. Am J Pathol 2003;162:1361–71.

22. Warth A, Kloor M, Schirmacher P, et al. Genetics and epigenetics of small bowel adenocarcinoma: the interactions of CIN, MSI, and CIMP. Mod Pathol 2011;24: 564–70.

23. Bläker H, von Herbay A, Penzel R, et al. Genetics of adenocarcinomas of the small intestine: frequent deletions at chromosome 18q and mutations of the SMAD4 gene. Oncogene 2002;21:158–64.

24. Laforest A, Aparicio T, Zaanan A, et al. ERBB2 gene as a potential therapeutic target in small bowel adenocarcinoma. Eur J Cancer 2014;50:1740–6.

25. McCarthy DM, Hruban RH, Argani P, et al. Role of the DPC4 tumor suppressor gene in adenocarcinoma of the ampulla of Vater: analysis of 140 cases. Mod Pathol 2003;16:272–8.

26. Santini D, Fratto ME, Spoto C, et al. Cetuximab in small bowel adenocarcinoma: a new friend? Br J Cancer 2010;103:1305.
27. De Dosso S, Molinari F, Martin V, et al. Molecular characterisation and cetuximab-based treatment in a patient with refractory small bowel adenocarcinoma. Gut 2010;59:1587–8.
28. Falcone R, Roberto M, Filetti M, et al. Anti epidermal growth factor receptor therapy in small bowel adenocarcinoma: case report and literature review. Medicine 2018;97:e9672.
29. Wang Y, Jiang CQ, Guan J, et al. Molecular alterations of EGFR in small intestinal adenocarcinoma. Int J Colorectal Dis 2013;28:1329–35.
30. Bang YJ, Van Cutsem E, Feyereislova A, et al. Trastuzumab in combination with chemotherapy versus chemotherapy alone for treatment of HER2-positive advanced gastric or gastro-oesophageal junction cancer (ToGA): a phase 3, open-label, randomised controlled trial. Lancet 2010;376:687–97.
31. Thota R, Gonzalez RS, Berlin J, et al. Could the PD-1 pathway be a potential target for treating small intestinal adenocarcinoma? Am J Clin Pathol 2017;148: 208–14.
32. Straker RJ, Gunasekaran S, Brady PG. Adenocarcinoma of the jejunum in association with celiac sprue. J Clin Gastroenterol 1989;11:320–3.
33. Bergmann F, Singh S, Michel S, et al. Small bowel adenocarcinomas in celiac disease follow the CIM-MSI pathway. Oncol Rep 2010;24:1535–9.
34. Brcic I, Cathomas G, Vanoli A, et al. Medullary carcinoma of the small bowel. Histopathology 2016;69:136–40.
35. Bosman FT. Molecular pathology of colorectal cancer [Chapter 1]. In: Cheng L, Eble J, editors. Molecular surgical pathology. New York: Springer; 2013. p. 1–16.
36. Svrcek M, Piton G, Cosnes J, et al. Small bowel adenocarcinomas complicating Crohn's disease are associated with dysplasia: a pathological and molecular study. Inflamm Bowel Dis 2014;20:1584–92.
37. Hechtman JF, Liu W, Sadowska J, et al. Sequencing of 279 cancer genes in ampullary carcinoma reveals trends relating to histologic subtypes and frequent amplification and overexpression of ERBB2 (HER2). Mod Pathol 2015;28:1123–9.
38. Sandhu V, Wedge DC, Bowitz Lothe IM, et al. The genomic landscape of pancreatic and periampullary adenocarcinoma. Cancer Res 2016;76:5092–102.
39. Chandrasegaram MD, Gill AJ, Samra J, et al. Ampullary cancer of intestinal origin and duodenal cancer: a logical clinical and therapeutic subgroup in periampullary cancer. World J Gastrointest Oncol 2017;9:407–15.
40. Demeure MJ, Craig DW, Sinari S, et al. Cancer of the ampulla of Vater: analysis of the whole genome sequence exposes a potential therapeutic vulnerability. Genome Med 2012;4:56.
41. Schultz NA, Werner J, Willenbrock H, et al. MicroRNA expression profiles associated with pancreatic adenocarcinoma and ampullary adenocarcinoma. Mod Pathol 2012;25:1609–22.
42. Saraggi D, Galuppini F, Remo A, et al. PD-L1 overexpression in ampulla of Vater carcinoma and its pre-invasive lesions. Histopathology 2017;71:470–4.
43. Yao JC, Hassan M, Phan A, et al. One hundred years after "carcinoid": epidemiology of and prognostic factors for neuroendocrine tumors in 35,825 cases in the United States. J Clin Oncol 2008;26:3063–72.
44. Hashemi J, Fotouhi O, Sulaiman L, et al. Copy number alterations in small intestinal neuroendocrine tumors determined by array comparative genomic hybridization. BMC Cancer 2013;13:505.

45. Francis JM, Kiezun A, Ramos AH, et al. Somatic mutation of CDKN1B in small intestine neuroendocrine tumors. Nat Genet 2013;45:1483–6.

46. Banck MS, Kanwar R, Kulkarni AA, et al. The genomic landscape of small intestine neuroendocrine tumors. J Clin Invest 2013;123:2502–8.

47. Chan J, Kulke M. Targeting the mTOR signaling pathway in neuroendocrine tumors. Curr Treat Options Oncol 2014;15:365–79.

48. Karpathakis A, Dibra H, Pipinikas C, et al. Prognostic impact of novel molecular subtypes of small intestinal neuroendocrine tumor. Clin Cancer Res 2016;22: 250–8.

49. Kidd M, Eick G, Shapiro M. Microsatellite instability and gene mutations in transforming growth factor-beta type II receptor are absent in small bowel carcinoid tumors. Cancer 2005;103:229–36.

50. Roberts JA, Gonzalez RS, Das S, et al. Expression of PD-1 and PD-L1 in poorly differentiated neuroendocrine carcinomas of the digestive system: a potential target for anti-PD-1/PD-L1 therapy. Hum Pathol 2017;70:49–54.

51. Cavalcanti E, Armentano R, Valentini AM, et al. Role of PD-L1 expression as a biomarker for GEP neuroendocrine neoplasm grading. Cell Death Dis 2017;8: e3004.

52. Turaga KK, Pappas SG, Gamblin T. Importance of histologic subtype in the staging of appendiceal tumors. Ann Surg Oncol 2012;19:1379–85.

53. Panarelli NC, Yantiss RK. Mucinous neoplasms of the appendix and peritoneum. Arch Pathol Lab Med 2011;135:1261–8.

54. Carr NJ, Sobin LH. Adenocarcinoma of the appendix. In: Bosman FT, Carneiro F, Hruban RH, et al, editors. WHO classification of tumours of the digestive system. Geneva (Switzerland): WHO Press; 2010. p. 122–5.

55. Overman M, Asare EA, Compton CC, et al. Appendix – carcinoma. In: Amin MB, editor. AJCC cancer staging manual. 8th edition. New York: Springer; 2016. p. 237–50.

56. Carr NJ, Cecil TD, Mohamed F, et al, Peritoneal Surface Oncology Group International. A consensus for classification and pathologic reporting of pseudomyxoma peritonei and associated appendiceal neoplasia: the results of the Peritoneal Surface Oncology Group International (PSOGI) Modified Delphi Process. Am J Surg Pathol 2016;40:14–26.

57. Cancer Genome Atlas Network. Comprehensive molecular characterization of human colon and rectal cancer. Nature 2012;487:330–7.

58. Shetty S, Thomas P, Ramanan B, et al. Kras mutations and p53 overexpression in pseudomyxoma peritonei: association with phenotype and prognosis. J Surg Res 2013;180:97–103.

59. Raghav KP, Shetty AV, Kazmi SM, et al. Impact of molecular alterations and targeted therapy in appendiceal adenocarcinomas. Oncologist 2013;18:1270–7.

60. Zauber P, Berman E, Marotta S, et al. Ki-ras gene mutations are invariably present in low-grade mucinous tumors of the vermiform appendix. Scand J Gastroenterol 2011;46:869–74.

61. Vilar E, Gruber SB. Microsatellite instability in colorectal cancer-the stable evidence. Nat Rev Clin Oncol 2010;7:153–62.

62. Maru D, Wu TT, Canada A, et al. Loss of chromosome 18q and DPC4 (Smad4) mutations in appendiceal adenocarcinomas. Oncogene 2004;23:859–64.

63. Borazanci E, Millis SZ, Kimbrough J, et al. Potential actionable targets in appendiceal cancer detected by immunohistochemistry, fluorescent in situ hybridization, and mutational analysis. J Gastrointest Oncol 2017;8:164–72.

64. Austin F, Manavur A, Magesh S, et al. Aggressive management of peritoneal carcinomatosis from mucinous appendiceal neoplasm. Ann Surg Oncol 2012; 19:1386–93.

65. Kabbani W, Houlihan PS, Luthra R, et al. Mucinous and nonmucinous appendiceal adenocarcinomas: different clinicopathological features but similar genetic alterations. Mod Pathol 2002;15:599–605.

66. Pietrantonio F, Maggi C, Fanetti G, et al. FOLFOX-4 chemotherapy for patients with unresectable or relapsed peritoneal pseudomyxoma. Oncologist 2014;19: 845–50.

67. Nishikawa G, Sekine S, Ogawa R, et al. Frequent GNAS mutations in low-grade appendiceal mucinous neoplasms. Br J Cancer 2013;108:951–8.

68. Nummela P, Saarinen L, Thiel A, et al. Genomic profile of pseudomyxoma peritonei analyzed using next-generation sequencing and immunohistochemistry. Int J Cancer 2015;136:E282–9.

69. Singhi AD, Davison JM, Choudry HA, et al. GNAS is frequently mutated in both low-grade and high-grade disseminated appendiceal mucinous neoplasms but does not affect survival. Hum Pathol 2014;45:1737–43.

70. Alakus H, Babicky ML, Ghosh P, et al. Genome-wide mutational landscape of mucinous carcinomatosis peritonei of appendiceal origin. Genome Med 2014; 6:43.

71. Liu X, Mody K, de Abreu FB, et al. Molecular profiling of appendiceal epithelial tumors using massively parallel sequencing to identify somatic mutations. Clin Chem 2014;60:1004–11.

72. Noguchi R, Yano H, Gohda Y, et al. Molecular profiles of high-grade and low-grade pseudomyxoma peritonei. Cancer Med 2015;4:1809–16.

73. Davison JM, Hartman DA, Singhi AD, et al. Loss of SMAD4 protein expression is associated with high tumor grade and poor prognosis in disseminated appendiceal mucinous neoplasms. Am J Surg Pathol 2014;38:583–92.

74. Hara K, Saito T, Hayashi T, et al. A mutation spectrum that includes GNAS, KRAS and TP53 may be shared by mucinous neoplasms of the appendix. Pathol Res Pract 2015;211:657–64.

75. Davison JM, Choudry HA, Pingpank JF, et al. Clinicopathologic and molecular analysis of disseminated appendiceal mucinous neoplasms: identification of factors predicting survival and proposed criteria for a three-tiered assessment of tumor grade. Mod Pathol 2014;27:1521–39.

76. Pietrantonio F, Perrone F, Mennitto A, et al. Toward the molecular dissection of peritoneal pseudomyxoma. Ann Oncol 2016;27:2097–103.

77. Saarinen L, Nummela P, Thiel A, et al. Multiple components of PKA and TGF-β pathways are mutated in pseudomyxoma peritonei. PLoS One 2017;12: e0174898.

78. Pape UF, Niederle B, Costa F, et al, Vienna Consensus Conference participants. ENETS consensus guidelines for neuroendocrine neoplasms of the appendix (excluding goblet cell carcinomas). Neuroendocrinology 2016;103:144–52.

79. D'adda T, Pizzi S, Azzoni C, et al. Different patterns of 11q allelic losses in digestive endocrine tumors. Hum Pathol 2002;33:322–9.

80. Stancu M, Wu TT, Wallace C, et al. Genetic alterations in goblet cell carcinoids of the vermiform appendix and comparison with gastrointestinal carcinoid tumors. Mod Pathol 2003;16:1189–98.

81. Paraskevakou H, Saetta A, Skandalis K, et al. Morphological-histochemical study of intestinal carcinoids and K-ras mutation analysis in appendiceal carcinoids. Pathol Oncol Res 1999;5:205–10.

82. Ramnani DM, Wistuba II, Behrens C, et al. K-ras and p53 mutations in the pathogenesis of classical and goblet cell carcinoids of the appendix. Cancer 1999;86: 14–21.

83. Dimmler A, Geddert H, Faller G. EGFR, KRAS, BRAF-mutations and microsatellite instability are absent in goblet cell carcinoids of the appendix. Pathol Res Pract 2014;210:274–8.

84. Modlin IM, Kidd M, Latich I, et al. Genetic differentiation of appendiceal tumor malignancy: a guide for the perplexed. Ann Surg 2006;244:52–60.

85. Kidd M, Modlin IM, Mane SM, et al. The role of genetic markers–NAP1L1, MAGE-D2, and MTA1–in defining small-intestinal carcinoid neoplasia. Ann Surg Oncol 2006;13:253–62.

86. Jesinghaus M, Konukiewitz B, Foersch S, et al. Appendiceal goblet cell carcinoids and adenocarcinomas ex-goblet cell carcinoid are genetically distinct from primary colorectal-type adenocarcinoma of the appendix. Mod Pathol 2018. https://doi.org/10.1038/modpathol.2017.184.

87. Shenoy S. Goblet cell carcinoids of the appendix: tumor biology, mutations and management strategies. World J Gastrointest Surg 2016;8:660–9.

88. Yantiss RK, Panczykowski A, Misdraji J, et al. A comprehensive study of nondysplastic and dysplastic serrated polyps of the vermiform appendix. Am J Surg Pathol 2007;31:1742–53.

89. Bellizzi AM, Rock J, Marsh WL, et al. Serrated lesions of the appendix: a morphologic and immunohistochemical appraisal. Am J Clin Pathol 2010;133:623–32.

90. Pai RK, Hartman DJ, Gonzalo DH, et al. Serrated lesions of the appendix frequently harbor KRAS mutations and not BRAF mutations indicating a distinctly different serrated neoplastic pathway in the appendix. Hum Pathol 2014;45: 227–35.

Molecular Diagnostics in Esophageal and Gastric Neoplasms: 2018 Update

Muhammad Zulfiqar, MD[a],*, Martin H. Bluth, MD, PhD[a,b,c],
Amarpreet Bhalla, MBBS, MD[d]

KEYWORDS

- Esophagus • Squamous cell carcinoma • Adenocarcinoma • Gastric carcinoma
- Molecular genetics • HER-2 • Trastuzumab • Next-generation sequencing

KEY POINTS

- Esophageal cancer (EC) is rapidly increasing in incidence in the United States. Genetic changes associated with the development of EC involve the p16, p53, and APC genes. Human epidermal growth factor 2 (HER-2) overexpression is seen in gastroesophageal junction carcinoma and a subset, gastric carcinoma (GC).
- Trastuzumab is the first Food and Drug Administration–approved target agent for treatment of patients with HER-2 amplified cancers.
- Up to 50% cases of GC are related to *Helicobacter pylori* infection and up to 16% are related to Epstein-Barr virus infection.
- Microsatellite instability (MSI) is observed in up to 39% of GC. American Joint Committee on Cancer *AJCC Cancer Staging Manual* recommends MSI testing on GC.
- Other genetic changes seen in GC include chromosome gains and losses, MSI, changes in expression of vascular endothelial growth factor expression, cyclin E, retinoblastoma, p53, and protection of telomeres 1.

INTRODUCTION

Esophageal carcinoma (EC) is the most rapidly increasing tumor in incidence in the United States. It has an established association with a precursor lesion (Barrett esophagus). Gastric carcinoma (GC) is the second leading cause of cancer death in the world. Most genetic alterations reported in esophageal carcinoma do not show significant differences compared with GC.

This article has been updated from a version previously published in *Clinics in Laboratory Medicine*, Volume 33, Issue 4, December 2013.

[a] Southeastern Pathology Associates (SEPA Labs), 203 Indigo Drive, Brunswick, GA 31525, USA;
[b] Department of Pathology, Wayne State University School of Medicine, 540 East Canfield Street, Detroit, MI 48201, USA; [c] Pathology Laboratories, Michigan Surgical Hospital, 21230 Dequindre Road, Warren, MI 48091, USA; [d] Department of Pathology and Anatomical Sciences, Jacobs School of Buffalo, 955 Main Street, Buffalo, NY 14203, USA
* Corresponding author.
E-mail addresses: mzulfiqar@sepalabs.com; muhammad.zulfiqar@bmcjax.com

Clin Lab Med 38 (2018) 357–365
https://doi.org/10.1016/j.cll.2018.02.009
0272-2712/18/© 2018 Elsevier Inc. All rights reserved.

Up to half of the cases of GC are related to *Helicobacter pylori* infection.[1–5] The prognosis for patients with advanced stage GC and EC is poor. Human epidermal growth factor 2 (HER-2) overexpression is seen in gastroesophageal junction (GEJ) carcinoma and a subset of GC. HER-2 overexpressing tumors are eligible for HER-2–targeted therapies, which leads to a better survival in these patients.

EPIDEMIOLOGY

EC is the sixth leading cause of cancer death worldwide.[6] Two subtypes of EC, squamous cell carcinoma and adenocarcinoma (ADC), differ in the incidence and distribution of disease.[6] Squamous cell EC is more prevalent in the Asia-Pacific region, whereas ADC is more common in the Western world. EC is common in men more than 50 years of age, with a strong prevalence in whites.

Squamous cell EC is related to smoking and alcohol, whereas Barrett esophagus, caused by gastroesophageal reflux disease, is the risk factor for ADC.[7] The tumors evolve through a pathway from metaplasia (Barrett esophagus) to dysplasia and finally to cancer.[7]

The incidence of GC is the highest in Eastern Asia, Eastern Europe, and South America.[8] Distal stomach tumors are more common in Asia and tend to have a favorable outcome with surgery[9] compared with gastric cardia tumors, which are more common in US patients.[8]

Diffuse GC has a hereditary form and results from cadherin 1 or E-cadherin (CDH1) deregulation, whereas occurrence of intestinal type is associated with environmental factors, such as obesity, dietary factors, and cigarette smoking as well as with infection by *H pylori*.

CLINICAL FEATURES

EC presents with obstructive symptoms, including dysphagia and odynophagia. Weight loss is also common. Most patients with GC are asymptomatic. Epigastric pain and dyspepsia are the most frequent symptoms. Most tumors are located on the lesser curvature and are 2 cm to 5 cm in size. Multiple tumors are associated with a worse prognosis.[10]

PATHOPHYSIOLOGY AND MOLECULAR GENETICS

The evolution of ADC of the esophagus involves earlier losses of the p16 and p53 genes and later losses of the APC gene.[11] Aneuploidy occurs early and can be found before cancer occurs.

A multistep process has been proposed for GC starting with chronic gastritis to atrophic gastritis, intestinal metaplasia, and dysplasia before resulting in intestinal-type GC.[12] Premalignant counterparts are not seen in diffuse-type cancers.

Helicobacter pylori

H pylori is implicated with atrophic gastritis, intestinal metaplasia, and dysplasia leading to intestinal-type GC.[13,14] A positive association is demonstrated in regions where high-risk CagA (1) *H pylori* strains are endemic.[15] Bacterial virulence factors contributing to GC risk include vacA, babA2, OipA, and CagA.[16] Single-nucleotide polymorphisms in interleukin (IL)-1b and endogenous receptor antagonists (IL-1RN) are associated with increased susceptibility to *H pylori*–induced GC.[17,18]

EPSTEIN-BARR VIRUS

EBV has been demonstrated in 2% to 16% of conventional gastric ADC. EBV-positive GC has a tendency to show CpG island methylator phenotype of cancer-related genes (CIMP) but does not show MSI-H phenotype or HMLH1 hypermethylation.[19] Morphologically, EBV-positive GC has characteristic abundant lymphoid stroma. Recent studies have supported the relationship between the presence of EBV and aberrant immune checkpoint protein expression, as demonstrated by high PD-L1 protein expression in EBV-positive GC.[20,21] Although EBV and MSI are mutually exclusive in GC, microsatellite unstable GC also shows lymphocyte-rich histology.[22] To determine the EBV status of GC patients, EBV can be detected in newly diagnosed GC patients by EBER in situ hybridization (ISH) (gold standard for EBV detection and localization of latent EBV in tissue samples) on paraffin sections from biopsy, surgical excision, or cytology specimens. Nonspecific positivity in cytoplasm of scattered normal epithelial cells and scattered EBER-positive memory B cells must be taken into consideration when interpreting EBER ISH results.

Chromosomal Instability

Intestinal-type GC shows copy number gains at 8q, 17q, and 20q and losses at 3p and 5q.[23,24] Diffuse-type GC show copy number gains at 12q and 13q and losses at 4q, 15q, 16q, and 17p.[25–27]

Microsatellite Instability

MSI is observed in 8% to 39% of GC.[28–33] Most studies have shown that MSI is associated with less aggressive behavior and favorable survival, whereas other studies have indicated no prognostic impact.[34]

Microsatellite unstable GC is associated with older age, female gender, expanding growth pattern, antral location, intestinal-type histology, and a lower incidence of lymph node metastasis. Hypermethylation of MLH1 promotor is associated with the development of sporadic GC with MSI[35,36] and is detected in 20% to 30% of nondiffuse, distal GC. The new *AJCC Cancer Staging Manual* recommends MSI testing on GC.[37]

Vascular Endothelial Growth Factor

In GC, vascular endothelial growth factor (VEGF) expression is associated with advanced stage and poor survival.[38] Plasma VEGF-A and tumor neuropilin-1 are strong biomarker candidates for predicting clinical outcome in patients with advanced GC treated with VEGF inhibitor, bevacizumab.[39]

Human Epidermal Growth Factor 2

HER-2 has been shown to be overexpressed/amplified in 6% to 35% of gastric tumors.[39–43] This overexpression/amplification is associated with GEJ tumors more than with GC[44]; 20% of intestinal-type cancers have HER-2 overexpression/amplification compared with 5% of diffuse-type cancers. In the ToGA study, the addition of trastuzumab, a monoclonal antibody targeting HER-2, to palliative chemotherapy led to an overall survival benefit specifically in patients with HER-2 overexpression or amplification.[45] Trastuzumab-based combination therapy is now the standard treatment of patients with HER-2 amplified GC. HER-2 immunohistochemistry (IHC) should be performed on in all inoperable locally advanced GC and GEJ cancer at initial diagnosis as well as recurrent and metastatic setting. If the HER-2 IHC results are equivocal, HER-2 testing by fluorescence ISU (FISH) or ISH Is recommended.

Additionally HER-2 testing should be performed at relapse in patients with previously HER-2–negative tumors.

Human Epidermal Growth Factor 2 Testing

To date, HER-2 is the only validated therapeutic target in GC. The guidelines for HER2 testing of gastric or GEJ tumors were established by the ToGA trial.

Immunohistochemistry and Fluorescence In Situ Hybridization

HER2 expression may be assessed by IHC, with scoring ranging from 0 to 3, or by gene amplification using FISH or silver ISU (SISH). The survival benefit associated with trastuzumab is seen greatest in IHC 3 or IHC 2 and FISH-positive patients with high HER-2–expressing tumors.

Because of the heterogeneous nature of HER-2 overexpression/amplification in GC, and because gastric tumor cells may only show HER-2 staining at the basolateral or lateral membrane regions, complete membranous staining is not a prerequisite for IHC 2 or IHC 3 scores in GC as it is for breast cancer.[46]

A 10% cutoff of positive cells is defined for assessment of both breast cancer and gastric cancer. Small biopsy specimens or tumor cell clusters, however, are assessed regardless of the percentage of the cells staining.[46]

ISU in cancer tissue samples is considered the gold standard for gene amplification. SISH is preferred because of the ability to use bright field microscopy, considering HER-2 tumor heterogeneity. SISH slides can be stored for a longer period of time without bleaching than FISH slides. ISU results are generally not acceptable if 20 invasive tumor cells are not found, greater than 25% of signals are not scorable (due to weak signal), greater than 10% of signals occur over cytoplasm, nuclear resolution is poor, auto-fluorescence is strong, or controls are not expected. For GC or GEJ cancers, the presence of more than 4 copies of the HER-2 gene per tumor cell (if no chromosome 17 control is used) is not a positive result, a difference from breast cancer guidelines.[46]

Other Abnormalities

CDH1 is involved in the initiation and progression of both sporadic and hereditary forms of GC.[47,48] Serum-soluble CDH1 is a prognostic marker for GC, and a high concentration predicts extensive tumor invasion.[49] Cyclin E gene is amplified in 15% to 20% of GC and this overexpression of cyclin E correlates with the aggressiveness of the cancer. Reduced p27 expression is a negative prognostic factor for patients with a cyclin E–positive tumor.[50] Reduced expression of retinoblastoma is associated with worse overall survival.[33] Abnormal expression of p53 significantly affects cumulative survival and p53 status may also influence response to chemotherapy.[51,52] Protection of telomeres 1 expression levels are significantly higher in GC of advanced stage.

Next-generation sequencing

Based on genomic sequencing data, The Cancer Genome Atlas (TCGA) research network has divided GC into hypermutated and nonhypermutated tumor. The nonhypermutated tumor includes genomically stable and unstable subtypes. The hypermutated tumor includes EBV-positive and MSI-H subtypes and has frequent mutations in the PIK3CA and ARID1A genetic pathways. TCGA data have highlighted genetic mutations relevant to GC. Multigene panels should be able to identify clinically significant genetic aberrations for targeted therapy, treatment response and prognostication. Such panels are undergoing laboratory validation for clinical practice.

TREATMENT

The treatment of EC is esophagectomy, which carries a high morbidity.[6] Surgical resection is the mainstay of treatment of early-stage GC. The prognosis for patients with advanced stage GC and GEJ cancers is poor despite new treatment strategies.[53,54] HER-2–overexpressing tumors are eligible for HER-2–targeted therapies, including monoclonal antibodies (ie, trastuzumab) or tyrosine kinase inhibitors (lapatinib).[46] Trastuzumab-based combination therapy is now the standard treatment of patients with HER-2 amplified GC.[36]

MORPHOLOGY

Two main histologic subtypes of EC include squamous cell carcinoma and ADC. According to the World Health Organization and the Laurén classifications, 2 main histologic types of GC include the diffuse and intestinal subtypes.[55–57] Readers are referred to gastrointestinal pathology literature for further reading.[10,58]

Circulating Tumor Cells and Cell Free Nucleic Acid Analysis

Although solid tissue–based analysis has been the mainstay of esophageal and gastric cancer diagnosis, analysis of fluid samples via interrogation of circulating micro-RNA, circulating tumor cells (CTCs), and cell-free DNA in fluids, including serum, plasma, urine, and spinal fluid, has proved beneficial for diagnosis and prognosis of these disease states.[59,60] To this end, micro-RNA, including miR-21, miR-25, miR-92, and miR-223, were found up-regulated whereas miR-195 and miR-326 and miR-148a have been found down-regulated in gastric cancer cells and could be associated with disease prognosis.[61–64] Various genetic alterations, such as copy number, chromosomal instability, and mutations, have been detected in circulating tumor DNA, including TP53, SMAD4, and PIK3CA, which have been detected in gastroesophageal carcinoma.[65] CTCs have also been shown as potentially useful prognostic indicators in EC where CTCs obtained from peripheral blood increased as the disease stage advanced (88.0% in stages III–IV, 58.9% in stages I–II). CTC counts were also correlated with the degree of tumor differentiation, tumor infiltration, and lymph node and distant metastases.[66] Cell-freeDNA analysis of 5-hydroxymethylcytosine has also been reported to be useful for the detection of gastric cancer and showed a trend of increasing cancer call rate with cancer clinical stage.[67] Further studies will help elucidate the ideal application of circulating nucleic acid utilization in gastrointestinal cancers.

REFERENCES

1. de Vries AC, Haringsma J, Kuipers EJ. The detection, surveillance and treatment of premalignant gastric lesions related to Helicobacter pylori infection. Helicobacter 2007;12:1–15.

2. Garcia-Gonzalez MA, Lanas A, Quintero E, et al. Gastric cancer susceptibility is not linked to pro- and anti-inflammatory cytokine gene polymorphisms in whites: a Nationwide Multicenter Study in Spain. Am J Gastroenterol 2007;102:1878–92.

3. Rad R, Prinz C, Neu B, et al. Synergistic effect of Helicobacter pylori virulence factors and interleukin-1 polymorphisms for the development of severe histological changes in the gastric mucosa. J Infect Dis 2003;188:272–81.

4. Machado JC, Pharoah P, Sousa S, et al. Interleukin 1B and interleukin 1RN polymorphisms are associated with increased risk of gastric carcinoma. Gastroenterology 2001;121:823–9.

5. Forman D, Newell DG, Fullerton F, et al. Association between infection with Helicobacter pylori and risk of gastric cancer: evidence from a prospective investigation. BMJ 1991;302:1302–5.

6. Holmes RS, Vaughan TL. Epidemiology and pathogenesis of esophageal cancer [review]. Semin Radiat Oncol 2007;17(1):2–9.

7. Montgomery E, Goldblum JR, Greenson JK, et al. Dysplasia as a predictive marker for invasive carcinoma in Barrett esophagus: a follow-up study based on 138 cases from a diagnostic variability study. Hum Pathol 2001;32(4):379–88.

8. Siegel R, Ward E, Brawley O, et al. Cancer statistics, 2011: the impact of eliminating socioeconomic and racial disparities on premature cancer deaths. CA Cancer J Clin 2011;61(4):212–36.

9. Strong VE, Song KY, Park CH, et al. Comparison of gastric cancer survival following R0 resection in the United States and Korea using an internationally validated nomogram. Ann Surg 2010;251(4):640–6.

10. Lauwers GY. Epithelial neoplasms of the stomach. In: Odze RD, Goldblum JR, editors. Surgical pathology of the GI tract, liver, biliary tract and pancreas. Philadelphia: Saunders Elsevier; 2009. p. 563–79.

11. Maley CC, Galipeau PC, Finley JC, et al. Genetic clonal diversity predicts progression to esophageal adenocarcinoma. Nat Genet 2006;38(4):468–73.

12. Correa P. Helicobacter pylori and gastric carcinogenesis. Am J Surg Pathol 1995; 19(Suppl 1):S37–43.

13. Correa P. Human gastric carcinogenesis: a multistep and multifactorial process–First American Cancer Society Award Lecture on Cancer Epidemiology and Prevention. Cancer Res 1992;52(24):6735–40.

14. Correa P, Haenszel W, Cuello C, et al. A model for gastric cancer epidemiology. Lancet 1975;2(7924):58–60.

15. Cavaleiro-Pinto M, Peleteiro B, Lunet N, et al. Helicobacter pylori infection and gastric cardia cancer: systematic review and meta-analysis. Cancer Causes Control 2011;22(3):375–87.

16. Tan IB, Ng I, Tai WM, et al. Understanding the genetic basis of gastric cancer: recent advances. Expert Rev Gastroenterol Hepatol 2012;6(3):335–41.

17. El-Omar EM, Carrington M, Chow WH, et al. Interleukin-1 polymorphisms associated with increased risk of gastric cancer. Nature 2000;404(6776):398–402.

18. Persson C, Canedo P, Machado JC, et al. Polymorphisms in inflammatory response genes and their association with gastric cancer: a HuGE systematic review and meta-analyses. Am J Epidemiol 2011;173(3):259–70.

19. Bass A, Thorsson V, Shmulevich I, et al. Comprehensive molecular characterization of gastric adenocarcinoma. Nature 2014;513(7517):202–9.

20. Ma C, Patel K, Singhi A. Programmed death-ligand 1 expression is common in castric cancer associated with epstein-barr virus or microsatellite instability. Am J Surg Pathol 2016;40(11):1496–506.

21. Kawazoe A, Kuwata T, Kuboki Y, et al. Clinicopathological features of programmed death ligand 1 expression with tumor-infiltrating lymphocyte, mismatch repair, and Epstein-Barr virus status in a large cohort of gastric cancer patients. Gastric Cancer 2017;20:407–15.

22. Chetty R. Gastrointestinal cancers accompanied by a dense lymphoid component: an overview with special reference to gastric and colonic medullary and lymphoepithelioma-like carcinomas. J Clin Pathol 2012;65:1062–5.

23. Kokkola A, Monni O, Puolakkainen P, et al. 17q12-21 amplicon, a novel recurrent genetic change in intestinal type of gastric carcinoma: a comparative genomic hybridization study. Genes Chromosomes Cancer 1997;20(1):38–43.

24. Wu MS, Chang MC, Huang SP, et al. Correlation of histologic subtypes and replication error phenotype with comparative genomic hybridization in gastric cancer. Genes Chromosomes Cancer 2001;30(1):80–6.

25. Weiss MM, Kuipers EJ, Postma C, et al. Genomic alterations in primary gastric adenocarcinomas correlate with clinicopathological characteristics and sur- vival. Cell Oncol 2004;26(5–6):307–17.

26. Tsukamoto Y, Uchida T, Karnan S, et al. Genome-wide analysis of DNA copy number alterations and gene expression in gastric cancer. J Pathol 2008;216(4): 471–82.

27. Han HJ, Yanagisawa A, Kato Y, et al. Genetic instability in pancreatic cancer and poorly differentiated type of gastric cancer. Cancer Res 1993;53:5087–9.

28. Lee HS, Choi SI, Lee HK, et al. Distinct clinical features and outcomes of gastric cancers with microsatellite instability. Mod Pathol 2002;15(6):632–40.

29. Beghelli S, de Manzoni G, Barbi S, et al. Microsatellite instability in gastric cancer is associated with better prognosis in only stage II cancers. Surgery 2006; 139(3):347–56.

30. Seo HM, Chang YS, Joo SH, et al. Clinicopathologic characteristics and outcomes of gastric cancers with the MSI-H phenotype. J Surg Oncol 2009;99(3): 143–7.

31. Corso G, Pedrazzani C, Marrelli D, et al. Correlation of microsatellite instability at multiple loci with long-term survival in advanced gastric carcinoma. Arch Surg 2009;144(8):722–7.

32. Gu M, Kim D, Bae Y, et al. Analysis of microsatelliteinstability, protein expression and methylation status of hMLH1 and hMSH2 genes in gastric carcinomas. Hepatogastroenterology 2009;56(91–92):899–904.

33. Yasui W, Oue N, Aung PP, et al. Molecular-pathological prognostic factors of gastric cancer: a review. Gastric Cancer 2005;8(2):86–94.

34. Nakajima T, Akiyama Y, Shiraishi J, et al. Age-related hypermethylation of the hMLH1 promoter in gastric cancers. Int J Cancer 2001;94(2):208–11.

35. Guo RJ, Arai H, Kitayama Y, et al. Microsatellite instability of papillary subtype of human gastric adenocarcinoma and hMLH1 promoter hypermethylation in the surrounding mucosa. Pathol Int 2001;51(4):240–7.

36. Janjigian YY, Kelsen DP. Genomic dysregulation in gastric tumors. J Surg Oncol 2013;107(3):237–42.

37. Amin MB, Edge S, Greene F, et al. AJCC cancer staging manual. 8th edition. New York: Spinger; 2017. p. 203–74.

38. Van Cutsem E, de Haas S, Kang YK, et al. Bevacizumab in combination with chemotherapy as first-line therapy in advanced gastric cancer: a biomarker evaluation from the AVAGAST randomized phase III trial. J Clin Oncol 2012;30(17): 2119–27.

39. Gravalos C, Jimeno A. HER2 in gastric cancer: a new prognostic factor and a novel therapeutic target. Ann Oncol 2008;19(9):1523–9.

40. Beltran Gárate B, Yabar Berrocal A. HER2 expression in gastric cancer in Peru. Rev Gastroenterol Peru 2010;30(4):324–7 [in Spanish].

41. Hofmann M, Stoss O, Shi D, et al. Assessment of a HER2 scoring system for gastric cancer: results from a validation study. Histopathology 2008;52(7): 797–805.

42. Im SA, Kim JW, Kim JS, et al. Clinicopathologic characteristics of patients with stage III/IV (M(0)) advanced gastric cancer, according to HER2 status assessed by immunohistochemistry and fluorescence in situ hybridization. Diagn Mol Pathol 2011;20(2):94–100.

43. Tanner M, Hollmén M, Junttila TT, et al. Amplification of HER-2 in gastric carcinoma: association with Topoisomerase II alpha gene amplification, intestinal type, poor prognosis and sensitivity to trastuzumab. Ann Oncol 2005;16(2): 273–8.
44. Albarello L, Pecciarini L, Doglioni C. HER2 testing in gastric cancer. Adv Anat Pathol 2011;18(1):53–9.
45. Bang YJ, Van Cutsem E, Feyereislova A, et al, ToGA Trial Investigators. Trastuzumab in combination with chemotherapy versus chemotherapy alone for treatment of HER2-positive advanced gastric or gastro-oesophageal junction cancer (ToGA): a phase 3, open-label, randomised controlled trial. Lancet 2010;376(9742):687–97.
46. Bang YJ. Advances in the management of HER2-positive advanced gastric and gastroesophageal junction cancer. J Clin Gastroenterol 2012;46(8):637–48.
47. Birchmeier W, Behrens J. Cadherin expression in carcinomas: role in the formation of cell junctions and the prevention of invasiveness. Biochim Biophys Acta 1994;1198(1):11–26.
48. Christofori G, Semb H. The role of the cell-adhesion molecule E-cadherin as a tumour-suppressor gene. Trends Biochem Sci 1999;24(2):73–6.
49. Chan AO, Lam SK, Chu KM, et al. Soluble E-cadherin is a valid prognostic marker in gastric carcinoma. Gut 2001;48(6):808–11.
50. Xiangming C, Natsugoe S, Takao S, et al. The cooperative role of p27 with cyclin E in the prognosis of advanced gastric carcinoma. Cancer 2000;89(6):1214–9.
51. Fondevila C, Metges JP, Fuster J, et al. p53 and VEGF expression are independent predictors of tumor recurrence and survival following curative resection of gastric cancer. Br J Cancer 2004;90(1):206–15.
52. Pinto-de-Sousa J, Silva F, David L, et al. Clinicopathological significance and survival influence of p53 protein expression in gastric carcinoma. Histopathology 2004;44(4):323–31.
53. Cunningham D, Allum WH, Stenning SP, et al, MAGIC Trial Participants. Perioperative chemotherapy versus surgery alone for resectable gastroesophageal cancer. N Engl J Med 2006;355(1):11–20.
54. Macdonald JS, Smalley SR, Benedetti J, et al. Chemoradiotherapy after surgery compared with surgery alone for adenocarcinoma of the stomach or gastroesophageal junction. N Engl J Med 2001;345(10):725–30.
55. Milne AN, Carneiro F, O'Morain C, et al. Nature meets nurture: molecular genetics of gastric cancer. Hum Genet 2009;126(5):615–28.
56. Lauren P. The two histological main types of gastric carcinoma: diffuse and so-called intestinal-type carcinoma. An attempt at a histo- clinical classification. Acta Pathol Microbiol Scand 1965;64:31–49.
57. Hudler P. Genetic aspects of gastric cancer instability. ScientificWorldJournal 2012;2012:761909.
58. Glickman JN. Epithelial neoplasms of the esophagus. In: Odze RD, Goldblum JR, editors. Surgical pathology of the GI tract, liver, biliary tract and pancreas. Philadelphia: Saunders Elsevier; 2009. p. 535–62.
59. Traver S, Assou S, Scalici E, et al. Cell-free nucleic acids as non-invasive biomarkers of gynecological cancers, ovarian, endometrial and obstetric disorders and fetal aneuploidy. Hum Reprod Update 2014;20(6):905–23.
60. Nordgård O, Tjensvoll K, Gilje B, et al. Circulating tumour cells and DNA as liquid biopsies in gastrointestinal cancer. Br J Surg 2018;105:e110–20.
61. Shrestha S, Hsu S, Huang W, et al. A systematic review of microRNA expression profiling studies in human gastric cancer. Cancer Med 2014;3(4):878–88.

62. Ye R, Wei B, Li S, et al. Expression of miR-195 is associated with chemotherapy sensitivity of cisplatin and clinical prognosis in gastric cancer. Oncotarget 2017; 8(57):97260–72.

63. Li Y, Gao Y, Xu Y, et al. Down-regulation of miR-326 is associated with poor prognosis and promotes growth and metastasis by targeting FSCN1 in gastric cancer. Growth Factors 2015;33(4):267–74.

64. Xia J, Guo X, Yan J, et al. The role of miR-148a in gastric cancer. J Cancer Res Clin Oncol 2014;140(9):1451–6.

65. Openshaw M, Richards C, Guttery D, et al. The genetics of gastroesophageal adenocarcinoma and the use of circulating cell free DNA for disease detection and monitoring. Expert Rev Mol Diagn 2017;17(5):459–70.

66. Qiao Y, Li J, Shi C, et al. Prognostic value of circulating tumor cells in the peripheral blood of patients with esophageal squamous cell carcinoma. Onco Targets Ther 2017;10:1363–73.

67. Li W, Zhang X, Lu X, et al. 5-Hydroxymethylcytosine signatures in circulating cell-free DNA as diagnostic biomarkers for human cancers. Cell Res 2017;27: 1243–57.

Molecular Diagnostics in the Neoplasms of the Pancreas, Liver, Gallbladder, and Extrahepatic Biliary Tract

2018 Update

Lei Zhang, MD, PhD[a], Martin H. Bluth, MD, PhD[b,c],
Amarpreet Bhalla, MBBS, MD[d],*

KEYWORDS

- Pancreatic neoplasms • Liver • Hepatic adenoma • Hepatocellular carcinoma
- Cholangiocarcinoma • Molecular diagnostics • Cell free nucleic acid

KEY POINTS

- Pancreatic neoplasms, including ductal adenocarcinoma, solid pseudopapillary neoplasm, pancreatic endocrine neoplasms, acinar cell carcinoma, and pancreatoblastoma, are associated with different genetic abnormalities.
- Hepatic adenomas with β-catenin exon 3 mutation are associated with a high risk of malignancy.
- Hepatic adenoma with arginosuccinate synthetase 1 expression or sonic hedgehog mutations are associated with a risk of bleeding.
- Hepatocellular carcinoma and cholangiocarcinoma display heterogeneity at both morphologic and molecular levels.
- Cholangiocellular carcinoma is most commonly associated with IDH 1/2 mutations.

Disclosure: The authors have nothing to disclose.

This article has been updated from a version previously published in *Clinics in Laboratory Medicine*, Volume 33, Issue 4, December 2013.

[a] Department of Pathology and Anatomical Sciences, Jacobs School of Medicine and Biomedical Sciences, University at Buffalo, Buffalo General Hospital, 100 High Street, Buffalo, NY 14203, USA; [b] Department of Pathology, Wayne State University School of Medicine, 540 East Canfield Street, Detroit, MI 48201, USA; [c] Pathology Laboratories, Michigan Surgical Hospital, 21230 Dequindre Road, Warren, MI 48091, USA; [d] Department of Pathology and Anatomical Sciences, Jacobs School of Medicine and Biomedical Sciences, University at Buffalo-SUNY, Buffalo General Hospital A-701, 100 High Street, Buffalo, NY 14203, USA
* Corresponding author.
E-mail address: ABhalla@KaleidaHealth.org

Clin Lab Med 38 (2018) 367–384
https://doi.org/10.1016/j.cll.2018.03.003
0272-2712/18/© 2018 Elsevier Inc. All rights reserved.

PANCREATIC NEOPLASMS
Epidemiology

Pancreatic cancer has become the fourth leading cause of cancer related death in both men and women in the United States.[1] There will be an estimated 55,440 new cases, and 44,330 affected individuals are expected to die from the disease in 2018.[1] As the incidence of pancreatic cancer gradually increases, little progress has been made in the early detection and effective treatment of pancreatic cancer. Most patients are diagnosed at an advanced stage. The prognosis remains poor with a 5-year relative survival rate of only 6% to 8%. More than 90% of patients die within 1 year.[2] It has been projected that pancreatic cancers will be second leading causes of cancer deaths by 2030.[2] Although a variety of risk factors have been consistently related to pancreatic cancer, including chronic pancreatitis, diabetes mellitus, physical inactivity, obesity, smoking, alcohol abuse, high intake of saturated fat and sugar, aspirin use, and occupational exposure to pesticides,[3,4] an increased incidence has been observed in patients with certain hereditary syndromes such as Peutz-Jeghers syndrome, Lynch syndrome, familial breast cancer, hereditary pancreatitis, familial atypical mole malignant melanoma, familial pancreatic cancer, Li–Fraumeni syndrome, and familial adenomatous polyposis.[5–7]

Clinical Features

The pancreatic neoplasms are classified by differentiation of the neoplastic cells as ductal, acinar, or neuroendocrine, and by the macroscopic appearance as solid or cystic lesions. Pancreatic ductal adenocarcinoma is the most common type and comprises around 90% of all pancreatic neoplasms. Other pancreatic neoplasms such as pancreatic neuroendocrine neoplasms, solid pseudopapillary neoplasm, acinar cell carcinoma (ACC), and pancreatoblastoma comprise about 5% to 10% of pancreatic malignant tumors.[8] At their early stage, pancreatic cancers usually do not cause any signs or symptoms. However, by the time patients are symptomatic, the tumors may often have already metastasized. Common signs and symptoms include anorexia, malaise, nausea, fatigue, jaundice, and midepigastric or back pain. Significant weight loss is a characteristic feature of pancreatic cancer. Malabsorption with diarrhea and malodorous, greasy, or pale colored stools may also be present.[8]

Pathophysiology and Molecular Genetics

Ductal adenocarcinoma

Currently, 3 neoplasms—pancreatic intraepithelial neoplasia, intraductal papillary mucinous neoplasms (IPMNs), and mucinous cystic neoplasms, have been recognized as precursor lesions for invasive ductal adenocarcinoma. Several recent large-scale sequencing studies have identified multiple combinations of genetic mutations that are commonly found in pancreatic ductal adenocarcinomas as well as in these precursor lesions.[9–12] The most common genetic changes in ductal adenocarcinoma include KRAS codon 12 mutations seen in 90%, p16/CDKN2A inactivation in approximately 95%, loss of Smad4/DPC4 in 55%, and TP53 mutations seen in 50% of cases.[11–15] Genetic alterations seen in pancreatic intraepithelial neoplasia are KRAS at early stages, p16/CDKN2A inactivation during the middle stages, and Smad4/DPC4 and p53 during later stages.[16–18] The prevalence of these mutations increases with increasing degrees of dysplasia in the noninvasive precursor lesions. IPMNs show molecular alterations similar to that of ductal adenocarcinoma; mutations in KRAS and TP53 are not as frequent as they are in ductal adenocarcinoma.[19] Loss of Smad4/DPC4 within IPMN was the best marker for the presence of invasive carcinoma. Smad4/DPC4 mutations are rarely seen in IPMNs compared with ductal adenocarcinoma.[18,20,21] In addition, somatic *GNAS* oncogene mutations (codon 201) are seen in 58% to 60% of IPMNs.[22] Somatic *RNF43* mutations are also seen in IPMN and mucinous cystic neoplasms.[23,24] Loss of heterozygosity (LOH) of numerous tumor suppressor genes in pancreatic cyst fluid is used to diagnose pancreatic malignancy with a 83% sensitivity and 100% specificity for all malignant cysts and 83.3% sensitivity and 90.6% specificity for IPMN.[22,25–27] DNA mismatch repair genes are mutated in 2% to 3% of pancreatic cancers.[28–30] Pancreatic cancers with high levels of microsatellite instability seem to have a better prognosis than standard ductal adenocarcinomas.[31]

Pancreatic neuroendocrine neoplasms

Pancreatic neuroendocrine neoplasms are epithelial tumors with endocrine differentiation that are currently classified into well-differentiated neuroendocrine tumors (PanNETs; World Health Organization grades 1 and 2), and poorly differentiated neuroendocrine carcinoma (PanNECs; World Health Organization grade 3) based on mitotic count and Ki67 index.[3] Pancreatic neuroendocrine neoplasms are mostly sporadic (90%), but may be associated with hereditary syndromes including most frequently with multiple endocrine neoplasia type 1 and, more rarely, with von Hippel-Lindau (VHL) syndrome, neurofibromatosis type 1, and tuberous sclerosis complex (TSC).[3,32,33] In patients with sporadic PanNETs, 45% show *DAXX* and *ATRX* gene mutations, 15% show alterations in the mammalian target of rapamycin (mTOR) pathway, which involves somatic mutations in *PIK3CA*, *PTEN*, and *TSC2*, 45% show somatic *MEN1* mutations or LOH at the *MEN1* locus, and 25% show deletion of the VHL gene.[34–37] In patients with germline mutations, 65% of patients with multiple endocrine neoplasia type 1 syndrome develop PanNETs,[38–40] and 17% of patients with VHL syndrome develop PanNETs.[40,41] PanNETs lack *KRAS*, p16/*CDKN2A*, or *SMAD4* mutations, and only rarely show *TP53* mutation or microsatellite instability.[42] Chromosomal gains and losses have also been identified in PanNETs, and when frequent are associated with worse prognosis.[43,44] As for PanNECs, more than 95% of cases are associated with *TP53* mutations, and more than 50% of cases show retinoblastoma (*RB-1*) gene mutations. Rb-1 mutation seems to be mutually exclusive with p16/CDKN2A inactivation in PanNECs.[34,35,37]

Acinar Cell Carcinoma

ACC of the pancreas is a rare tumor of acinar differentiation that is often seen in older adults. Unlike other pancreatic cancers, ACC lacks KRAS, SMAD4, and p16 alterations,[45] and bears distinct genetic mutations with APC, TP53 alterations, SND1-BRAF fusions, or allelic loss on chromosome 11p.[28,46–48] Interestingly, the presence of RAF rearrangements in ACC is mutually exclusive with inactivation of DNA repair genes; ACCs without RAF fusion were significantly enriched for genomic alterations and have been associated with sensitivity to platinum-based therapies and PARP inhibitors.[28]

Solid Pseudopapillary Neoplasms

The most frequent genetic alterations seen in SPN is the activating somatic mutations of β-catenin gene (*CTNNB1*).[49,50] *CTNNB1* alterations lead to aberrant E-cadherin overexpression, resulting in the characteristic and diagnostic pseudopapillary growth pattern of discohesive tumor cells.[51] Solid pseudopapillary neoplasms show nuclear accumulation of β-catenin in 95%, activating β-catenin mutation in 90%, cyclin D1 in 74%, and overexpression of p53 in 15.8% of cases.[49,50,52]

Pancreatoblastoma

Pancreatoblastoma is an extremely rare childhood primary pancreatic neoplasm that often shows acinar, ductal, and/or neuroendocrine differentiation. The most common molecular alteration of pancreatoblastoma is allelic loss of chromosome 11p.[53,54] Somatic alterations of *CTNNB1* and *APC* are less common, but have also been reported.[53] The major genetic alterations of these pancreatic tumors are summarized in **Table 1**.

INTRADUCTAL PAPILLARY MUCINOUS NEOPLASMS

KRAS and GNAS mutations together possess high specificity and sensitivity for mucinous differentiation. Otherwise, KRAS mutation is more prevalent in invasive IPMN. The malignant transformation is a multistep carcinogenesis involving numerous other genes inclusive of CDKN2A/p16, p53, reprimo, and SMAD4. IPMN with high-grade dysplasia is associated with CDKN2A abnormalities, p53 mutations, and aberrant methylation patterns. Plectin-1 is also a marker for high-grade dysplasia and adenocarcinoma in IPMN. The strongest association with malignant progression of IPMN involves hTERT, Shh, and MUC1 genes. MiR-21, MiR-155, and miR-708 are also involved.[55–58]

Treatment

For advanced pancreatic ductal adenocarcinoma, surgical resection with gemcitabine-based chemotherapy is the mainstay of systemic treatment with a modest therapeutic benefit.[59,60] Recent studies showed that FOLFIRINOX and gemcitabine plus albumin-bound paclitaxel (nab-paclitaxel), have become the standard of care for metastatic pancreatic cancer with improved overall and progression-free survival compared with gemcitabine alone.[61,62] Single agent immunotherapy with anti–CTLA-4 or anti–PD-1/anti–PD-1 pathway (anti–PD-L1) were largely ineffective in pancreatic cancer.[63–65] Ipilimumab failed to induce tumor response in patients with advanced pancreatic cancer in a phase II study.[64] Another anti–PD-L1 monoclonal antibody (BMS-936559) failed to show any activity in a phase I study.[63] Multiple clinical trials combining immunotherapy with other chemotherapy or radiation modalities are currently ongoing and the outcomes of these trials are keenly anticipated.[66] For pancreatic endocrine neoplasms, ACC, SPN, and pancreatoblastoma, surgical resection is still the mainstay to resolve the mass effect and other associated symptoms with necessary follow-ups.

Table 1	
Pancreatic neoplasms with their key genetic alterations	
	Major Genetic Alterations
Pancreatic ductal adenocarcinoma	KRAS, CDNK2A, GNAS, RNF43, SMAD4, TP53,
Pancreatic neuroendocrine tumor/carcinoma	MEN1, ATRX, DAXX, TSC2, PTEN, Rb, TP53, VHL
Solid pseudopapillary neoplasm	CTNNB1
Acinar cell carcinoma	TP53, APC, SND1-BRAF, allelic loss on chromosome 11p
Pancreatoblastoma	Loss of chromosome 11p, CTNNB1, APC

Data from Refs.[67–70]

Summary
Recent large-scale profiling of pancreatic neoplasms has not only provided insight into the carcinogenesis of pancreatic tumors, but has also unraveled many clinically relevant somatic mutations, potential actionable drug targets, novel noncoding alterations, and more mutational signatures. The genetic alterations identified in these studies are beginning to be integrated into early tumor detection, diagnosis, classification, treatment, and patient prognosis. However, their diagnostic and prognostic usefulness are still in the early developing stage and additional prospective validation studies are needed before any molecular screening test can be recommended for routine clinical practice.

LIVER NEOPLASMS
Hepatic Adenoma

Epidemiology
Hepatic adenomas (HCAs) arise in women of childbearing age, with long-term contraceptive use as a risk factor.

Pathophysiology and molecular genetics
HCAs are monoclonal tumors with several recurrent mutations. They are divided into 6 groups according to molecular genetic abnormalities (**Fig. 1, Table 2**). The significant characteristics for each group are described.

Group 1 (H-HCA): Hepatocyte nuclear factor 1 alpha mutations, either somatic or germline steatosis; There is strong association with younger age at presentation, history of diabetes and familial adenomatous polyposis. The tumors reveal loss of expression of liver fatty acid binding protein. These neoplasms have significant steatosis and may be classified on radiologic imaging.

Group 2 (β-HCA): β-Catenin (CTNNB1) mutations in exon 3. It is more common in men and patients with vascular liver disease. There is strong homogenous expression of glutamine synthetase, leucine rich repeat containing G-protein coupled receptor-5 (LGR5) and nuclear expression of β-catenin. The tumors often reveal mild cytologic abnormalities, pseudogland formation, and cholestasis. They are relatively larger and associated with low exposure to estrogen. They are more frequently associated with the development of hepatocellular carcinoma (HCC).

Percentage

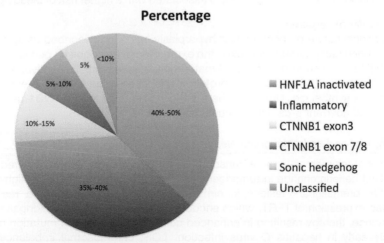

Fig. 1. Subtypes of hepatic adenoma. (*Data from* Refs.[67–70])

Table 2
Molecular aberrations in hepatic adenomas

Type of Hepatoma	Genes Involved	Immunohistochemistry
H-HCA	HNF1A/mTOR	LFABP loss
B-HCA exon 3	β-catenin exon 3	β-catenin/GS, LGR5 +++
B-HCA exon 7/8	β-catenin 7/8	β-catenin/GS, LGR5 +
I-HCA	JAK-STAT	SAA/CRP
Sh-HCA	INHBE-GLI1	Not known
Unclassified	Not specified	LFABP+, SAA/CRP-,GS- β-catenin -

Abbreviations: B-HCA, β-catenin mutated hepatic adenoma; CRP, C-reactive protein; GS, glutamine synthetase; H-HCA, HNF 1 alpha mutated hepatic adenoma; I-HCA, inflammatory-type hepatic adenoma; INHBE-GLI1, focal deletions fuse promoter of INHBE gene with GLI1 gene; LFABP, liver fatty acid binding protein; LGR5, leucine rich repeat containing G protein coupled receptor 5; mTOR, mammalian target of rapamycin; SAA, serum amyloid A; Sh, sonic hedgehog pathway.
Data from Refs.[67–70]

Group 3 (β-HCA): β-Catenin (CTNNB1) mutations; exons 7 and 8 harbor mutations in CTNNB1 gene in the respective exons. There is weak activation of β-catenin, glutamine synthetase, and leucine-rich repeat containing G-protein coupled receptor-5 (LGR5).

Group 4 (I-HCA): Inflammatory type is associated with activation of JAK/STAT pathway, and neoplasms may also harbor β-catenin mutations. High exposure to estrogen and obesity are major risk factors. There is clinical association with inflammatory syndrome, anaemia and fever. They are often misdiagnosed as focal nodular hyperplasia.

Group 5 (sh-HCA): Sonic hedgehog type is characterized by activation of sonic hedgehog signaling. Obesity and estrogen exposure are major risk factors. They are associated with a higher risk of bleeding.

Group 6 (unclassified HCA): Cases that do not fit into groups 1 through 5.

In addition, adenomas of the unclassified and inflammatory types (groups 4 and 6) may reveal immunohistochemical expression of arginosuccinate synthetase 1 and arginosuccinate lyase. These tumors are associated with a higher risk of bleeding.[67–70]

Focal nodular hyperplasia

The polyclonal nature of focal nodular hyperplasia has been described using the human androgen receptor test. However, the expression of angiopoietin genes ANGPT1 and ANFPT2 involved in blood vessel maturation is increased. The activation of the β-catenin pathway at the RNA and protein levels leads to an increased expression of glutamine synthetase. However, there is no mutation of the CTNNB1 gene and, therefore, no aberrant β-catenin immunostaining.[70]

Premalignant and Early Malignant Hepatocellular Lesions

Mutations of telomerase reverse transcriptase (TERT promoter) are considered to be the earliest genetic change in tumorigenesis. They are found in low- and high-grade dysplasia, premalignant lesions in cirrhosis, and in HCC. There is a resultant, increased expression of TERT, which encodes enzymes for telomere elongation and maintenance, thereby resulting in enhanced cell survival. β-Catenin mutation occurs relatively early in hepatitis C virus infection. LOH, chromosomal imbalance, and DNA methylation occur at an earlier stage and at a lower level than in HCC.[70]

Hepatocellular Carcinoma

Epidemiology

HCC usually develops in the setting of chronic liver disease, particularly in patients with chronic hepatitis B and C virus infection.[4]

Pathophysiology and molecular genetics

HCC is heterogenous and variable at morphologic, genetic, and molecular levels, and defies sole reliability on molecular findings for precise classification. The current approach of staging, grading, and morphologic subtyping provides reliable information required by various management guidelines. Two major mutually exclusive subtypes of HCC are classified by CTNNB1 and p53 mutations. Tumors with CTNNB1 mutations are associated with nuclear β-catenin staining, high glutamate synthetase expression, and downregulation of the interleukin (IL)-6/JAK-STAT pathway. They are larger well-differentiated tumors with microtrabecular and pseudoglandular architecture. The tumors are cholestatic and are not associated with significant inflammatory infiltrate. Tumors with p53 mutations are associated with activation of the PI3K/AKT pathway. They are poorly differentiated, highly proliferative, massive tumors with macrotrabecular architecture, and pleomorphic histology, often with sarcomatous and multinucleated components. They have a high propensity for both macrovascular and microvascular invasion. In addition, somatic mutations involving TERT are frequent genetic alterations in dysplastic nodules and HCC.[71,72]

The molecular findings in various subtypes of HCC are described.

Scirrhous HCC: TSC1 and TSC2 genes are involved, along with pathway for epithelial to mesenchymal transition (transforming growth factor-β, VIM) and PI3/AKT pathway activation. There is upregulation of cancer stem cell genes (CD24, KRT19, Thy1, CD133). CK19 expression is enhanced. There is a lack of CTNNB1 activation.

Steatohepatitic HCC: There is IL-6/JAK-STAT involvement along with immunohistochemical expression of C-reactive protein. Also, it is characterized by lack of Wnt/ β-catenin pathway activation.

Macrotrabecular massive variant of HCC: There are Tp53 mutations, FGF19 amplifications, ATM mutations, angiogenesis activation consisting of upregulation of ANGPT2, and vascular endothelial growth factor A expression.

Carcinosarcoma: There is Tp53 involvement in both carcinoma and sarcoma part, PIK3CA involvement in HCC, and FGFR3 involvement in sarcoma.

Fibrolamellar HCC: There is activation of protein kinase A resulting from microdeletion on Chr 19. It leads to fusion between the DNAJB1 gene and the PRKACA gene.

Chromophobe HCC: It is associated with alternative lengthening of telomeres, where tumor cells maintain telomeres by a telomere-independent mechanism that involves homologous recombination of telomeres.

HCC–cholangiocarcinoma (CCA): Wnt/β -catenin and transforming growth factor- β signaling are reported to be significantly activated in mixed HCC–CCA when compared with progenitor-like HCC. It shares higher frequency of TERT promoter mutations and lower frequency of KRAS and IDH 1/2 mutations with HCC. High level amplifications of 11q13 harboring oncogenes CCND1 and FGF19 have been reported. CXCL12-CXCR4 pathway for chemoattraction of myeloid and lymphoid cells is upregulated. Pathways enriched in intrahepatic CCA component-associated aberrations include promitotic DNA replication related signaling, proliferative signals MYC and mTOR, proinflammatory pathway interferon-γ and downstream IL2/STAT5.

HCC with stem cell features: Stem cell subclass is associated with MYC, mTOR, and NOTCH signaling pathway. Other upregulated pathway includes insulin-like growth factor 2 and genes implicated in liver progenitor cells (PROX1, HNF-1β, FOXA1, FOXA3).[71–73]

Role of PD-L1 in immunotherapy of hepatocellular carcinoma

PD-L1 tumoral expression is observed in 16% of HCC in accordance with recent reports. Accurate scoring of PD-L1 protein expression is complex owing to technical and biological pitfalls. Also, objective responses to immune check point inhibitors in clinical trials are not related to PD-L1 expression on tumor cells. The identification of accurate predictive markers and/or immune classifiers to select ideal candidates for immunotherapy are still in the pipeline, because multiple cancer pathways interact to modulate the immune profiles of tumors.[74]

Role of microRNA in hepatocellular carcinoma

Differential expression of microRNA (miRNA) in HCC have varied significance. Hepatitis B virus infection in HCC is associated with differential expression of miR-106a. miR-515, -518a, -3p, -520f, -525 and -3p are selectively overexpressed in HCC in comparison with cirrhosis. miR-519d and -525-3p are overexpressed in HCC versus dysplasia. miR-214 is downregulated in HCC versus non-tumor tissue. The lower expression of miR-21 and -148a is associated with better patient outcomes, with miR-21 being an independent prognostic factor for the same. Low levels of expression of miR-3607 and high levels of expression of miR-182, miR-18a, miR-21, miR-221, and miR-25 are associated with a poor prognosis. Downregulation of miR-214 is associated with early recurrence, shorter overall survival, stem cell-like traits, and cancer cell invasion. A reduction in the expression of miR-122 and -29a-5p is associated with early tumor recurrence. High expression of miR-155, -15a, -486-3p, -15b and -30b is associated with shorter recurrence-free survivals.[75,76]

Treatment

HCAs are treated with resection. The only curative therapy for HCC is surgical resection or liver transplantation. For advanced stage disease, survival remains limited. Newer targeted therapies are being developed with an increasing understanding of the molecular mechanisms of the disease.

Hepatoblastoma

There are numerous complex genetic alterations in hepatoblastomas, the most common of which is Wnt/β-catenin signaling among the sporadic tumors. The cell cycle and check point control perturbations include polo like kinase-1 (PLK1 oncogene), p16, p27, and p53. Additionally identified mutations include CAPRIN2, and the tumor suppressors SPOP, OR5I1, and CDC20B. There is alteration in the insulin-like growth factor 2 regulator PLAG1 as well.[77]

Cholangiocarcinoma

Epidemiology

CCA is the second most common primary hepatic neoplasm, and its incidence has increased within the past 3 decades. Worldwide, the average age at presentation is 50 years, with the highest prevalence seen in Southeast Asia. Although several risk factors have been identified, including primary sclerosing cholangitis and chronic biliary tract inflammation, most patients with CCA have no identifiable risk factors.[4]

Clinical features

Cholangiocarcinomas become symptomatic when the tumor obstructs the biliary system, causing painless jaundice, pruritus, right upper quadrant abdominal pain, weight loss, and fever.

Molecular aberrations

The most common alterations in CCA include the epidermal growth factor receptor–mitogen-activated protein kinase–PI3K pathway. KRAS mutations are also highly prevalent. BRAF are mutually exclusive with RAS alterations and less frequent. PIK3CA are more common in ECC (extrahepatic CCA) and gallbladder carcinoma. HER-2 amplification is most common in gallbladder cancer (**Fig. 2**).[78] The tumors otherwise are heterogenous and lack stereotype signatures. The distinct stem cell niches and variable risk factors contribute to the variability and make therapeutic targeting extremely challenging. Critical epigenetic events and deficient apoptosis have significant contributory role. IL-6 signaling is one of the major pathways involved in the proliferation of cells and progression of malignancy. The IL-6 receptor subunit gp130 is overexpressed by the CCA cells. Stimulation by IL-6 upregulates the antiapoptotic proteins bcl-2 and mcl-1, enhances telomerase activity to evade cell senescence, and activates p44/p42 and p38 MAP kinases. There is significant upregulation of p53 and mdm-2, leading to loss of cell cycle control. Increased expression of the cell cycle modulating proteins p16, p21, and p27 is associated with aggressive cholangiocarcinomas. Differential expression of p16, bcl-2, and p53 between intrahepatic and extrahepatic CCA is reported, with p16 and bcl-2 being significantly expressed in intrahepatic tumors, whereas p53 is

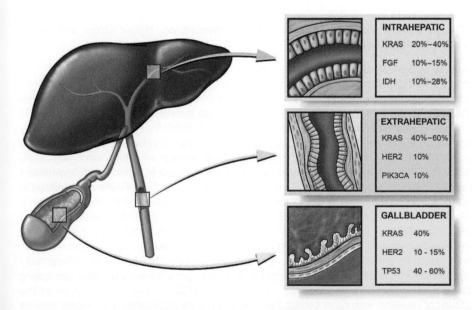

INTRAHEPATIC	
KRAS	20%–40%
FGF	10%–15%
IDH	10%–28%

EXTRAHEPATIC	
KRAS	40%–60%
HER2	10%
PIK3CA	10%

GALLBLADDER	
KRAS	40%
HER2	10 - 15%
TP53	40 - 60%

CCF
2015

Fig. 2. Molecular aberrations in biliary cancer. (*From* Sohal DPS, Shrotriya S, Abazeed M, et al. Molecular characteristics of biliary tract cancer. Crit Rev Oncol Hematol 2016;107:113; with permission.)

more frequently expressed in extrahepatic tumors. In addition, p16 has significant prognostic value, regulates the cyclin D1 pathway, and shows a relationship with lymph node metastasis.[78–84]

Pathophysiology and molecular genetics of intrahepatic cholangiocarcinoma

The other frequent mutations in intrahepatic CCA include BAP1, ARID1A, and PBRM1 involved in chromatin remodeling. Isocitrate dehydrogenase 1 (IDH1) or IDH2 (IDH1/2) mutations are significantly higher (10%–23%) in cholangiocellular carcinoma than in other mass forming or non–mass-forming intrahepatic tumors, extrahepatic or gallbladder cholangiocarcinomas. Mutant IDH genes block liver progenitor cells from undergoing hepatocytic differentiation and drive cholangiocytic differentiation through production of 2-hydroxyglutarate and suppression of HNF 4α. The liver fluke-associated CCAs are most commonly associated with p53 mutation. Fibroblast growth factor receptor produce fibroblast growth factor receptor fusion genes in both intrahepatic CCA and ECC, but are more frequent in intrahepatic CCA (6%–50%) than ECC (0%–6%). The fusion protein is constitutively activated leading to downstream signaling through mitogen activated protein kinase and PI3K/mTOR pathways. Angiogenesis-associated vascular endothelial growth factor expression is reported in around 30% to 40% of CCA and correlates with increased lymph node metastasis and poor survival. ROS1 mutations are associated with 8% to 9%, KRAS with 9% to 47% and BRAF with 0% to 22% tumors.[81–83] Downregulation of β-catenin, seen in high-grade tumors, correlates with reduced immunohistochemical staining. Decreased p27 is associated with more aggressive tumor behavior and increased risk of vascular invasion. Downregulation of BCL2 is also associated with more aggressive tumors.[84–88]

PD-L1 expression in cholangiocarcinoma

PD-L1 expression is associated with poor differentiation, higher stage, and higher levels of CD8+ T cells.[83]

Role of microRNA in cholangiocarcinoma

miR-21, -141, -200b, -150 are overexpressed in CCA cells. miRNA-148 and -152 regulate DNA methyltransferase expression, result in DNA hypermethylation, and promote the silencing of tumor suppressor genes. Reduced expression of miR-29b results in the upregulation of the antiapoptotic protein MCL-1. miRNA-494 induces G1/S transition through the downregulation of CDK6. miRNA levels can be used to discriminate patients with CCA from controls. miR-150 is a biomarker with high accuracy. miR-192 and -21 together have a stronger diagnostic significance. Differentially expressed miRNA in blood include miR-21, -26a, −122, and −150. A few miRNAs are involved in epithelial-mesenchymal transition, the key factor in metastases with validated targets. They include miR-34a (SMAD4), miR-221, -92a, −19a −21 (PTEN), miR-200b, −200c (ROCK2, ZEB1), miR-204 (Slug), miR-214 (Twist), and miR-29a (HDAC4). A microvesicle-based panel consisting of miR-191, miR-486-3p, miR-16, and miR-484 was used to evaluate bile for the presence of CCA. Other miRNA differentially expressed in the bile of patients with CCA versus patients with primary sclerosing cholangitis include miR-412, -640, −1537, and −3189. Lower miRNA levels in the serum of patients with CCA versus those with primary sclerosing cholangitis include miR-1281, -126, −26a, −30b, and −122. miR-21 is increased in patients with CCA and associated with a more advanced clinical stage. miR-192 is also associated with advanced disease and poor prognosis. miR-106a is downregulated in intrahepatic CCA and associated with advanced disease and a poor prognosis. Resistance to gemcitabine is associated with miR-21, -200b, −21, Let-7a, −29b, −205, −221,

−664b, −3651, −6087, and −181c. Resistance to 5-fluoracil is associated with differential expression of miR-200b and −320. Resistance to TRAIL is associated with the differential expression of miR-25 and -29b.[88-92]

Summary

Although the described genetic changes can lead to detectable phenotypic changes, the diagnostic or prognostic usefulness of these developments is unclear, and molecular profiling does not yet have an established clinical role in patients with CCA.

GALLBLADDER AND EXTRAHEPATIC BILIARY TRACT NEOPLASMS
Epidemiology

Gallbladder carcinoma, the most frequent malignancy of the biliary tract, has a female predominance. The mean age at diagnosis is 72 years. Gallstones and inflammation are responsible for most biliary tract abnormalities.[93]

Clinical features

Gallbladder adenomas produce symptoms when they are multiple, large, or detached. Adenomas of the extrahepatic biliary tract are usually discovered incidentally, or patients may present with symptoms of obstruction. Advanced stage gallbladder carcinoma presents with right upper quadrant pain, weight loss, and anorexia, but for early stage tumors, symptoms at presentation can mimic those of chronic cholecystitis. Jaundice is not common at presentation.[4]

Pathophysiology and Molecular Genetics

Adenoma

Alterations in adenomas are distinct from those observed in conventional dysplasia carcinoma sequence of the gallbladder. β-Catenin mutations are detected in 58% of adenomas, and are rare in invasive cancer. TP53 mutations are rare in adenomas but are common in flat dysplasia and invasive carcinoma. KRAS mutations are detected in approximately 25% of adenomas.[93,94]

Dysplasia/carcinoma in situ

LOH of 5q is an early change, and LOH of 3p and 9p is related to progression of gallbladder carcinoma. LOH of 13q and 18q is likely to be a late event.[88] Decreased fragile histidine triad and LOH occurs at higher frequencies with increasing severity of histologic changes.[95]

Adenocarcinoma

Data support the hypothesis that adenomas and carcinomas of the gallbladder arise from distinct molecular pathways. Protein p53 overexpression is detected in approximately 50% of cases, with the highest frequency in distal common bile duct tumors.[95] KRAS and DPC4 mutations increase in frequency from low in proximal to high in distal bile duct tumors, and lower than in pancreatic tumors.[96,97] Her-2/neu (c-erB2) amplification is noted in 70% of biliary cancers with no known correlation with prognosis.[79] Epidermal growth factor receptor is found to be a negative predictor of overall survival in CCA. Human epidermal growth factor receptor 2 (Her-2) is rare in intrahepatic CCA but may be present in 20% of ECC.[83]

Data suggest that methylation is a frequent event in cholangiocarcinomas; the methylation status of the markers mentioned earlier may serve as a prognostic marker. Overall survival was reported poorer in patients with CpG island methylation of APC, p16, and TIMP3 than in those without methylation.[98,99]

Cell-free nucleic acid analysis Although solid tissue based analysis has been the mainstay of gastrointestinal cancer diagnosis, interrogation of cell-free DNA in fluids including serum, plasma, urine, and spinal fluid has proven beneficial for diagnosis and prognosis of these disease states.[100–103] Promoter hypermethylation analysis of 28 genes and TNM tumor staging for pancreatic cancer were assessed and showed that select genes (SEPT9v2, SST, ALX4, CDKN2B, HIC1, MLH1, NEUROG1, and BNC1) enabled the differentiation of stage IV from stage I through III disease (area under the curve of 0.87; cutpoint of 0.55; sensitivity of 74%; specificity of 87%) in pancreatic adenocarcinoma.[101] Other hypermethylated genes reported included (BMP3, RASSF1A, BNC1, MESTv2, TFPI2, APC, SFRP1, and SFRP2).[102] Gene panel analysis rather than single gene interrogation seem to have improved statistical power as potential disease predictors.[104] KRAS mutation in pancreatic cancer had poorer overall survival.[105] Circulating noncoding miRNA have also been assessed for their diagnostic value in pancreatic adenocarcinoma. To this end, plasma miRNA including miR-210, miR-21, miR-155, and miR-196a among others were found to be upregulated, whereas miR-375 has been found to be downregulated in pancreatic cancer cells and could be associated disease diagnosis and/or prognosis.[106] Interestingly, serum-derived miR-155, and miR-196a were found to be downregulated in contrast with plasma[106]; whether these differences were due to specimen type, methodology, and/or patient cohort is not clear. Hu and colleagues[107] reported that loss of miR-1258 contributes to carcinogenesis and progression of liver cancer and poor patient survival. Further studies into the development of liquid biopsy such as cell-free nucleic acid analysis could provide many benefits for patients with pancreatic cancer in addition to other malignancies.

SUMMARY

Although the described genetic changes in the neoplasms of the pancreas, liver, gallbladder, and extrahepatic biliary tract lead to detectable phenotypic changes, their diagnostic and prognostic significance, and usefulness for targeted therapy are still under investigation. PD-L1 expression and immunotherapy do not play a significant role in patient management to date.

REFERENCES

1. Siegel RL, Miller KD, Jemal A. Cancer statistics, 2018. CA Cancer J Clin 2018; 68(1):7–30.
2. Matrisian LM, Berlin JD. The past, present, and future of pancreatic cancer clinical trials. Am Soc Clin Oncol Educ Book 2016;35:e205–215.
3. Hruban RH, Boffetta P, Hiraoka N, et al. Ductal adenocarcinoma of the pancreas. In: Bosman FT, Carneiro F, Hruban RH, et al, editors. World Health Organization classification of tumours of the digestive system. 4th edition. Lyon (France): International Agency for Research on Cancer; 2010. p. 279–337.
4. Klimstra DS, Adsay NV. Tumors of the pancreas. In: Odze RD, Goldblum JR, editors. Odze and Goldblum surgical pathology of the GI tract, liver, biliary tract and pancreas. 3rd edition. Philadelphia: Expertconsult, Saunders Elsevier; 2014. p. 1081–119.
5. Klein AP. Genetic susceptibility to pancreatic cancer. Mol Carcinog 2012;51(1): 14–24.
6. Amundadottir LT. Pancreatic cancer genetics. Int J Biol Sci 2016;12(3): 314–25.
7. Petersen GM. Familial pancreatic cancer. Semin Oncol 2016;43(5):548–53.

8. Flejou JF. WHO classification of digestive tumors: the fourth edition. Ann Pathol 2011;31(5 Suppl):S27–31 [in French].

9. Biankin AV, Waddell N, Kassahn KS, et al. Pancreatic cancer genomes reveal aberrations in axon guidance pathway genes. Nature 2012;491(7424):399–405.

10. Cancer Genome Atlas Research Network. Electronic address: andrew_aguir-re@dfci.harvard.edu, Cancer Genome Atlas Research Network. Integrated genomic characterization of pancreatic ductal adenocarcinoma. Cancer Cell 2017;32(2):185–203.e13.

11. Jones S, Zhang X, Parsons DW, et al. Core signaling pathways in human pancreatic cancers revealed by global genomic analyses. Science 2008; 321(5897):1801–6.

12. Waddell N, Pajic M, Patch AM, et al. Whole genomes redefine the mutational landscape of pancreatic cancer. Nature 2015;518(7540):495–501.

13. Almoguera C, Shibata D, Forrester K, et al. Most human carcinomas of the exocrine pancreas contain mutant c-K-ras genes. Cell 1988;53(4):549–54.

14. Hruban RH, van Mansfeld AD, Offerhaus GJ, et al. K-ras oncogene activation in adenocarcinoma of the human pancreas. A study of 82 carcinomas using a combination of mutant-enriched polymerase chain reaction analysis and allele-specific oligonucleotide hybridization. Am J Pathol 1993;143(2):545–54.

15. Bailey P, Chang DK, Nones K, et al. Genomic analyses identify molecular sub-types of pancreatic cancer. Nature 2016;531(7592):47–52.

16. Moskaluk CA, Hruban RH, Kern SE. p16 and K-ras gene mutations in the intraductal precursors of human pancreatic adenocarcinoma. Cancer Res 1997;57(11):2140–3.

17. Jimenez RE, Warshaw AL, Z'Graggen K, et al. Sequential accumulation of K-ras mutations and p53 overexpression in the progression of pancreatic mucinous cystic neoplasms to malignancy. Ann Surg 1999;230(4):501–9.

18. Wilentz RE, Iacobuzio-Donahue CA, Argani P, et al. Loss of expression of Dpc4 in pancreatic intraepithelial neoplasia: evidence that DPC4 inactivation occurs late in neoplastic progression. Cancer Res 2000;60(7):2002–6.

19. Biankin AV, Biankin SA, Kench JG, et al. Aberrant p16(INK4A) and DPC4/Smad4 expression in intraductal papillary mucinous tumours of the pancreas is associ-ated with invasive ductal adenocarcinoma. Gut 2002;50(6):861–8.

20. Lacobuzio-Donahue CA, Klimstra DS, Adsay NV, et al. Dpc-4 protein is ex-pressed in virtually all human intraductal papillary mucinous neoplasms of the pancreas: comparison with conventional ductal adenocarcinomas. Am J Pathol 2000;157(3):755–61.

21. Lacobuzio-Donahue CA, Wilentz RE, Argani P, et al. Dpc4 protein in mucinous cystic neoplasms of the pancreas: frequent loss of expression in invasive carci-nomas suggests a role in genetic progression. Am J Surg Pathol 2000;24(11): 1544–8.

22. Springer S, Wang Y, Dal Molin M, et al. A combination of molecular markers and clinical features improve the classification of pancreatic cysts. Gastroenterology 2015;149(6):1501–10.

23. Lee JH, Kim Y, Choi JW, et al. KRAS, GNAS, and RNF43 mutations in intraductal papillary mucinous neoplasm of the pancreas: a meta-analysis. Springerplus 2016;5(1):1172.

24. Sakamoto H, Kuboki Y, Hatori T, et al. Clinicopathological significance of so-matic RNF43 mutation and aberrant expression of ring finger protein 43 in intra-ductal papillary mucinous neoplasms of the pancreas. Mod Pathol 2015;28(2): 261–7.

25. DiMaio CJ, Kim MK. Adjunctive molecular analysis of pancreatic cyst fluid to determine malignant potential. Gastroenterology 2015;149(1):249–51.
26. Li F, Malli A, Cruz-Monserrate Z, et al. Confocal endomicroscopy and cyst fluid molecular analysis: comprehensive evaluation of pancreatic cysts. World J Gastrointest Endosc 2018;10(1):1–9.
27. Shen J, Brugge WR, Dimaio CJ, et al. Molecular analysis of pancreatic cyst fluid: a comparative analysis with current practice of diagnosis. Cancer 2009;117(3): 217–27.
28. Chmielecki J, Hutchinson KE, Frampton GM, et al. Comprehensive genomic profiling of pancreatic acinar cell carcinomas identifies recurrent RAF fusions and frequent inactivation of DNA repair genes. Cancer Discov 2014;4(12): 1398–405.
29. Jiao L, Bondy ML, Hassan MM, et al. Selected polymorphisms of DNA repair genes and risk of pancreatic cancer. Cancer Detect Prev 2006;30(3):284–91.
30. Zhao F, Shang Y, Zeng C, et al. Association of single nucleotide polymorphisms of DNA repair genes in NER pathway and susceptibility to pancreatic cancer. Int J Clin Exp Pathol 2015;8(9):11579–86.
31. Cloyd JM, Katz MG, Wang H, et al. Clinical and genetic implications of DNA mismatch repair deficiency in patients with pancreatic ductal adenocarcinoma. JAMA Surg 2017;152(11):1086–8.
32. Capelli P, Martignoni G, Pedica F, et al. Endocrine neoplasms of the pancreas: pathologic and genetic features. Arch Pathol Lab Med 2009;133(3):350–64.
33. Maia MCDF, Muniz Lourenço D Jr, Riechelmann R. Efficacy and long-term safety of everolimus in pancreatic neuroendocrine tumor associated with multiple endocrine neoplasia type I: case report. Oncol Res Treat 2016;39(10):643–5.
34. Jiao Y, Shi C, Edil BH, et al. DAXX/ATRX, MEN1, and mTOR pathway genes are frequently altered in pancreatic neuroendocrine tumors. Science 2011; 331(6021):1199–203.
35. Klimstra DS, Modlin IR, Coppola D, et al. The pathologic classification of neuroendocrine tumors: a review of nomenclature, grading, and staging systems. Pancreas 2010;39(6):707–12.
36. Marinoni I, Kurrer AS, Vassella E, et al. Loss of DAXX and ATRX are associated with chromosome instability and reduced survival of patients with pancreatic neuroendocrine tumors. Gastroenterology 2014;146(2):453–60.e5.
37. Yachida S, Vakiani E, White CM, et al. Small cell and large cell neuroendocrine carcinomas of the pancreas are genetically similar and distinct from well-differentiated pancreatic neuroendocrine tumors. Am J Surg Pathol 2012; 36(2):173–84.
38. Gortz B, Roth J, Krahenmann A, et al. Mutations and allelic deletions of the MEN1 gene are associated with a subset of sporadic endocrine pancreatic and neuroendocrine tumors and not restricted to foregut neoplasms. Am J Pathol 1999;154(2):429–36.
39. Hessman O, Lindberg D, Einarsson A, et al. Genetic alterations on 3p, 11q13, and 18q in nonfamilial and MEN 1-associated pancreatic endocrine tumors. Genes Chromosomes Cancer 1999;26(3):258–64.
40. Komminoth P. Review: multiple endocrine neoplasia type 1, sporadic neuroendocrine tumors, and MENIN. Diagn Mol Pathol 1999;8(3):107–12.
41. Moore PS, Missiaglia E, Antonello D, et al. Role of disease-causing genes in sporadic pancreatic endocrine tumors: MEN1 and VHL. Genes Chromosomes Cancer 2001;32(2):177–81.

42. Arnold CN, Sosnowski A, Schmitt-Gräff A, et al. Analysis of molecular pathways in sporadic neuroendocrine tumors of the gastro-entero-pancreatic system. Int J Cancer 2007;120(10):2157–64.

43. de Wilde RF, Edil BH, Hruban RH, et al. Well-differentiated pancreatic neuroendocrine tumors: from genetics to therapy. Nat Rev Gastroenterol Hepatol 2012; 9(4):199–208.

44. Pea A, Hruban RH, Wood LD. Genetics of pancreatic neuroendocrine tumors: implications for the clinic. Expert Rev Gastroenterol Hepatol 2015;9(11): 1407–19.

45. Hoorens A, Lemoine NR, McLellan E, et al. Pancreatic acinar cell carcinoma. An analysis of cell lineage markers, p53 expression, and Ki-ras mutation. Am J Pathol 1993;143(3):685–98.

46. Abraham SC, Wu T-T, Hruban RH, et al. Genetic and immunohistochemical analysis of pancreatic acinar cell carcinoma. Am J Pathol 2002;160(3):953–62.

47. Furlan D, Sahnane N, Bernasconi B, et al. APC alterations are frequently involved in the pathogenesis of acinar cell carcinoma of the pancreas, mainly through gene loss and promoter hypermethylation. Virchows Arch 2014; 464(5):553–64.

48. La Rosa S, Bernasconi B, Frattini M, et al. TP53 alterations in pancreatic acinar cell carcinoma: new insights into the molecular pathology of this rare cancer. Virchows Arch 2016;468(3):289–96.

49. Tanaka Y, Kato K, Notohara K, et al. Frequent beta-catenin mutation and cytoplasmic/nuclear accumulation in pancreatic solid-pseudopapillary neoplasm. Cancer Res 2001;61(23):8401–4.

50. Abraham SC, Klimstra DS, Wilentz RE, et al. Solid-pseudopapillary tumors of the pancreas are genetically distinct from pancreatic ductal adenocarcinomas and almost always harbor beta-catenin mutations. Am J Pathol 2002;160(4):1361–9.

51. Chetty R, Serra S. Membrane loss and aberrant nuclear localization of E-cadherin are consistent features of solid pseudopapillary tumour of the pancreas. An immunohistochemical study using two antibodies recognizing different domains of the E-cadherin molecule. Histopathology 2008;52(3):325–30.

52. Wu J, Jiao Y, Dal Molin M, et al. Whole-exome sequencing of neoplastic cysts of the pancreas reveals recurrent mutations in components of ubiquitin-dependent pathways. Proc Natl Acad Sci U S A 2011;108(52):21188–93.

53. Abraham SC, Wu T-T, Klimstra DS, et al. Distinctive molecular genetic alterations in sporadic and familial adenomatous polyposis-associated pancreatoblastomas. Am J Pathol 2001;159(5):1619–27.

54. Sullivan MJ. Beckwith-Wiedemann syndrome, pancreatoblastoma, and the Wnt signaling pathway. Am J Pathol 2002;160(4):1541–2.

55. Kuboki Y, Shimizu K, Hatori T, et al. Molecular biomarkers for progression of intraductal papillary mucinous neoplasm of the pancreas. Pancreas 2015;44: 227–35.

56. Nissim S, Idos GE, Wu B. Genetic markers of malignant transformation in intraductal papillary mucinous neoplasm of pancreas: a meta-analysis. Pancreas 2012;41:1195–205.

57. Moris M, Dawson DW, Jiang J, et al. Plectin as a biomarker of malignant progression in intraductal papillary mucinous neoplasms. Pancreas 2016;45: 1353–8.

58. Nakazato T, Suzuki Y, Tanaka R, et al. Effect of reprimo down-regulation on malignant transformation of intraductal papillary mucinous neoplasm. Pancreas 2018;47:291–5.

59. Burris HA 3rd, Moore MJ, Andersen J, et al. Improvements in survival and clinical benefit with gemcitabine as first-line therapy for patients with advanced pancreas cancer: a randomized trial. J Clin Oncol 1997;15(6):2403–13.
60. Sun C, Ansari D, Andersson R, et al. Does gemcitabine-based combination therapy improve the prognosis of unresectable pancreatic cancer? World J Gastroenterol 2012;18(35):4944–58.
61. Conroy T, Desseigne F, Ychou M, et al. FOLFIRINOX versus gemcitabine for metastatic pancreatic cancer. N Engl J Med 2011;364(19):1817–25.
62. Von Hoff DD, Ervin T, Arena FP, et al. Increased survival in pancreatic cancer with nab-paclitaxel plus gemcitabine. N Engl J Med 2013;369(18):1691–703.
63. Brahmer JR, Tykodi SS, Chow LQM, et al. Safety and activity of anti–PD-L1 antibody in patients with advanced cancer. N Engl J Med 2012;366(26):2455–65.
64. Royal RE, Levy C, Turner K, et al. Phase 2 trial of single agent Ipilimumab (anti-CTLA-4) for locally advanced or metastatic pancreatic adenocarcinoma. J Immunother 2010;33(8):828–33.
65. Winograd R, Byrne KT, Evans RA, et al. Induction of T-cell immunity overcomes complete resistance to PD-1 and CTLA-4 blockade and improves survival in pancreatic carcinoma. Cancer Immunol Res 2015;3(4):399–411.
66. Thind K, Padrnos LJ, Ramanathan RK, et al. Immunotherapy in pancreatic cancer treatment: a new frontier. Therap Adv Gastroenterol 2017;10(1):168–94.
67. Zucman-Rossi J, Jeannot E, Nhieu JT, et al. Genotype-phenotype correlation in hepatocellular adenoma: new classification and relationship with HCC. Hepatology 2006;43(3):515–24.
68. Henriet E, Abou Hammoud A, Dupuy JW, et al. Arginosuccinate synthetase 1 (ASS1): a marker of unclassified hepatocellular Adenoma and high bleeding risk. Hepatology 2017;66(6):2016–28.
69. Nault JC, Paradis V, Cherqui D, et al. Molecular classification of hepatocellular adenoma in clinical practice. J Hepatol 2017;67:1074–83.
70. Bioulac-Sage P, Frulio N, Balabaud CP. Benign hepatocellular tumors. In: Saxena R, editor. Practical hepatic pathology: a diagnostic approach. 2nd edition. Philadelphia: Elsevier; 2018. p. 507–27.
71. Calderaro J, Couchy G, Imbeaud S, et al. Histological subtypes of hepatocellular carcinoma are related to gene mutations and molecular tumor classification. J Hepatol 2017;67:727–38.
72. Torbenson MS. Morphologic subtypes of hepatocellular carcinoma. Gastroenterol Clin North Am 2017;46:365–91.
73. Moeini A, Sia D, Zhang Z, et al. Mixed hepatocellular cholangiocarcinoma tumors: cholangiocellular carcinoma is a distinct molecular entity. J Hepatol 2017;66:952–61.
74. Sia D, Jiao Y, Martinez-Quetglas I, et al. Identification of an immune specific class of Hepatocellular Carcinoma, Based on molecular features. Gastroenterology 2017;153:812–26.
75. Tang S, Wu WK, Li X, et al. Stratification of digestive cancers with different pathological features and survival outcomes by MicroRNA expression. Sci Rep 2016;6:24466.
76. Lee SC, Tan HT, Chung MC. Prognostic biomarkers for prediction of recurrence of hepatocellular carcinoma: current status and future prospects. World J Gastroenterol 2014;20(12):3112–24.
77. Zimmerman A. Liver tumors of childhood. In: Saxena R, editor. Practical hepatic pathology: a diagnostic approach. 2nd edition. Philadelphia: Elsevier; 2018. p. 555–82.

78. Sohal DP, Shrotriya S, Abazeed M, et al. Molecular characteristics of biliary tract cancer. Crit Rev Oncol Hematol 2016;107:111–8.
79. Brandi G, Farioli A, Astolfi A, et al. Genetic heterogeneity in cholangiocarcinoma: a major challenge for targeted therapies. Oncotarget 2015;6(17):14744–53.
80. Rizvi S, Borad MJ, Patel T, et al. Cholangiocarcinoma: molecular pathways and therapeutic opportunities. Semin Liver Dis 2014;34(4):456–64.
81. Goodman ZD, Terracciano LM, Wee A. Tumors and tumor like lesions of the liver. In: Burt AD, Portmann BC, Ferrell LD, editors. MacSween's pathology of the liver. 6th edition. Philadelphia: Churchill Livingstone, Elsevier; 2012. p. 761–851.
82. Maemura K, Natsugoe S, Takao S. Molecular mechanism of cholangiocarcinoma carcinogenesis. J Hepatobiliary Pancreat Sci 2014;21(10):754–60.
83. Kayhanian H, Smyth EC, Braconi C. Emerging molecular targets and therapy for cholangiocarcinoma. World J Gastrointest Oncol 2017;9(7):268–80.
84. Karamitopoulou E, Tornillo L, Zlobec I, et al. Clinical significance of cell cycle- and apoptosis-related markers in biliary tract cancer: a tissue microarray-based approach revealing a distinctive immunophenotype for intrahepatic and extrahepatic cholangiocarcinomas. Am J Clin Pathol 2008;130(5):780–6.
85. Sugimachi K, Taguchi K, Aishima S, et al. Altered expression of beta-catenin without genetic mutation in intrahepatic cholangiocarcinoma. Mod Pathol 2001;14(9):900–5.
86. Ashida K, Terada T, Kitamura Y, et al. Expression of E-cadherin, alpha-catenin, beta-catenin, and CD44 (standard and variant isoforms) in human cholangiocarcinoma: an immunohistochemical study. Hepatology 1998;27(4):974–82.
87. Taguchi K, Aishima S, Asayama Y, et al. The role of p27kip1 protein expression on the biological behavior of intrahepatic cholangiocarcinoma. Hepatology 2001;33(5):1118–23.
88. Ito Y, Takeda T, Sasaki Y, et al. Bcl-2 expression in cholangiocellular carcinoma is inversely correlated with biologically aggressive phenotypes. Oncology 2000;59(1):63–7.
89. Li L, Masica D, Ishida M, et al. Human bile contains microRNA-laden extracellular vesicles that can be used for cholangiocarcinoma diagnosis. Hepatology 2014;60:896–907.
90. Voigtländer T, Gupta SK, Thum S, et al. MicroRNAs in serum and bile of patients with primary sclerosing cholangitis and/or cholangiocarcinoma. PLoS One 2015;10:e0139305.
91. Zhou J, Liu Z, Yang S, et al. Identification of microRNAs as biomarkers for cholangiocarcinoma detection: a diagnostic meta-analysis. Clin Res Hepatol Gastroenterol 2017;41:156–62.
92. Puik JR, Meijer LL, Large Le, et al. miRNA profiling for diagnosis, prognosis, and stratification of cancer treatment in cholangiocarcinoma. Pharmacogenomics 2017;18(14):1343–58.
93. Volkan Adsay N, Klimstra DS. Benign and malignant tumors of the gallbladder and extrahepatic biliary tract. In: Odze RD, Goldblum JR, editors. Surgical pathology of the GI tract, liver, biliary tract and pancreas. 2nd edition. Philadelphia: Saunders/Elsevier; 2009. p. 1021–54.
94. Chang HJ, Jee CD, Kim WH. Mutation and altered expression of beta-catenin during gallbladder carcinogenesis. Am J Surg Pathol 2002;26(6):758–66.
95. Chang HJ, Kim SW, Kim YT, et al. Loss of heterozygosity in dysplasia and carcinoma of the gallbladder. Mod Pathol 1999;12(8):763–9.

96. Wistuba II, Ashfaq R, Maitra A, et al. Fragile histidine triad gene abnormalities in the pathogenesis of gallbladder carcinoma. Am J Pathol 2002;160(6):2073–9.
97. Batheja N, Suriawinata A, Saxena R, et al. Expression of p53 and PCNA in cholangiocarcinoma and primary sclerosing cholangitis. Mod Pathol 2000;13(12): 1265–8.
98. Argani P, Shaukat A, Kaushal M, et al. Differing rates of loss of DPC4 expression and of p53 overexpression among carcinomas of the proximal and distal bile ducts. Cancer 2001;91(7):1332–41.
99. Nagahashi M, Ajioka Y, Lang I, et al. Genetic changes of p53, K-ras, and microsatellite instability in gallbladder carcinoma in high-incidence areas of Japan and Hungary. World J Gastroenterol 2008;14(1):70–5.
100. Vietsch EE, Graham GT, McCutcheon JN, et al. Circulating cell-free DNA mutation patterns in early and late stage colon and pancreatic cancer. Cancer Genet 2017;218-219:39–50.
101. Henriksen SD, Madsen PH, Larsen AC, et al. Promoter hypermethylation in plasma-derived cell-free DNA as a prognostic marker for pancreatic adenocarcinoma staging. Int J Cancer 2017;141:2489–97.
102. Henriksen SD, Madsen PH, Larsen AC, et al. Cell-free DNA promoter hypermethylation in plasma as a diagnostic marker for pancreatic adenocarcinoma. Clin Epigenetics 2016;8:117.
103. Shi XQ, Xue WH, Zhao SF, et al. Dynamic tracing for epidermal growth factor receptor mutations in urinary circulating DNA in gastric cancer patients. Tumour Biol 2017;39. 1010428317691681.
104. Henriksen SD, Madsen PH, Krarup H, et al. DNA hypermethylation as a blood-based marker for pancreatic cancer: a literature review. Pancreas 2015;44: 1036–45.
105. Zhuang R, Li S, Li Q, et al. The prognostic value of KRAS mutation by cell-free DNA in cancer patients: a systematic review and meta-analysis. PLoS One 2017;12:e0182562.
106. Imamura T, Komatsu S, Ichikawa D, et al. Liquid biopsy in patients with pancreatic cancer: circulating tumor cells and cell-free nucleic acids. World J Gastroenterol 2016;22:5627–41.
107. Hu M, Wang M, Lu H, et al. Loss of miR-1258 contributes to carcinogenesis and progression of liver cancer through targeting CDC28 protein kinase regulatory subunit 1B. Oncotarget 2016;7:43419–31.

An Update Regarding the Molecular Genetics of Melanocytic Neoplasms and the Current Applications of Molecular Genetic Technologies in Their Diagnosis and Treatment

Katrin Kiavash, MD[a,b], Martin H. Bluth, MD, PhD[a,c,d],
Andrew David Thompson, MD, PhD[a,b],*

KEYWORDS

- Melanoma • Spitz tumor • Fluorescence in situ hybridization
- Comparative genomic hybridization • Next-generation sequencing
- Cell-free nucleic acid analysis • Programmed death receptor

KEY POINTS

- Molecular genetic technologies are currently used to aid in the diagnosis and treatment of borderline melanocytic tumors as an adjuvant tool to the gold standard histopathologic evaluation.
- New melanoma probe cocktails targeting RREB1 (6p25), C-MYC (8q24), CDKN2A (9p21), and CCND1 (11q13) have revealed increased sensitivity and specificity in ambiguous melanocytic cases.
- Cutting-edge technologies, including next-generation sequencing and cell-free nucleic acid analysis, are promising time-effective and cost-effective biomarker applications for mutation detection.
- DNA sequence analysis allows personalized use of the newest generation of antimelanoma therapies, including inhibitory molecules targeting the mitogen-activated protein kinase pathway and monoclonal antibodies targeting immune checkpoint molecules.

This article has been updated from a version previously published in Clinics in Laboratory Medicine, Volume 33, Issue 4, December 2013.
[a] Department of Pathology, Wayne State University, 4160 John R Street, Detroit, MI 48201, USA; [b] Department of Pathology and Laboratory Medicine, Detroit Medical Center University Laboratories, 4160 John R Street, Detroit, MI 48201, USA; [c] Department of Pathology, Wayne State University, School of Medicine, 540 East Canfield Street, Detroit, MI 48201, USA; [d] Pathology Laboratories, Michigan Surgical Hospital, 21230 Dequindre Road, Warren, MI 48091, USA
* Corresponding author. Department of Pathology, Wayne State University, 4160 John R Street, Detroit, MI 48201.
E-mail address: athompso2@dmc.org

Clin Lab Med 38 (2018) 385–399
https://doi.org/10.1016/j.cll.2018.02.002
0272-2712/18/© 2018 Elsevier Inc. All rights reserved.

INTRODUCTION

Neoplastic transformation of cells results in part from genetic mutations that lead to abnormal proliferation and clonal expansion. Genetic changes continue to accumulate and ultimately lead to invasion of surrounding tissues and metastasis to distant organs. Genes involved in neoplastic transformation usually regulate cell proliferation and survival, cellular motility, and differentiation.

Melanocytes are pigment-producing cells in the skin that, after embryologic migration, are normally located at the dermoepidermal junction and within hair follicles. Nevi is the accepted nomenclature for benign melanocytic neoplasms. Melanomas, on the other hand, are highly aggressive cancers. There are other melanocytic lesions that are not as clear-cut and have clinical or/and histopathologic features of both melanoma and nevi, causing diagnostic uncertainty. Dysplastic nevi and atypical nevi are terms used to describe lesions with concerning histologic and/or clinical features. Diagnostic controversies are especially common regarding a subgroup of melanocytic neoplasms called Spitzoid tumors, which can be viewed as a spectrum extending from Spitz nevus to Spitzoid melanoma, with intermediate stages, including atypical Spitzoid tumors of uncertain malignant potential (STUMPs).[1]

Melanoma is a heterogeneous disease genetically; it is associated with various combinations of genomic alterations that allow deregulated melanocytic proliferation. Since identification of NRAS as the first oncogene in melanoma in 1984,[2] significant progress has been made in understanding genetic changes in melanocytic neoplasia. These genetic alterations include point mutations, genetic deletion or amplification, and structural rearrangements, such as chromosomal translocations. In the past 15 years, molecular profiling of melanoma has been gaining increasing interest with the goals of improving the diagnosis and prognostication of melanoma and providing optimal personalized treatments of patients.

There are different methods to detect these molecular genetic changes. The current molecular techniques include fluorescence in situ hybridization (FISH), comparative genomic hybridization (CGH), genomic expression profiling (GEP) using reverse transcriptase (RT)–polymerase chain reaction (PCR), and different methods of DNA sequencing. These techniques are used for diagnosis of melanocytic lesions with ambiguous histology, for stratifying the prognosis of melanoma, and as a guide for treatment purposes.

In CGH, the entire genomic DNAs of tumor cells and reference cells are isolated and differentially labeled and then hybridized to metaphase chromosomes or microarrays (array CHG [aCGH]). Hybridization intensity of DNA of tumor cells and reference cells is compared. Increases or decreases in intensity ratio indicate relative DNA copy number variation in the genome of tumor cells. Overall, approximately one-third of the tumor should harbor copy number changes to be clearly identifiable on CGH.

FISH targets individual chromosomes or specific regions within a chromosome. Fluorescence-labeled oligonucleotide probes bind to their complementary DNA sequence and label that region, which can then be visualized under a fluorescence microscope. Currently, 2 types of probes are relevant in melanoma work-up. Centromere probes identify the centromere region of a specific chromosome and help establish the number of copies of that chromosome, and allele-specific probes adhere to a specific target sequence corresponding or adjacent to an oncogene. FISH allows detection of abnormal subpopulations of cells within a heterogeneous tissue mix and much smaller amounts of tissue are needed compared with CGH. It only detects, however, aberrations in preselected target areas.

CGH and FISH evaluate genomic DNA. RT-PCR is a variant of PCR that entails cloning expressed genes and allows a functional evaluation of genome.[3] It starts with reverse transcribing the RNA of interest into its DNA complement by RT and then amplifying the newly synthesized cDNA using PCR.

Point mutations are detected using DNA sequence analysis. Different methods of sequencing include direct (Sanger) sequencing and pyrosequencing. Single nucleotide extension assays are used for detecting a specific point mutation. Two commonly used techniques include iPlex (Agena Bioscience, San Diego, CA) and SNaPshot (Thermo Fisher Sientific, Ann Arbor, MI). Next-generation sequencing (NGS), or massively parallel sequencing, refers to a group of technologies that can capture data from millions of sequencing reactions simultaneously. It can be used for whole-genome sequencing, only the exons of the known genes, or only a limited number of genes.[4]

THE GENETICS OF MELANOCYTIC NEOPLASMS

Nevi can be subcategorized based on clinical and histologic characteristics into groups including congenital melanocytic nevi (CMN), common acquired melanocytic nevi, blue nevi, and Spitz nevi. Studies have showed different genetic alterations in different types of nevi. In 2003, it was found that *BRAF*-activating mutations, which were already known to be present in melanoma, were also present in nevi.[5] Most studies have shown that *BRAF* is mutated in approximately 80% of acquired nevi. A single amino acid substitution (V600E) accounts for approximately 80% of these mutations.[6] The V600E mutation alters the 600 amino acid position on the *BRAF* protein from valine to glutamic acid. Additional activating mutations, such as the BRAFV600K and BRAFV600R mutations, have also been identified in melanomas.[6] *NRAS* mutation has been found in approximately 6% to 18% of acquired melanocytic nevi.[7] Both these genes are involved in the mitogen-activated protein kinase (MAPK) pathway, a central activator of cellular proliferation, and tend to occur in a mutually exclusive fashion in melanocytic neoplasms.

Results of genetics studies suggest *NRAS* mutations and, to a lesser extent, *BRAF* mutations, contribute to the development of CMN. A consistent relationship between the size of lesion and mutation status has been found, with an inverse relationship between the prevalence of *BRAF* mutations and the size of CMN lesion.[8] Most blue nevi have a somatic mutation of either GNAQ or GNA11, which are 2 G protein alpha units.[9] These mutations cause a loss of GTPase activity, leading to constitutive activation and subsequent up-regulation of MAPK pathway signaling.

Although individual MAPK pathway mutations may initiate inappropriate proliferation resulting in nevus formation, they are not sufficient for melanoma formation. The initial growth of a melanocytic nevus is followed by loss of proliferative activity and stabilization of size. Mechanisms involved in growth arrest are complex. Although there are some similarities to replicative senescence, important differences exist, and the term, *stable clonal expansion*, rather than oncogene-induced senescence, has been suggested.[7]

Although a majority of nevi remain benign over time, a small proportion progresses to melanoma. There has been controversy whether or not progression from benign nevi to melanoma goes through an intermediate stage. Although earlier studies failed to show genetic difference between common and dysplastic nevi, a recent study by Shain and colleagues[10] has showed that melanocytic lesions with intermediate histopathologic findings have a genetically distinct signature different from both simple nevi and melanoma. They found that whereas banal nevi typically had *BRAFV600E* mutation only, ambiguous lesions tended to have NRAS mutations and BRAF non-V600E mutations as well as telomerase RT (TERT) promoter mutations. Other studies have also found relatively lower rates (approximately 60%) of BRAFV600E mutation in dysplastic nevi.[8] These data suggest that histologic dysplasia may be a true intermediate lesion but also imply that dysplastic nevi are often likely not derived from previously banal nevi. These findings await confirmation.

Studies have showed distinct patterns of genetic alterations in different groups of primary melanomas.[11] The Cancer Genome Atlas Network has proposed to classify melanoma into 4 categories based on the pattern of the most prevalent significantly mutated genes: mutant BRAF, mutant RAS, mutant neurofibromatosis (NF1), and triple wild-type (WT).[12] Mutations in BRAF can be identified in approximately 50% of melanomas. BRAF-mutated melanomas are most often found on nonchronically sun-damaged skin and are believed to arise from nevi with BRAF mutation. Focal amplifications of BRAF, the melanocyte lineage-specific oncogene microophthalmia-associated transcription factor, and the ligand for the coinhibitory immune checkpoint protein programmed death-1 (PD-1), PD-L1 gene (CD274) are observed at significant frequencies in the BRAF mutant subtype.

NF1 loss has been described in up to 10% to 15% of melanomas. NRAS amplifications co-occurs in tumors with NRAS mutations. Significant 4q12 focal amplification containing the oncogene KIT only has been found in the triple-WT cohort. Two other adjacent oncogenes, platelet-derived growth factor receptor alpha polypeptide (PDGFRA) and KDR, were frequently coamplified with KIT. There are also observed high-level focal copy number alterations containing the oncogenes CDK4 as well as MDM2 and TERT in triple-WT melanomas. This classification is based on potential implications for prognosis and therapy and recent advances in immunotherapy.[12]

Bastian[13] has proposed classification of melanoma based on genetic alterations that arise early during progression, clinical or histologic features, characteristics of the host, and the role of environmental factors, such as UV radiation. Melanomas on sun-exposed skin without cumulative sun-induced damage (CSD) usually originate from acquired or Spitz nevi, with (possible) intermediate stages of dysplastic nevi and atypical Spitz tumor, respectively. Melanomas associated with high UV exposure are melanomas on skin with CSD and include desmoplastic melanomas. CSD melanomas have infrequent BRAF mutations (more often V600K than V600E), inactivating mutations of NF1 (30% of cases), copy number increase of CCND1 (20% of cases), and activating mutations of KIT (approximately 10% of cases). Acral melanoma and mucosal melanoma are not associated with UV exposure. It has been shown that non–UV-related activating mutations in KIT and alterations in platelet-derived growth factor receptor alpha polypeptide (PDGFRA) lead to tumor proliferation in these sites.[11]

As melanomas progress, point mutation burden increases steadily, finally stabilizing once melanomas became invasive. By contrast, copy number alterations only became prevalent at the transition to invasive melanoma. Progressive telomere attrition with end-to-end fusion of chromatids during crisis could explain the frequent chromosomal aberrations in melanoma.[14] Numerous recurrent chromosomal gains and deletions have been described in melanomas.[15] Gains in 6p25 (RREB1) are highly sensitive in the detection of melanoma (73% sensitive overall). Losses of 6q23 are identified in 24% of melanomas overall. Copy number gains at 11q13 are 36% sensitive in the detection of melanoma overall. They are least frequently seen in superficial spreading type (22%) and most frequently seen in nodular type (55%). This gain was found most frequently in melanomas associated with chronic sun damage. Melanomas with 8q24 copy number gains, the locus that codes for the MYC gene, are associated with an amelanotic appearance and a nodular growth pattern and frequently occur on nonchronically sun-damaged skin. A deletion at 9p, the same chromosome locus implicated in hereditary melanoma syndromes, has been found in approximately 80% of melanomas.

Spitz Tumors

Genetic studies of Spitz nevi have demonstrated an absence of mutations involved in common acquired nevi. In total, *BRAF* and *NRAS* mutations have been detected in 6.4% (21/330) and 2.2% (4/178) of Spitz nevi, respectively.[8]

The most frequently observed genetic alterations in Spitz nevi involve the *HRAS* gene. Approximately 20% of cases show oncogenic mutations of *HRAS*, typically accompanied by copy number increases of the entire short arm of chromosome 11 as the only chromosomal aberration.[16] *HRAS* mutation seems to occur almost exclusively in Spitz nevi and it has not been identified in Spitzoid melanomas.

Another variant has a combination of *BRAF V600E* mutations and biallelic loss of the tumor suppressor *BAP1* on chromosome 3p21.[17] This category is called melanocytic *BAP-1*–associated intradermal tumors, also called Wiesner nevus or BAPoma, and may represent a progression from an acquired nevus.[18] Intact BAP1 has a tumor suppressive function and BAP1 deficiency leads to genomic instability.

Recently, gene rearrangements of ROS1, NTRK1, ALK, *BRAF*, and RET, resulting in in-frame kinase fusions, were reported through genomic analysis of 140 Spitzoid neoplasms.[19] No fusions were detected in tumors with *HRAS* mutations. Each of the fusions was identified across the spectrum of Spitzoid neoplasms, implying that translocation is an early event in tumorigenesis.

Homozygous deletion of 9p21 (CDKN2A), which has been found in melanomas, also happens in Spitzoid tumors and is an important (although not unequivocal) indicator of aggressive behavior and poor prognosis among Spitzoid neoplasms.[20] Another indicator of clinically aggressive disease among STUMPs is TERT promoter mutations. TERT encodes the catalytic subunit for the telomerase complex, which maintains telomere length during DNA replication. Lee and colleagues[21] have proposed that TERT mutations can be a marker of aggressive Spitzoid neoplasms. Additional prospective studies are necessary, however, to assess the absolute correlation of TERT promoter mutations with aggressive clinical behavior.[22] **Table 1** summarizes common genes involved in different melanocytic lesions.

Table 1
Common genes involved in cutaneous melanocytic neoplasms

Melanocytic Neoplasm	Common Genes
Common acquired melanocytic nevi	*BRAFV600E* (80%), *NRAS* (6%–18%)
CMN	*NRAS* (>80%)
Spitzoid melanocytic tumors	*HRAS* (20%), *BAP1*, rearrangement of kinase in 60% of cases (*ALK, ROS1, RET, NTRK1, BRAF*)
Blue nevi, nevus of Ota, nevus of Ito	*GNAQ, GNA11*
Malignant melanoma (sun exposed, CSD)	*BRAFV600K, NRAS, KIT, NF1* (30%) *CCND1* (20%), *KIT* (10%), *TP53, ARID2*
Malignant melanoma (sun exposed, non-CSD)	*BRAFV600E, NRAS*
Acral/mucosal melanoma (non–sun-exposed)	*KIT, PDGFRA* (4q12), *CCND1* (11q13), *hTERT* (5p15), *CDK4* (12q14), *NRAS*
Desmoplastic melanoma	*NF1* (25%)

USE OF CYTOGENETIC TESTS IN DIAGNOSIS OF MELANOCYTIC NEOPLASMS

Histopathologic analysis of hematoxylin-eosin–stained tissue sections and correlation with the clinical context remains the gold standard for diagnosing melanoma. A subset of lesions, however, has unusual or atypical histopathologic features.

In 2003, Bastian and colleagues[14] evaluated 132 melanomas and 54 benign nevi with CGH and found that 96.2% of the melanomas had some type of chromosomal copy number aberration. Among the 54 nevi evaluated, only 7 lesions (13%), all Spitz nevi, showed aberrations. Except 1 case, these aberrations were restricted to copy number increase of the entire short arm of chromosome 11. Remarkably, this aberration was not seen in any of the 132 melanomas. Wang and colleagues[23] have reported positive aCGH findings in 92% of melanomas but in no benign nevi. Overall, detection of multiple copy number changes represents strong evidence in favor of malignant melanoma. Exceptions include subtypes of Spitz nevus/tumor characterized by gains of 11p or loss of chromosome 3. Unfortunately, a rare melanoma (4%–8%) may be CGH negative. Other disadvantages to aCGH include the requirement for more tissue (relative to FISH), its inability to identify small clones of aberrant cells, and its inability to detect point mutations and balanced chromosomal translocations. The greatest current disadvantages to aCGH are its cost and complexity that, for the time being, limit its use mostly to investigative studies in a small number of laboratories, where it mainly is used in diagnosis of Spitz tumors.[24]

In FISH, short DNA probes are hybridized to formalin-fixed paraffin-embedded (FFPE) tissue. Because of overlapping wavelength spectra, the number of probes that can be used together in a single experiment is limited to 4.[25] Based on CGH results, Gerami and colleagues[26] selected a group of 4 probes and then combined numerical cutoffs of parameters for single probes and pairs of probes to yield the best combination of sensitivity and specificity. The probes and corresponding genes were 6p25 (RREB1), centromere 6, 6q23 (MYB1), and 11q13 (CCND1). Centromeric portion of chromosome 6 (CEP6) is not used by itself as a marker for melanoma, but it is used as a reference when detecting 6p25 gains and 6q23 losses in melanoma FISH panels. These probes were applied to a cohort of melanocytic lesions and showed sensitivity of 86.7% and a specificity of 95.4% in the differentiation of nevi from melanomas. As a final test, the probes were applied to a group of 27 ambiguous melanocytic tumors, and all 6 of the primary tumors that had eventually metastasized were positive by this FISH assay.[26]

Although using these has permitted test sensitivity of 86% and specificity of 95% for histopathologically obvious/noncontroversial benign and malignant lesions, results for diagnostically ambiguous melanocytic neoplasms have been variable. Although in some studies, all lesions proved to be melanoma were FISH positive, other groups have reported a specificity of only 50% for metastasis and a sensitivity of 60%. In 2011, Gerami and Zembowicz[25] reviewed experiences of the dermatopathology community with FISH for the diagnosis of melanocytic neoplasms and concluded that the sensitivity and specificity, discussed previously, are not satisfactory for the diagnosis of melanoma, and "thus melanoma FISH must not be used as a stand-alone test and has to be considered as a diagnostic adjunct."[25] They noted that NeoGenomics data (from the time of publication of their review article) demonstrate only 75% sensitivity for melanoma. They also pointed out that the use of the current FISH test results in as low as a 50% sensitivity for certain types of melanomas. Another review cites a sensitivity lower than 70% for the use of FISH in thin conventional melanomas.[27] Sensitivity of standard FISH probes in unequivocal Spitzoid melanomas has been estimated at approximately 70%.[28]

To overcome these problems, additional probes are currently being incorporated into clinical utility, such as those targeting 9p21 (CDKN2A), which are useful for diagnosing both conventional and Spitzoid melanomas by increasing sensitivity and specificity. Probes targeting 8q24 are useful for nodular, amelanotic, and nevoid melanomas.[29] More recently a new melanoma FISH probe cocktail targeting RREB1 (6p25), C-MYC (8q24), CDKN2A (9p21), and CCND1 (11q13) has been proposed by Ferrara and De Vanna[30] These investigators have proposed implementation of a FISH algorithm; starting with the standard 4-probe test and followed by either C-MYC or CDKN2A/centromere 9.

The other technique in use for melanoma diagnosis is GEP. This technique analyzes mRNA, in contrast to FISH or CGH, which uses DNA, and is a functional genome evaluation. Clarke and colleagues[31] have used quantitative PCR on a selected set of 23 genes on 464 samples. This group developed a gene expression signature that differentiates benign nevi from malignant melanoma with sensitivity of 89% and specificity of 93%. More recently, a GEP assay consisting of 31 genes, which has been approved by Food and Drug Administration (FDA), has been developed for cutaneous melanoma as a prognostication assay to classify melanoma to low risk (class 1) and high risk (class 2)[32] and may have the potential to reduce the costs. Recently, Gerami and colleagues[33] demonstrated that 31-gene GEP results are a more accurate predictor of metastasis in 5 years, compared with sentinel lymph node biopsy (SLNB). In addition, combination of GEP results with SLNB have improved prognostication.

RT-PCR has also been used in the past 2 decades for detection of circulating tumor cells (CTCs) in blood. Based on the theory of epithelial-to-mesenchymal transition of melanoma cells and invasion of the malignant cells into the vascular system and spread to the solid tissues, CTCs are the subject of great interest and research among oncologists and clinical pathologists. Detection of melanoma cells in peripheral blood by RT-PCR was first reported by Smith and colleagues[34] in 1991. Khoja and colleagues[35] used a melanoma Cell Search CTC kit with CD146 MelCAM (BD Horizon, San Jose, CA) for CTC capture, costaining with CD45 and CD34 to differentiate CTCs from leukocytes and vasculature, respectively. They proposed that CTCs may be prognostic in patients with stage III melanoma. Clinical utility of CTCs in melanoma is limited, however, by heterogeneity of melanoma cells, sparseness of released cells into the blood stream, and discrepancies between studies regarding method of detection and lack of validated detection methods and lack of quality control assays. Additional research and clinical trials is warranted to investigate whether CTCs could be used as liquid biopsy for exploring mutational profile of melanoma cells as a guide for targeted immunotherapies.

NEXT-GENERATION SEQUENCING AND CELL-FREE NUCLEIC ACID ANALYSIS

Conventional gene sequencing for mutation analysis is not only relevant for treatment selection but also can be useful for diagnostic purposes. The detection of a GNAQ/GNA11 mutation in a sclerosing melanocytic tumor with a differential diagnosis of amelanotic sclerosing blue nevus versus desmoplastic melanoma supports a diagnosis of a blue nevus.[36] Currently, there is a tendency toward testing with NGS methods. The sensitivity of NGS is higher than other common available techniques in mutation detection and is applicable in FFPE specimens. Moreover, the amount of DNA that is needed for the analysis of a gene panel is low in comparison to Sanger sequencing.[37]

NGS offers the unique opportunity to provide detailed information of the mutational profile, allowing the sequencing of multiple melanoma-driving genes in a single assay. Not only can the driver mutations (BRAF, NRAS, and KIT) be identified but also mutations that are less common and potentially actionable, which lead the tumor cells to escape targeted therapy, revealed. NGS has the capacity to detect not only the DNA mutational profile but also the mRNA expression profile, copy number aberrations, translocations, and methylation status.[38] The cost-effectiveness and feasibility of a custom-designed targeted NGS panel suggest implementation of targeted NGS into routine daily practice.[39]

Analysis of tumor characterization via cell-free DNA (cfDNA) analysis has also been recently reported as a surrogate marker. Valpione and colleagues[40] have shown that baseline cfDNA concentration obtained from 43 patients with melanoma correlated with pretreatment tumor burden, hazard of death, and overall survival (OS). A cutoff value of greater than or equal to 89 pg/μL prognosticated a shorter OS. In addition, McEvoy and colleagues[41] reported that a droplet digital PCR assay designed for the concurrent detection of chr5:1,295,228 C > T and chr5:1,295,250 C > T TERT promoter mutations demonstrated a 68% concordance between matched plasma and tumor tissue, with a sensitivity of 53% (95% CI, 27%–79%) and a specificity of 100% (95% CI, 59%–100%). Additional utility of cfDNA as well as circulating tumor cell DNA (ctDNA) mutations and concentrations have also been reported, suggesting that cfDNA and ctDNA analysis may serve as novel biomarkers for melanoma patients.[42,43]

These molecular techniques are rapidly emerging as important tools in evaluation of melanocytic neoplasms. **Table 2** highlights the relative advantages and disadvantages of each molecular technique.

THERAPEUTIC APPROACHES FOR METASTATIC MELANOMA IN THE MOLECULAR ERA

Metastatic melanoma is an aggressive malignancy. It shows poor response to single-agent and multiagent chemotherapy. Dacarbazine (DTIC), interleukin 2, and interferon alpha have been standard chemotherapeutic and immunotherapeutic agents for melanoma for many years, despite an absence of or limited survival advantage in clinical trials.[44] Recently, a new generation of antimelanomas therapies has been developed. These include targeted inhibitors of the MAPK pathway and mutated KIT as well as immune checkpoint blockade by monoclonal antibodies targeting cytotoxic T-lymphocyte antigen 4 (CTLA-4).[45] Coupled with detection of the mutational status of the BRAF and KIT, these therapies and increasingly combinations of these therapies are showing great promise for the treatment of advanced metastatic melanomas.

BRAF Inhibitors

Activating mutations of the gene encoding for BRAF are found in 40% to 60% of melanomas. Although BRAF inhibition has improved OS, it has been associated with cutaneous squamous cell carcinoma. The mechanism of squamous cell carcinoma development in these patients has been attributed to upstream RAS mutation along with paradoxic activation of MAPK signaling.[46] Recently, β-genus human papillomavirus 17 and Merkel cell polyomavirus have been reported in these lesions.[47]

Vemurafenib

Vemurafenib is an orally delivered, FDA-approved drug available for the treatment of melanoma patients with the BRAFV600E mutation. A large phase 2 second-line trial in 132 patients confirmed a high response rate and longer median progression free-survival (PFS).[48] Treatment with vemurafenib is discouraged in WT BRAF melanomas, as studies have demonstrated that BRAF inhibitors can enhance rather than down-regulate the MAPK pathway in tumor cells with WT BRAF and upstream RAS mutations.[49–52]

Table 2
Molecular techniques in cutaneous melanoma diagnosis

Technique	Advantages	Disadvantages
CGH	Detects genome-wide DNA aCGH is more sensitive than traditional CGH	Larger amount of tissue is needed than for FISH False-negative results when less than adequate tumor cells represented in the sample False-negative results in 4%–8% of melanoma False-positive results in Spitz nevi with 11p gain or chromosome 3 loss Inability to detect point mutations and balanced chromosomal translocations High cost and more complexity Limited availability
Sanger sequencing	FFPE specimens Simple Low cost Fast turnaround time	Low sensitivity Detects 15%–25% allele frequency vs 2%–10% detection rate for NGS Laborious process
RT(PCR)/ GEP/mRNA	FFPE specimens High (90%) sensitivity and (91%) specificity 31-gene GEP is more sensitive than SLNB for prognosis	Difficulty in maintaining linearity Slight DNA contamination leads to inaccurate results
FISH	Less amount of tissue needed than CGH New FISH probe set (targeting chromosomal loci 11q13, 8q24, 6p25 and 9p21) with sensitivity and specificity of 94% and 98%, respectively	Only detects genes and chromosomes targeted by specific probes Enumeration needs experience Polyploidy including tetraploidy in Spitz nevi can lead to false-positive results Low sensitivity and specificity in certain types of melanoma and atypical Spitzoid neoplasms with the traditional 4-probe assay
NGS	FFPE specimens Requires very low input DNA/RNA High sensitivity and accuracy Screens variety of genomic alteration simultaneously (small and large deletions/insertions, copy number variations, fusion transcripts) Quick turnaround time	Availability High cost of whole-genome sequencing
cfDNA/ctDNA	Requires blood, serum or plasma Low cost Quick turn-around time	Variable specificity and sensitivity depending on tumor types Early stage in adaptation/Emerging technology

Dabrafenib

Dabrafenib is a newer drug undergoing testing and has shown efficacy in patients with the *BRAFV600E* mutation.[53] When compared with DTIC in the BREAK-2 trial, dabrafenib showed longer PFS. OS data were limited by the median duration of follow-up. Partial response and complete response were also higher in patients receiving dabrafenib versus DTIC.

MEK Inhibitors

MEK inhibitors are recently FDA-approved drugs that inhibit MAPKs MEK1 and MEK 2, which are downstream from *BRAF* in the MAPK pathway. MEK inhibitors are currently used for treatment of *BRAF*-mutated melanoma.

Trametinib

Trametinib dimethyl sulfoxide was the first MEK inhibitor approved by the FDA for treatment of *BRAF*-mutated metastatic melanoma. It is also approved in combination with the *BRAF* inhibitor dabrafenib. Combination of *BRAF* and MEK inhibitors have shown significant improvement in response rates, PFS and OS in addition to fewer side effects related to paradoxic activation of MAPK pathway.[54]

Cobimetinib

Cobimetinib is another MEK inhibitor, approved in 2015 for treatment of *BRAF*-mutated metastatic melanoma in combination with the *BRAF* inhibitor vemurafenib.[54]

KIT Inhibitors

Approximately one-third of melanomas arising in non–sun-exposed areas, such as the mucosal surfaces and acral areas, have amplifications or activating mutations of the receptor tyrosine kinase KIT. The most clinically tested drug thus far in patients with KIT-mutant melanoma is imatinib.

Imatinib

Imatinib was demonstrated to have a remarkable tumor response in metastatic melanomas with a mutated KIT gene in a phase 2 study.[55] Numerous phase 2 studies, however, using imatinib to treat unselected groups of patients with metastatic melanoma showed inconsistent tumor response.[56–58] Other studies have demonstrated the value of imatinib in selected groups of patients with metastatic melanomas with KIT alterations.[59,60]

Nilotinib

The introduction of second-generation tyrosine kinase inhibitors, such as nilotinib, sunitinib, and dasatinib, is expanding the interest in inhibiting mutated KIT in metastatic melanomas. A recent global phase II Tasigna Efficacy in Advanced Melanoma (TEAM) trial has shown efficacy and safety of nilotinib in KIT-mutated metastatic melanoma.[61]

Ipilimumab

Ipilimumab, a humanized IgG1 monoclonal antibody targeting the CTLA-4, was the first drug to demonstrate an improvement OS compared with the standard of care for melanoma. It augments T-cell activation.[62–65]

When given in combination with the glycoprotein vaccine gp100, the antibody showed improved OS when compared with vaccine alone. In patients with previously treated metastatic melanoma, an improvement in OS was seen when ipilimumab was used in combination with chemotherapy compared with chemotherapy alone.

PD-1 Inhibitors

PD-1 is an inhibitory receptor and is a member of the CD28 family. PD-1 is expressed on B and T lymphocytes and, on ligation to PDL-1 and PDL-2 on macrophages and dendritic cells, inhibits immune cell activation and induces T-cell apoptosis. Monoclonal antibodies against PD-1 and PDL-1 cause T cells to be activated and become more efficient in tumor surveillance. PD-1 antibodies have been approved by the FDA for advanced melanoma treatment. It has demonstrated significant activity against melanoma with durable response along with a manageable toxicity profile and less serious adverse complications compared with common immunotherapies.[45]

Nivolumab

Nivolumab is an FDA-approved PD-1 checkpoint inhibitor. In 1 open-label, phase II trial in Japan, approximately one-quarter of patients with previously treated stage III/IV melanoma achieved a partial tumor response when given intravenous nivolumab, 2 mg/kg every 3 weeks.[66] A phase III trial of nivolumab had a response rate of 40% with a 72.9% 1-year survival rate.[66]

Pembrolizumab

Pembrolizumab is safe, tolerable, and effective in the treatment of melanoma. It has been reported to increase OS and prolonged PFS rates. It has a lower incidence of adverse reactions in comparison to other melanoma treatments and has shown a favorable pharmacokinetics profile with minimal undesired side effects.

Pembrolizumab is administered for patients with advanced unresectable melanoma or metastatic melanomas with a mutated BRAFV600E/K gene that are unresponsive to treatment with BRAF inhibitors. Pembrolizumab has shown remarkable improvement in OS.[67] Immunotherapy combination therapy trials are under way to investigate the efficacy of different combined treatments, and the addition of an anti–PD1/PDL-1

Table 3
Summary of melanoma treatment drugs

Drug	Class or Mechanism of Action	Common Side Effects
DTIC	Chemotherapy	Photosensitivity, anemia, leukopenia, thrombocytopenia
Interferon	Immunotherapy	Flulike symptoms, low blood cell counts
Interleukin-2	Immunotherapy	Fluid retention
Ipilimumab (Yervoy)	Anti–CTLA-4 antibody, IgG1 monoclonal antibody, augments T-cell activation	Colitis, hepatitis, numbness and tingling, skin sensitivity eruptions
Vemurafenib (Zelboraf)	Targets cells with BRAFV600E mutation	Fatigue, hair loss, blurred vision, squamous cell carcinoma
Dabrafenib	Targets cells with BRAFV600E mutation	Hyperglycemia, hyponatremia, night sweats, squamous cell carcinoma
Imatinib (Gleevec)	Targets cells with KIT mutation	Low blood counts, edema, skin rash, muscle cramps, diarrhea, fever
Nilotinib (Tasigna)	Targets cells with KIT mutation	Cold symptoms, hair loss, skin rash
Trametinib (Mekinist)	MEK inhibitor	Acne, rosacea, dry skin, itch, papulopustular eruption, dusky erythema
Cobimetinib (Cotellic)	MEK inhibitor	Diarrhea, fever, nausea, hypertension, papulopustular eruption, dusky erythema
Pembrolizumab (Keytruda, lambrolizumab)	PD-1 inhibitor	Fatigue, cough, pneumonitis, hepatitis, rash, itching, vitiligo, diarrhea, colitis, headache
Nivolumab (Opdivo)	PD-1 inhibitor	Fatigue, skin rash, cough, swelling of extremities, fever, upper respiratory tract infection, psoriasis

agent, such as pembrolizumab, to combined *BRAF* and MEK inhibitors has shown promising results.[45]

The future of antimelanoma therapy certainly lies in the detection of specific mutations in patient malignant melanomas and subsequent personalized treatment of these malignancies with various combinations of molecular inhibitors and immune therapies. **Table 3** summarizes current therapeutic drugs for melanoma treatment.

REFERENCES

1. Menezes FD, Mooi WJ. Spitz tumors of the skin. Surg Pathol Clin 2017;10(2): 281–98.
2. Padua RA, Barrass N, Currie GA. A novel transforming gene in a human malignant melanoma cell line. Nature 1984;311(5987):671–3.
3. Sellheyer K, Belbin TJ. DNA microarrays: from structural genomics to functional genomics. The applications of gene chips in dermatology and dermatopathology. J Am Acad Dermatol 2004;51(5):681–92.
4. Ilyas M. Next-generation sequencing in diagnostic pathology. Pathobiology 2017; 84(6):292–305.
5. Pollock PM, Harper UL, Hansen KS, et al. High frequency of BRAF mutations in nevi. Nat Genet 2003;33(1):19–20.
6. Davies H, Bignell GR, Cox C, et al. Mutations of the BRAF gene in human cancer. Nature 2002;417(6892):949–54.
7. Damsky WE, Bosenberg M. Melanocytic nevi and melanoma: unraveling a complex relationship. Oncogene 2017;36(42):5771–92.
8. Roh MR, Eliades P, Gupta S, et al. Genetics of melanocytic nevi. Pigment Cell Melanoma Res 2015;28(6):661–72.
9. Van Raamsdonk CD, Bezrookove V, Green G, et al. Frequent somatic mutations of GNAQ in uveal melanoma and blue naevi. Nature 2009;457(7229):599–602.
10. Shain AH, Yeh I, Kovalyshyn I, et al. The genetic evolution of melanoma from precursor lesions. N Engl J Med 2015;373(20):1926–36.
11. Curtin JA, Fridlyand J, Kageshita T, et al. Distinct sets of genetic alterations in melanoma. N Engl J Med 2005;353(20):2135–47.
12. Cancer Genome Atlas Network. Genomic classification of cutaneous melanoma. Cell 2015;161(7):1681–96.
13. Bastian BC. The molecular pathology of melanoma: an integrated taxonomy of melanocytic neoplasia. Annu Rev Pathol 2014;9:239–71.
14. Bastian BC, Olshen AB, LeBoit PE, et al. Classifying melanocytic tumors based on DNA copy number changes. Am J Pathol 2003;163(5):1765–70.
15. Bradish JR, Cheng L. Molecular pathology of malignant melanoma: changing the clinical practice paradigm toward a personalized approach. Hum Pathol 2014; 45(7):1315–26.
16. Bastian BC, LeBoit PE, Pinkel D. Mutations and copy number increase of HRAS in Spitz nevi with distinctive histopathological features. Am J Pathol 2000;157(3): 967–72.
17. Wiesner T, Murali R, Fried I, et al. A distinct subset of atypical Spitz tumors is characterized by BRAF mutation and loss of BAP1 expression. Am J Surg Pathol 2012;36(6):818–30.
18. Wiesner T, Obenauf AC, Murali R, et al. Germline mutations in BAP1 predispose to melanocytic tumors. Nat Genet 2011;43(10):1018–21.
19. Wiesner T, He J, Yelensky R, et al. Kinase fusions are frequent in Spitz tumours andmelanomas. Nat Commun 2014;5:3116.

20. Tetzlaff MT, Reuben A, Billings SD, et al. Toward a molecular-genetic classification of spitzoid neoplasms. Clin Lab Med 2017;37(3):431–48.
21. Lee S, Barnhill RL, Dummer R, et al. TERT promoter mutations are predictive of aggressive clinical behavior in patients with spitzoid melanocytic neoplasms. Sci Rep 2015;5:11200.
22. Requena C, Heidenreich B, Kumar R, et al. TERT promoter mutations are not always associated with poor prognosis in atypical spitzoid tumors. Pigment Cell Melanoma Res 2017;30(2):265–8.
23. Wang L, Rao M, Fang Y, et al. A genome-wide high-resolution array-CGH analysis of cutaneous melanoma and comparison of array-CGH to FISH in diagnostic evaluation. J Mol Diagn 2013;15(5):581–91.
24. Braun-Falco M, Schempp W, Weyers W. Molecular diagnosis in dermatopathology: what makes sense, and what doesn't. Exp Dermatol 2009;18(1):12–23.
25. Gerami P, Zembowicz A. Update on fluorescence in situ hybridization in melanoma: state of the art. Arch Pathol Lab Med 2011;135(7):830–7.
26. Gerami P, Jewell SS, Morrison LE, et al. Fluorescence in situ hybridization (FISH) as an ancillary diagnostic tool in the diagnosis of melanoma. Am J Surg Pathol 2009;33(8):1146–56.
27. McCalmont TH. Fillet of FISH. J Cutan Pathol 2011;38(4):327–8.
28. Gammon B, Beilfuss B, Guitart J, et al. Enhanced detection of spitzoid melanomas using fluorescence in situ hybridization with 9p21 as an adjunctive probe. Am J Surg Pathol 2012;36(1):81–8.
29. Gerami P, Jewell SS, Pouryazdanparast P, et al. Copy number gains in 11q13 and 8q24 [corrected] are highly linked to prognosis in cutaneous malignant melanoma. J Mol Diagn 2011;13(3):352–8.
30. Ferrara G, De Vanna AC. Fluorescence in situ hybridization for melanoma diagnosis: a review and a reappraisal. Am J Dermatopathol 2016;38(4):253–69.
31. Clarke LE, Warf MB, Flake DD 2nd, et al. Clinical validation of a gene expression signature that differentiates benign nevi from malignant melanoma. J Cutan Pathol 2015;42(4):244–52.
32. Gerami P, Cook RW, Wilkinson J, et al. Development of a prognostic genetic signature to predict the metastatic risk associated with cutaneous melanoma. Clin Cancer Res 2015;21(1):175–83.
33. Gerami P, Cook RW, Russell MC, et al. Gene expression profiling for molecular staging of cutaneous melanoma in patients undergoing sentinel lymph node biopsy. J Am Acad Dermatol 2015;72(5):780–5.
34. Smith B, Selby P, Southgate J, et al. Detection of melanoma cells in peripheral blood by means of reverse transcriptase and polymerase chain reaction. Lancet 1991;338(8777):1227–9.
35. Khoja L, Lorigan P, Dive C, et al. Circulating tumour cells as tumour biomarkers in melanoma: detection methods and clinical relevance. Ann Oncol 2015;26(1): 33–9.
36. Gerami P, Busam KJ. Cytogenetic and mutational analyses of melanocytic tumors. Dermatol Clin 2012;30(4):555–66.
37. van Engen-van Grunsven AC, Kusters-Vandevelde H, Groenen PJ, et al. Update on molecular pathology of cutaneous melanocytic lesions: what is new in diagnosis and molecular testing for treatment? Front Med (Lausanne) 2014;1:39.
38. Lee CY, Gerami P. Molecular techniques for predicting behaviour in melanocytic neoplasms. Pathology 2016;48(2):142–6.

39. de Unamuno Bustos B, Murria Estal R, Pérez Simó G, et al. Towards personalized medicine in melanoma: implementation of a clinical next-generation sequencing panel. Sci Rep 2017;7(1):495.
40. Valpione S, Gremel G, Mundra P, et al. Plasma total cell-free DNA (cfDNA) is a surrogate biomarker for tumour burden and a prognostic biomarker for survival in metastatic melanoma patients. Eur J Cancer 2017;88:1–9.
41. McEvoy AC, Calapre L, Pereira MR, et al. Sensitive droplet digital PCR method for detection of promoter mutations in cell free DNA from patients with metastatic melanoma. Oncotarget 2017;8(45):78890–900.
42. Calapre L, Warburton L, Millward M, et al. Circulating tumour DNA (ctDNA) as a liquid biopsy for melanoma. Cancer Lett 2017;404:62–9.
43. Busser B, Lupo J, Sancey L, et al. Plasma circulating tumor DNA levels for the monitoring of melanoma patients: landscape of available technologies and clinical applications. Biomed Res Int 2017;2017:5986129.
44. Ives NJ, Stowe RL, Lorigan P, et al. Chemotherapy compared with biochemotherapy for the treatment of metastatic melanoma: a meta-analysis of 18 trials involving 2,621 patients. J Clin Oncol 2007;25(34):5426–34.
45. Jazirehi AR, Lim A, Dinh T. PD-1 inhibition and treatment of advanced melanoma-role of pembrolizumab. Am J Cancer Res 2016;6(10):2117–28.
46. Su F, Viros A, Milagre C, et al. RAS mutations in cutaneous squamous-cell carcinomas in patients treated with BRAF inhibitors. N Engl J Med 2012;366(3):207–15.
47. Falchook GS, Rady P, Hymes S, et al. Merkel cell polyomavirus and HPV-17 associated with cutaneous squamous cell carcinoma arising in a patient with melanoma treated with the BRAF inhibitor dabrafenib. JAMA Dermatol 2013;149(3):322–6.
48. Ribas A, Kim K, Schuchter L. BRIM-2: an open label, multicenter phase II study of vemurafenib in previously treated patients with BRAF V600E mutation-positive metastatic melanoma. J Clin Oncol 2011;29 [abstract: 8509].
49. Schwartzentruber DJ, Lawson DH, Richards JM, et al. gp100 peptide vaccine and interleukin-2 in patients with advanced melanoma. N Engl J Med 2011;364(22):2119–27.
50. Heidorn SJ, Milagre C, Whittaker S, et al. Kinase-dead BRAF and oncogenic RAS cooperate to drive tumor progression through CRAF. Cell 2010;140(2):209–21.
51. Hatzivassiliou G, Song K, Yen I, et al. RAF inhibitors prime wild-type RAF to activate the MAPK pathway and enhance growth. Nature 2010;464(7287):431–5.
52. Poulikakos PI, Zhang C, Bollag G, et al. RAF inhibitors transactivate RAF dimers and ERK signalling in cells with wild-type BRAF. Nature 2010;464(7287):427–30.
53. Ascierto PA, Minor D, Ribas A, et al. Phase II trial (BREAK-2) of the BRAF inhibitor dabrafenib (GSK2118436) in patients with metastatic melanoma. J Clin Oncol 2013;31(26):3205–11.
54. Grimaldi AM, Simeone E, Festino L, et al. MEK Inhibitors in the treatment of metastatic melanoma and solid tumors. Am J Clin Dermatol 2017;18(6):745–54.
55. Hodi FS, Friedlander P, Corless CL, et al. Major response to imatinib mesylate in KIT-mutated melanoma. J Clin Oncol 2008;26(12):2046–51.
56. Wyman K, Atkins MB, Prieto V, et al. Multicenter phase II trial of high-dose imatinib mesylate in metastatic melanoma: significant toxicity with no clinical efficacy. Cancer 2006;106(9):2005–11.
57. Kim KB, Eton O, Davis DW, et al. Phase II trial of imatinib mesylate in patients with metastatic melanoma. Br J Cancer 2008;99(5):734–40.

58. Ugurel S, Hildenbrand R, Zimpfer A, et al. Lack of clinical efficacy of imatinib in metastatic melanoma. Br J Cancer 2005;92(8):1398–405.
59. Carvajal RD, Antonescu CR, Wolchok JD, et al. KIT as a therapeutic target in metastatic melanoma. JAMA 2011;305(22):2327–34.
60. Guo J, Si L, Kong Y, et al. Phase II, open-label, single-arm trial of imatinib mesylate in patients with metastatic melanoma harboring c-Kit mutation or amplification. J Clin Oncol 2011;29(21):2904–9.
61. Guo J, Carvajal RD, Dummer R, et al. Efficacy and safety of nilotinib in patients with KIT-mutated metastatic or inoperable melanoma: final results from the global, single-arm, phase II TEAM trial. Ann Oncol 2017;28(6):1380–7.
62. O'Day SJ, Hamid O, Urba WJ. Targeting cytotoxic T-lymphocyte antigen-4 (CTLA-4): a novel strategy for the treatment of melanoma and other malignancies. Cancer 2007;110(12):2614–27.
63. Fong L, Small EJ. Anti-cytotoxic T-lymphocyte antigen-4 antibody: the first in an emerging class of immunomodulatory antibodies for cancer treatment. J Clin Oncol 2008;26(32):5275–83.
64. Robert C, Ghiringhelli F. What is the role of cytotoxic T lymphocyte-associated antigen 4 blockade in patients with metastatic melanoma? Oncologist 2009;14(8):848–61.
65. Hodi FS, O'Day SJ, McDermott DF, et al. Improved survival with ipilimumab in patients with metastatic melanoma. N Engl J Med 2010;363(8):711–23.
66. Deeks ED. Nivolumab: a review of its use in patients with malignant melanoma. Drugs 2014;74(11):1233–9.
67. Poole RM. Pembrolizumab: first global approval. Drugs 2014;74(16):1973–81.

Breast Carcinoma
Updates in Molecular Profiling 2018

Sudeshna Bandyopadhyay, MD[a],*, Martin H. Bluth, MD, PhD[b,c],
Rouba Ali-Fehmi, MD[a]

KEYWORDS

- Carcinoma - Breast - Molecular subtyping - Genetic alterations

KEY POINTS

- Understanding the molecular heterogeneity underlying the clinical heterogeneity of breast cancer.
- Molecular and genetic variations in breast cancer with impact on treatment and prognosis.
- Correlation of the histologic variants of breast cancer and their molecular correlates.
- Introduction to progression of in situ carcinoma to invasive carcinoma.

Breast carcinoma is the most common malignancy affecting women in the United States, comprising almost 29% of all cancers occurring in women. Moreover, it is the second most common cause of mortality, responsible for 14% of cancer-related mortality.[1] It is estimated to increase both in this country and globally.

Traditionally, this tumor is classified based on morphologic features.[2] The most common subtype is invasive ductal carcinoma (IDC), not otherwise specified (NOS). This type accounts for approximately 60% to 75% of all breast carcinomas. Established prognostic factors associated with survival in breast cancer are clinicopathologic factors such as tumor size and grade, lymph node involvement, margin status, and lymph vascular invasion.[3] Predictive biological markers that are in use clinically are estrogen and progesterone receptors and Her-2/neu receptor status. Predictive markers are used to determine subsequent treatment options and estimate response to treatment.[4] Receptor expression is determined using validated immunohistochemical methods. In the case of Her-2/neu, fluorescence in situ hybridization assay is performed to evaluate gene amplification, in the event of equivocal Her-2/neu protein expression by immunohistochemistry. The testing methodology and protocols, cutoff values and reporting guidelines are based on College of American Pathologists/American Society of Clinical Oncology guidelines.[5]

[a] Department of Pathology, Detroit Medical Center, Harper University Hospital 3990 John R, Detroit, MI 48201, USA; [b] Department of Pathology, Wayne State University, School of Medicine, 540 East Canfield Street, Detroit, MI 48201, USA; [c] Pathology Laboratories, Michigan Surgical Hospital, 21230 Dequindre Road, Warren, MI 48091, USA
* Corresponding author.
E-mail address: SBandyop@dmc.org

Clin Lab Med 38 (2018) 401–420
https://doi.org/10.1016/j.cll.2018.02.006
labmed.theclinics.com

Over the past decades, the heterogeneity of breast carcinomas has been acknowledged and studied. Observations regarding variable outcome in patients with breast cancer have supported these theories. A landmark study by Perou and colleagues[6] showed that the heterogeneity of breast carcinoma was reflected in the molecular makeup of these tumors. Using complementary DNA technology, the investigators analyzed 65 tumors from 42 individuals, including 20 paired samples before and after chemotherapy. For the purpose of this study, 496 genes, nominated as the intrinsic gene subset, were included for analysis. Differences in specific signaling pathways, cellular components, and proliferation gene expressions were identified as variations in expression of different subsets of genes. Using hierarchical clustering to analyze these tumors, 2 main groups of tumors were identified based on the estrogen receptor status: estrogen-positive tumors and estrogen-negative tumors.[6–8] Estrogen-positive tumors corresponded with the luminal subtype, whereas the estrogen-negative group included the Her-2/neu-enriched and the basal groups.[6]

Also identified as a separate group was the normal breast subtype, which is characterized by genes normally characterizing adipose tissue and basal cell genes, with a low expression of genes characterizing luminal cells. It is thought that this group may represent contamination by the normal breast parenchyma and need further investigation.

A subsequent study by Sorlie and colleagues[7] extended the cohort to include 38 additional tumors (total of 78 cases). From the initial gene subset, 456 genes were selected for analysis. Expanding the size of the cohort allowed for identification of subclasses within the estrogen receptor–positive group.

Based on these molecular studies, breast carcinomas can be classified as follows:

a. Estrogen positive
   1. Luminal A
   2. Luminal B
b. Estrogen negative
   3. Her-2/neu
   4. Triple negative
   5. Normal breast–like

LUMINAL A

This subtype is characterized by upregulation of the estrogen receptor gene (ESR-1) and related genes such as GATA 3, FOX A1, and LIV 1. Her-2/neu gene amplification is not seen. By immunohistochemistry, these tumors are characterized as estrogen receptor positive (ER+) and Her-2/neu negative. They are positive for luminal cytokeratins such as CK8/18.

These tumors are generally well differentiated, more likely to be low stage (T1), with increased expression of progesterone receptor, low proliferation index, and negative Her-2/neu expression compared with luminal B tumors. These tumors are also associated with a significantly better recurrence-free survival and superior overall survival.[3,8–11] In addition, the level of progesterone receptor expression seems to be a significant prognosticator in luminal A tumors, in which levels higher than 20% are associated with a better survival,[9] compared with luminal B tumors. In the study by Sotirou and colleagues,[8] the 10-year relapse-free survival for luminal A tumors was 80%. Similarly, this subtype constitutes the largest group, comprising approximately 60% of all breast cancers and also shows a lower relapse rate (9% within 5 years).[3] Endocrine therapy alone is considered sufficient for this group of tumors.[12]

LUMINAL B

Increased expression for the estrogen receptor gene and related genes, expression of luminal cytokeratins (CK8/18), and increased expression of proliferation genes, such as CCNB1, MYBL2, and MKI67, characterize the luminal B subtype.[7] Compared with luminal A tumors, these tumors tend to have a lower expression of the estrogen receptor–related gene set. In addition, these tumors have higher proliferation rates, shown by Ki-67 nuclear labeling by immunohistochemistry, and also overexpress the Her-2/neu gene, at least in a subset of cases. Therefore, luminal B tumors seem to be a more heterogeneous group and can be defined as ER+/Her-2/neu-/Ki-67 ≥14% and ER+/Her-2/neu+.[12] Morphologically, they tend to be of a higher grade and have a worse outcome clinically with greater chances of relapse compared with luminal A tumors.[3,10,11,13] Incorporating the Ki-67 labeling index has been reported to have significant value in stratifying the luminal tumors and identifying different subgroups with poor prognosis.[14] Although a cutoff of 14% is used to stratify risk in these tumors,[14] it is important to remember that this cutoff value does not represent a true bimodal distribution because the expression of Ki-67 is a continuum,[15] leaving this cutoff to be debated and requiring further validating studies.[16,17] If left untreated, luminal B tumors have a relapse risk similar to that of basal-type tumors.[18] Accurately identifying these tumors is vital because treatment regimens are based on this. Additional chemotherapy and anti–Her-2–related drugs are indicated in these cases.[12]

Comparative genomic hybridization (CGH) studies have shown that recurrent chromosomal changes are present within the luminal group. Concurrent deletions of 16q and gains of 1q, which are considered hallmark changes associated with low-grade ductal carcinoma, are seen in most ER+ carcinoma, more frequent in the low-grade ER+ disease.[19] These chromosomal alterations are rare in ER-negative tumors, suggesting that progression from ER+ to ER-negative disease rarely happens, if ever.

One of the most common gene mutations present in luminal breast cancers involves the PIK3CA gene. In addition to adding prognostic significance, this may be important as a therapeutic target.

HER-2/NEU-ENRICHED (HER-2/NEU-POSITIVE) SUBTYPE

This subtype approximates 15% of all breast carcinomas. These tumors have a high histologic grade affecting approximately 75% of these tumors. By genomic analysis, these tumors show increased expression of the Her-2/neu gene and other genes related to the Her-2/neu amplicon, such as GRB 7 and TRAP 100 on chromosome 17q12. Genes related to proliferation also show increased expression. By immunohistochemistry, these tumors show estrogen receptor negativity and Her-2/neu protein positivity. However, it is important to understand that a substantial proportion of Her-2/neu protein expressing tumors belong in the luminal B subtype and not all of these tumors show gene amplification. Mutations related to the p53 gene are seen in a significant proportion of these tumors, estimated at 40%.

Her-2/neu-positive tumors, at presentation, seem to be associated significantly with multifocal/multicentric disease, positive lymph nodes, and high-volume nodal involvement (≥4 nodes) compared with luminal A disease.[20] Clinically, these tumors behave in an aggressive fashion. However, in the recent past, the outcome of these tumors has been modified by anti–Her-2 treatments, which has had a positive impact on survival.[21,22] In addition, these tumors reportedly show a better response to chemotherapeutic agents.[23–25] These tumors also have a better response to neoadjuvant therapy than the luminal subtypes, with complete pathologic response seen in a large proportion of these tumors.[26] Local recurrences are most commonly seen with Her-2/

neu-positive tumors, approximating 8% compared with 1.8% in luminal A tumors over a 5-year period following breast-conserving surgery.[27] Similarly significantly lower rates of regional relapse-free survival was seen in this group (along with the basal subtype)[28] compared with the Luminal A subtype. Bone and liver metastases are seen frequently with the Her-2/neu-positive subtype.[29]

BASAL-LIKE SUBTYPE

The basal phenotype is characterized by lack of expression of estrogen receptors and related genes and Her-2/neu-related genes, but shows increased expression of KRT5, KRT17, CX3CL1, Annexin 8, and TRIM29. As the name implies, there is increased expression of cytokeratins related to the basal/myoepithelial cells. Also seen is an increased expression of epidermal growth factor receptor. A large proportion of these tumors (approximately 75%) contain mutations in the p53 gene. By immunohistochemistry, these tumors are negative for estrogen, progesterone receptors, and Her-2/neu, although they are positive for basal cytokeratins and epidermal growth factor receptors. Common basal cytokeratins used to identify these tumors are CK5/6, CK17, and CK19 using immunohistochemical methods.

Morphologically, these tumors are high grade with a high mitotic rate, necrosis, pushing borders, and peritumoral lymphocytic infiltrate.[30] Clinically these tumors present at a younger age and are more common in the African American population, and present with larger tumors with a higher proportion of concomitant lymph node metastasis (reviewed in Ref.[31]). These tumors have a poor prognosis compared with luminal tumors, with a significantly shorter relapse-free survival with a high proportion of women relapsing in less than 3 years. Basal tumors also have a higher proportion of metastasis to the central nervous system.[29]

For routine clinical use, surrogate immunohistochemical markers are used to classify tumors into the intrinsic subtypes (**Table 1**).[32] This classification is important because subsequent treatment decisions are based on this categorization.

More recently, additional subtypes have been described.

Claudin Low Subtype

These tumors tend to cluster close to the triple-negative group. They have a low to negative expression of estrogen receptor–related genes and Her-2/neu and related genes. Also, basal cytokeratins are inconsistently expressed. In addition, the expression of proliferations markers is low in these tumors. This group of tumors, alternatively, seems to have an increased expression of genes related to the immune system, cell-cell communication, cell differentiation, cell migration, and angiogenesis. Decreased expression of genes related to cell-to-cell adhesion is also seen, such as

Table 1
Classification of breast carcinoma into intrinsic subtypes using immunohistochemistry

ER-Positive Tumors	ER-Negative Tumors
Luminal A: • ER positive/Her-2/neu negative	Her2/neu: • ER negative/Her-2/neu positive
Luminal B: • ER positive/Her-2/neu negative/Ki-67 ≥14% • ER positive/Her-2/neu positive	Basal phenotype: • ER negative/Her-2/neu negative • Positive for high-molecular-weight cytokeratins (eg, CK 5/6) and EGFR

From Bandyopadhyay S, Ali-Fehmi R. Breast carcinoma: molecular profiling and updates. Clin Lab Med 2013;33(4):895; with permission.

the claudin group (3,4 and 7) and E-cadherin. Morphologically, these tumors are heterogeneous, including metaplastic, medullary, and invasive ductal carcinoma, with no specific type in particular. Overall prognosis and survival in these tumors is worse than in the luminal A type and more akin to that of luminal B, Her-2/neu, and basal subtypes.[33]

Molecular Apocrine Subtype

Another group of breast carcinomas has been identified by Farmer and colleagues,[34] which include all ER-negative tumors (decreased expression of ESR1 gene), distinct from the basal-like group. These tumors overexpress ERRB2 genes and also show increased androgen receptor (AR) signaling. Other overexpressed genes include those related to metabolism (lipid synthesis). Correlation with apocrine morphology reveals a strong association between marked apocrine features and AR+/ER− phenotype. Similar associations between apocrine morphology, ER negativity, and ERRB2 positivity have been reported,[35] suggesting an overlap between the ERRB2 enriched group and the molecular apocrine group. Coexpression of AR and Her-2/neu has also been reported by immunohistochemistry in a subset of high-grade invasive carcinomas with apocrine features.[36] One of the proposed hypotheses to explain this association suggests that ERRB2 overexpression stabilizes, modifies, and affects AR function and expression.[37] Identifying genes that are overexpressed in molecular apocrine carcinomas, such as AR and 3-hydroxy, 3-methylgluryl glutaryl COa reductase(HMGCR), will help in the design and use of novel treatment options tailored in these patients.[34]

Interferon-Related Group

More recently, an additional possible subtype has been described, namely the interferon (IFN) group, which shows an increased proliferation of interferon-related genes, including STAT1.[18] STAT1 is considered to regulate the overexpression of the IFN-related genes.[38] Overexpression of these genes has been associated with poor prognosis.

Molecular correlates of histologic subtypes

As per the World Health Organization classification, 17 additional subtypes have been described based on specific morphologic features. Tumors in each of these categories are defined by a constellation of morphologic features (**Table 2**) that are unique to that special type. Together, these tumors approximate 25% of all breast cancers.[2] These morphologic subtypes have in the past intrigued researchers, and one of the questions that arise from morphologic categorization of these tumors is whether the morphology bears any independent prognostic and predictive significance. Also, the rarity of these subtypes hampers the study of these tumors in large cohorts to effectively determine outcomes.

Some morphologic variants have already been described to have characteristic clinical features. For example, tubular carcinomas are known to have an excellent prognosis with significantly longer disease-free and breast cancer–specific survival.[39] Similarly, cribriform carcinoma also has been reported to have a better disease-free survival[40] compared with grade 1 IDC-NOS. The morphologic variants within the triple-negative subtype also highlight the heterogeneity of this molecular subtype. Studies report the good prognosis of the adenoid cystic and medullary carcinoma compared with triple-negative IDC and, conversely, the worse outcome of metaplastic carcinoma.[41] Also, there is the pathologic response achieved among the different variants, further underscoring the importance of this knowledge.

Table 2	
Histologic subtypes and their molecular subtypes	
Histologic Subtype	**Molecular Subtype**
Invasive lobular carcinoma	–
Classic variant	Luminal A
Pleomorphic variant	Luminal A Her-2/neu enriched/molecular apocrine
Tubular carcinoma	Luminal A
Mucinous/neuroendocrine	Luminal A
Invasive papillary carcinoma	Luminal A
Micropapillary carcinoma	Luminal B/C ERRB2
Apocrine carcinoma	Her-2/neu enriched/molecular apocrine Triple negative
Metaplastic carcinoma	Triple negative
Medullary carcinoma	Triple negative
Adenoid cystic carcinoma	Triple negative
Secretory carcinoma	Triple negative

Data from Weigelt B, Horlings HM, Kreike B, et al. Refinement of breast cancer classification by molecular characterization of histological special types. J Pathol 2008;216:141–50.

Barring the usage of E-cadherin by immunohistochemistry, there are few identified and validated diagnostic markers that can be used appropriately to differentiate or characterize these subtypes. This scarcity brings forth another question: how different are these tumors at the molecular level and do these tumors bear any resemblance to the molecular subtypes thus far identified?

Weigelt and colleagues[42] undertook a study that included 113 cases of 11 pure histologic subtypes. Intrinsic genes that were analyzed were 1098 in number and hierarchical cluster analysis was performed. The investigators were able to identify molecular subtypes for most of the histologic types studied. Most histologic types seemed to be fairly homogenous and correlated with 1 molecular subtype; however, some of the histologic variants seemed to be more heterogeneous and corresponded with multiple intrinsic subtypes.

Some selected, more commonly encountered special histologic subtypes that are discussed in this article include:

1. Invasive lobular carcinoma
2. Tubular carcinoma/cribriform carcinoma
3. Invasive mucinous carcinoma/neuroendocrine carcinoma
4. Invasive papillary carcinoma
5. Invasive micropapillary carcinoma
6. Apocrine carcinoma
7. Metaplastic carcinoma
8. Medullary carcinoma
9. Secretory carcinoma
10. Adenoid cystic carcinoma.

Invasive lobular carcinoma Invasive lobular carcinoma accounts for 5% to 15% of all invasive carcinomas and is the most frequently encountered special type.[2] Discohesive cells characterize this histologic type morphologically, and may be singly dispersed or present as cords of cells in the stroma. Sometimes, these cells aggregate into small clusters (alveolar) and in a sheetlike pattern (solid). A definitive desmoplastic response is not associated with these neoplastic cells. In the classic variant, the nuclei are small (resembling a lymphocyte) and fairly uniform. The mitotic index is very low. Invasive lobular carcinoma seems to have distinct prognostic differences compared with ductal carcinoma, with an early survival advantage.[43] These tumors are positive for estrogen and progesterone receptors and negative for Her-2/neu. However, they are predominantly of the luminal These tumors are positive for estrogen and progesterone receptors (Luminal); however, they independently of Luminal A ductal carcinoma on unsupervised hiererchical clustering.[44,45] In the recent past, another subtype of lobular carcinoma, the pleomorphic variant, has been increasingly described in the literature.[46,47] This variant is characterized by a high-grade cytology with apocrine features and pleomorphic nuclei, and has a higher proliferation rate. Accurate identification of these tumors is of significant interest, because these tumors seem to have a worse prognosis with a higher rate of recurrence compared with high-grade ductal carcinoma and classic-type lobular carcinoma.[48,49] Almost all of these tumors are ER+ and Her-2/neu negative, whereas a small subset of the pleomorphic variant may be estrogen receptor negative and Her-2/neu positive by immunohistochemistry. At the molecular level, these tumors predominantly prove to be of the luminal A subtype; rare cases are luminal B, Her-2/neu enriched, and of the molecular apocrine subtype. Also, these tumors seem to be different at the molecular level from grade and molecular subtype–matched IDC-NOS. Downregulated genes in invasive lobular carcinoma compared with IDC are the CDH1 gene and genes associated with cell adhesion, cell cycle regulation, and cytoskeleton remodeling. Also downregulated differentially in lobular carcinoma is the TMSB10 gene, associated with cell growth and proliferation. Alternatively, genes that are upregulated include ESR2, genes involved in lipid metabolism, and the PLEKHA7 gene, which may play a role in invasion, among others.[42,44] Most of these tumors reveal 16q loss with gain of 1q by CGH analysis. Other alterations that differentiate them from ductal carcinoma are 13q and 22q losses, seen more frequently in lobular carcinoma, whereas losses in 11q are more common in ductal carcinoma.[45]

Tubular carcinoma/cribriform carcinoma These tumors, comprising approximately 4% of all breast carcinomas, are composed predominantly (>90%) of small round to oval or angulated tubular structures with open lumina.[2] The cells lining the tubules are cuboidal, cytologically bland cells with a low mitotic index. Cribriform carcinomas, often associated with tubular carcinoma, are histologically characterized by a predominant cribriform growth pattern.

By immunohistochemistry, both of these histologic subtypes are positive for estrogen receptor and negative for Her-2/neu.

Tubular carcinomas seem to have a significantly better prognosis compared with low-grade IDC-NOS,[39] with life expectancy approximating that of the general population. A similar good prognosis is also seen with cribriform carcinoma.[50]

At the molecular level, these tumors cluster with the luminal A subtype, indicating that they share similarities with these tumors at the genomic level.

Compared with grade and molecular subtype–matched IDC-NOS, these tumors show an upregulation of genes related to estrogen receptor, transcription, and apoptosis. Upregulation of the estrogen receptor signaling pathway seen in tubular carcinomas may explain the favorable prognosis that these tumors have compared with grade-matched IDC-NOS.[42]

By CGH analysis, loss of 16q has been documented in most tubular carcinoma cases studied (86%), with 52% of cases showing 2p loss and 48% of cases showing 9p loss. The most frequent (62%) chromosomal gains involve 11p and 13q.[51]

Mucinous and neuroendocrine carcinoma These tumors are estimated at 2% of all invasive breast carcinomas.[2] Morphologically, they are composed of tumor cell nests and clusters accompanied by large pools of extracellular mucin making up more than 90% of the tumor. They are noted to have a lower incidence of lymph nodal involvement and a better overall survival compared with invasive ductal carcinoma. These tumors have been divided into paucicellular and cellular groups (types A and B respectively).[52] The type A tumors have a lower cell to mucus ratio with 60% to 90% of the tumor being composed of mucus, whereas the hypercellular variant shows larger cell nests compared with the amount of mucin (30%–75% composed of mucin). These tumors are generally positive for estrogen receptor by immunohistochemistry and also for chromogranin and synaptophysin. The diagnosis of neuroendocrine carcinoma is made based on typical histologic features and when more than 50% of the cells are positive for neuroendocrine markers. On genomic analysis, these tumors correspond with the luminal A subtype.[42] Further hierarchical analysis concludes that, within this group, type A mucinous tumors tend to form a separate cluster, whereas the type B and neuroendocrine tumors are intermixed. Overall, they seem to be a distinct group compared with grade and molecular subtype–matched IDC-NOS.[53] At the transcript level, mucinous A tumors show downregulation of extracellular matrix genes compared with grade and subtype–matched IDC-NOS. Also downregulated are high molecular cytokeratin genes and Her-2/neu, whereas estrogen receptor–regulated genes, BCL2, luminal keratins, and genes of the fibroblast growth factor (FGF) family seem to be upregulated in these tumors. In the mucinous B subtype, the differences seen were similar to those in mucinous A; in addition, upregulation of the p53 and Wnt/β-catenin signaling pathway is seen. Considerable overlap is seen between the luminal B and neuroendocrine tumors.[53] By CGH analysis, mucinous tumors showed gains of 1q and 16p and losses of 16q and 22q less frequently than grade and ER–matched IDC-NOS. Also concurrent loss of 16q and gain of 1q, considered to be a characteristic feature of low-grade carcinomas, is not seen in pure mucinous tumors.[54]

Invasive papillary carcinoma Papillary carcinomas of the breast in addition to the encapsulated papillary carcinoma may be invasive and of the solid papillary subtype. Neoplastic epithelial cells lining a fibrovascular core and the lack of a myoepithelial cell layer characterize papillary carcinoma. In the solid papillary variant, the neoplastic cells form solid, nodular nests, surrounded by a fibrous capsule.

Most of these tumors are positive for estrogen receptor and negative for Her-2/neu (lumina A),[55,56] although lumina B, Her-2/neu overexpressing and triple-negative subtypes have been identified in smaller numbers.[56] Compared with matched cases of IDC-NOS, these tumors seem to have a better overall survival and disease-free survival. In addition, the subtype status also shows significant impact on survival.

These tumors do not cluster with grade and ER–matched IDC-NOS on unsupervised hierarchical cluster analysis. Although the pattern of genomic aberrations is similar to that seen in IDC-NOS, these changes are fewer and less complex.[55] Commonly seen are genomic alterations characteristic of ER+ low-grade breast cancer, such as loss of 16q and gains in 16p and 1q. The most commonly encountered amplification is CCND1 gene amplification, located on 11q13, seen in about one-tenth of the cases.[55] Also, PIK3CA mutations were more frequently seen in papillary carcinoma cases, compared with grade and ER–matched IDC-NOS.

In addition, the 3 variants of papillary carcinoma (encapsulated papillary carcinoma, solid papillary carcinoma, and invasive papillary carcinoma) do not cluster independently of each other on unsupervised hierarchical clustering and may represent variations of the same pathologic entity.

Invasive micropapillary carcinoma Pure or predominantly micropapillary carcinoma constitutes less than 2% of all breast cancer cases.[2] Morphologically, these tumors have a distinctive architectural pattern and are composed of nests of tumor cells with reversed polarity present within lacunar spaces. Abluminal staining pattern with epithelial membrane antigen (EMA) is useful in showing the reverse polarity of the cells. Micropapillary carcinomas are variably positive for estrogen receptor and Her-2/neu. They tend to have a higher rate of lymph node metastasis compared with IDC-NOS. Also, a worse prognosis has been attributed to these tumors.[57] These tumors tend to be predominantly of the luminal subtype with a smaller subset being of the Her-2 phenotype.[58] Also associated with these tumors is a high proliferation index, indicating that they belong to the luminal B subtype rather than luminal A.[58] Rare triple-negative cases have also been reported.[59]

Complex genomic alterations have been identified in this variant using CGH technology. The most frequent alteration seen is loss of 8p. Other chromosomal alterations include loss of 1p, 17p, and 16q. Also approximately two-thirds of these cases showed evidence of 6p gain and 6q loss.[58] Gains are seen in 16p, 1q, 17q, 13q, 8p, and 1p. Recurrent amplifications were reported in 4p, 8p, 8q, 11q, 17q, and 20q. Amplification of 8q has been significantly associated with micropapillary carcinoma,[58,60] compared with ductal carcinomas, and these amplified regions include the MYC gene. Amplification of the MYC gene has been reported in one-third of the cases and this has been linked to proliferation, metastasis, and aggressive behavior.[58]

Compared with grade and ER–matched IDC-NOS, micropapillary carcinomas tend to be genetically more complex more frequently and seem to be a distinct entity.

Apocrine carcinoma These are defined as carcinomas with more than 90% of the tumor showing apocrine differentiation, which includes eosinophilic cytoplasm, round nuclei, and prominent nucleoli. In some cases, the cytoplasm is finely vacuolated. They are rare and constitute 0.3% to 4% of all breast carcinomas.[2] These tumors are frequently positive for GCDFP 15 by immunohistochemistry. Most of these tumors are estrogen receptor negative, AR positive, and Her-2/neu negative, whereas the rest are estrogen receptor negative, AR and Her-2/neu receptor positive.[61,62] In addition, p53 overexpression is significantly associated with the triple-negative apocrine group.[62]

In addition to the morphologic features, this subtype has also been shown to exist as a distinct entity at the molecular level by gene expression profiling.[34]

Clinically, studies have shown that these tumors have a significantly worse overall disease-free survival compared with IDC. Also, reporting the AR status of these patients may be important because they could potentially benefit from targeted therapy.

Metaplastic carcinoma These are a morphologically heterogeneous group of tumors that constitute less than 1% of all breast carcinomas.[2] They are composed of an admixture of adenocarcinoma with a spindle cell, squamous, or mesenchymal component. In some cases, the spindle cell and squamous cell components may be pure, lacking an admixed adenocarcinoma component. These tumors are hormone receptor and Her-2/neu negative. Clinically, they are aggressive tumors and seem to be more chemoresistant than other triple-negative tumors.[63] With gene expression profiling and unsupervised hierarchical clustering, metaplastic carcinomas cluster with and are intermixed with basal-like ductal carcinoma. At the transcriptional level, differential expression of genes between the 2 groups is seen, clinically relevant among these being downregulation of PTEN and TOP2A genes in metaplastic carcinoma, which are targets for anthracyclines and therefore may explain chemoresistance to these agents.[42,64] Also, another study of the genomewide analysis of different components of these tumors reported genetic heterogeneity, which corresponds with the morphologic variations present.[65] A high proportion of alterations related to the PI3K (phosphatidylinositol-4,5-bisphosphate 3-kinase)/AKT(Protein kinase B) pathway have been identified in these tumors. In addition, these tumors show a high-level genomic instability based on the proportion of genetic alterations present. Gains in 1p, 11q, 12q, 14q, 22q, and 19p and increased loss of 1q, 2p, 3q, and 8q are seen. Gain in 1q and loss of 16q, alterations generally present in low-grade tumors, are not seen.[63] Although triple negative and seeming to cluster adjacent to the basal tumors by hierarchical clustering, at the transcriptional level, metaplastic tumors seem to be a distinct subset from the basal-like tumors.

Medullary carcinoma Tumors included in this histologic subtype have well-defined pushing borders, high-grade cytology with pleomorphic and vesicular nuclei and numerous mitoses and a syncytial growth pattern (at least 75%). Tubule formation and in situ components are not seen. A prominent tumoral lymphocytic infiltrate is present. These tumors comprise 1% to 7% of all breast carcinomas and this variation depends on the criteria used for diagnosis.[2] These tumors are predominantly estrogen receptor negative; however, cases that are estrogen positive have been described.[66] ER positivity seems to confer a poor prognosis on these patients. Although the rate of progesterone receptor positivity is low in these tumors, this seems to provide some survival benefit to these patients.[66] Overall, these tumors reportedly have a better overall survival compared with IDC-NOS.[66–68] However, numerous studies have documented lymph nodal involvement to significantly decrease overall survival.[66,69] Also, the size of the tumor and distant metastasis affect overall survival.[66,70]

At the molecular level, these tumors cluster with the basal tumors showing lack of expression of ESR and Her-2/neu genes.[42,71] However, some differences have been reported. Compared with basal-like tumors, medullary carcinomas showed increased expression of immune response genes, including T cell–associated genes, STAT1, and interferon regulating genes, such as IRF1, IRF7, IRF2, IRF4, and IRF8. Also seen was an overexpression of apoptosis-related genes such as tumor necrosis factor (TNF) receptor genes, TNF ligand superfamilies, and TNFα-induced proteins. Underexpressed genes included those related to maintenance of the cytoskeleton, including actins, myosin, and tropomyosin. Compared with basal-like cancers, there is a loss of expression of myoepithelial-related genes.[71] Medullary breast carcinomas show gains in chromosomes 1q, 8p, 10p, and 12p, which have not been reported in Basal Like Carcinoma (BLC).[72]

This tumor is also seen frequently in BRCA1 mutation–related tumors, approximating 11%.

Although these tumors are triple negative and appear similar to basal-like cancers at a glance, there are genetic/molecular differences between them, which may explain the good prognosis associated with them.

Secretory carcinoma These tumors are identified by the presence of eosinophilic secretions in intracellular vacuoles and spaces. They are extremely rare tumors and are comprise less than 0.15% of all breast cancers. Originally described in young patients, they were termed juvenile carcinomas[73]; however, with subsequent identification in adult patients, the terminology was changed to secretory carcinoma based on the characteristic morphology of these tumors.[74]

These tumors are typically slow growing with rare, if any, instances of lymph node metastasis. Most of these cases are triple negative, although rare cases with hormone receptor positivity have been reported. In addition, reports of these tumors document them to be positive for basal cytokeratins, C-KIT, and EGFR.[75,76] The occurrence of these indolent tumors as triple negative highlights the increasingly recognized heterogeneity of this group of tumors. Chromosomal translocation (t12; 15) resulting in fusion of ETSV6 and NTRK3 genes, although not consistently present, is considered characteristic for secretory carcinoma.[76,77]

Adenoid cystic carcinoma Adenoid cystic carcinoma of the breast is an extremely rare subtype and comprises about 0.1% of all breast carcinomas.[2] On histology, they mimic the adenoid cystic tumor of the salivary gland with the tumor cells resembling epithelial-myoepithelial cells. These cells are arranged in cords and cribriform and solid nests and are associated with eosinophilic hyaline basement membrane–like and mucoid material. Mitoses are rare. The basal cells express basal cytokeratins, p63, actin, calponin, and S 100, whereas the luminal cells express luminal cytokeratin, EMA, CEA, and C-KIT. Typically, these tumors are negative for estrogen receptors and Her-2/neu by immunohistochemistry.

Compared with IDC-NOS of similar grade, these tumors are reported to have a significantly better prognosis and overall survival. Axillary lymph node metastasis is rarely seen in these tumors and therefore axillary node dissection is not considered essential.

These tumors cluster with the basal subtype by gene expression profiling. However, there seems to be downregulation of genes involved in migration, proliferation, and invasion, possibly underlying the good prognosis in these patients.[42] The genomic alterations seem to differ from grade-matched IDC cases. A repeated genetic abnormality that has been detected in adenoid cystic carcinoma of both the breast and head and neck is fusion of MYB and NFIB transcription factors, which results from t(6;9). This abnormality has not been detected in grade-matched triple-negative breast carcinoma cases.[78–80]

Ductal carcinoma in situ

Since the institution of mammographic screening for breast cancer, the diagnosis of ductal carcinoma in situ (DCIS) has increased many fold, comprising approximately 20% of all breast carcinoma diagnoses. Although DCIS is a nonobligate precursor of invasive carcinoma, a diagnosis of DCIS increases the risk of subsequent invasive carcinoma 8 to 10 times. Without treatment, approximately half of the cases of DCIS transform to invasive carcinoma.[81] Traditionally, DCIS is classified by architectural growth pattern, nuclear grade, and the presence or absence of necrosis. Nuclear grade is considered to have prognostic significance, with DCIS of high nuclear grade having the highest recurrence rate (reviewed in Ref.[82]).

The biological markers, estrogen and progesterone receptors, are positive in approximately half to three-quarters of the in situ lesions and these hormone receptor–positive cases are associated with low nuclear grade and noncomedo carcinomas.[83–85] Her-2/neu expression has been reported in 30% to 55% of DCIS and has been associated with high nuclear grade. Provenzano and colleagues[86] reported that negative status of hormone receptors and positive Her-2 status were independent prognostic markers. In addition, p53 protein expression has been reported in high-grade DCIS.[87]

Studies that have analyzed gene expression at the RNA level have identified heterogeneity at the molecular level in these precursor lesions. Using 392 genes to identify the intrinsic subtypes, luminal, basal, and Her-2/neu subtypes were identified within the in situ lesions, which underscores the hypothesis that molecular abnormalities and alterations are acquired early in the neoplastic process.[88]

In situ to invasive carcinoma: molecular pathways

Two models of progression of DCIS to invasive cancer have been hypothesized. The first model is known as the theory of linear progression, which purports that low-grade DCIS progresses to high-grade DCIS and then transforms to invasive cancer. The second theory, also known as the theory of parallel disease, proposes that low-grade DCIS transforms into low-grade invasive carcinoma and high-grade DCIS progresses to high-grade invasive carcinoma (reviewed in Ref.[89]). A study by Gupta and colleagues[90] showed that the grade of DCIS and concurrent invasive carcinoma are correlated and this is also correlated with outcome. A more recent study by Wallis and colleagues[91] concluded that high-grade DCIS tends to recur earlier than low-grade DCIS. Also, in their study cohort of patients with low-grade DCIS, the investigators did not identify any high-grade recurrences, metastases, or deaths. Molecular studies also support this theory to be more likely involved in breast cancer progression. One such finding in support of this theory is that loss of chromosome 16q is seen more frequently in low-grade DCIS, whereas allelic imbalances of 13q, 17q, and 20q are more common in high-grade DCIS. These changes are recapitulated or maintained in concurrent invasive lesions.[92] Although these studies support the theory of parallel disease, they also imply that these 2 pathways may not be mutually exclusive, as exemplified in another study in which the investigators identified a subset of low-grade DCIS that eventually developed into high-grade DCIS.[93]

The tipping point in the progression of in situ carcinoma to invasive carcinoma is characterized by breach of the basement membrane and invasion of the stroma. Studies have shown differences at the molecular level when comparing stroma surrounding DCIS with stroma around invasive disease.[94,95] Considering cases of pure DCIS versus cases associated with invasive disease, upregulation of genes related to Epithelial mesenchymal transition and myoepithelial cells have been reported in the epithelial compartment of the latter compared with the epithelium of pure DCIS.[96] In contrast, the epithelial component of DCIS associated with invasive disease is very similar to the invasive component.[94,95] This similarity implies that pure DCIS might be a distinct disease compared with DCIS associated with invasion, at the molecular level.

Although the exact pathway of progression of DCIS is still under investigation and remains debatable, it seems that genetic/transcriptional changes in both epithelial and stromal compartments are essential to this process.

The Cancer Genome Atlas and breast carcinoma

The Cancer Genome Atlas (TCGA) Network was founded to research tumors from various organ systems at the genomic and epigenomic levels and subsequently provides open-access resources for breast cancer research worldwide.

Four-hundred and sixty-six breast carcinoma tumor samples were evaluated by 6 different platforms and used to identify changes in the genomic structure to provide comprehensive information regarding the same. These methods are (1) DNA methylation, (2) gene expression (3) microRNA (miRNA) sequencing, (4) single nucleotide polymorphism arrays, (5) exome sequencing, and (6) reverse phase protein arrays.[97]

The Cancer Genome Atlas and luminal carcinoma The luminal subtype of breast carcinoma is most diverse at the molecular level, when analyzing gene expression, mutations, and copy number changes.[98] The most significant findings within this subtype were increased messenger RNA (mRNA) and protein expression of the ER family of genes (ESR, GATA-3, FOX1A, XBP1, and cMYC).[97,98] It was also noted that mutations of GATA-3 and FOX1A were mutually exclusive; additionally ESR1 and XBP1 expression was increased.

One of the most frequently mutated genes in breast carcinoma is the PIK3CA gene, identified in approximately 45% of luminal A carcinomas and 29% of luminal B carcinomas.[97] However, although frequently mutated, subsequent markers of pathway expression were not identified by mRNA or protein assays in luminal carcinoma. Frequent possible inactivating mutations in MAP3K1 and MAP2K4 genes, part of the p38/JNK1pathway, were identified.

Another frequently mutated gene in luminal breast carcinoma was the TP53 gene (mainly missense mutations). The frequency of TP53 mutation in luminal A carcinoma was lower at 12% compared with luminal B carcinoma (29%). Luminal B tumors also showed associated pathway-related events such as ATM loss and MDM2 amplification, implying that the more aggressive luminal B subtype was more significantly affected by TP53 mutations.

RB1 gene expression was mostly intact in luminal A tumors as shown by both mRNA and protein expression.

The DNA hypermethylation phenotype was significantly enriched for the luminal B subtype[97]; however, this group showed a lower frequency of PIK3CA, MAP3K1, and MAP2K4 mutations. Characteristic methylation patterns were also noted in other studies[99]; when examining amplifications and deletions and arms-level gains and losses, characteristic 1q gain and/or 16q losses of luminal breast carcinomas was confirmed.[100,101] Protein assay analysis identified increased protein expression of ER, PR, AR, GATA-3, BCL2, and INPP4B.[97]

The Cancer Genome Atlas and HER2-enriched carcinoma The TCGA study confirmed the HER2/Her-2/neu gene amplification in the Her-2 intrinsic subtype of breast carcinoma. Approximately 50% of the clinically Her-2–positive group clustered within the Her-2–enriched group and the remainder clustered within the ER+ intrinsic subtype. Those tumors which were within the HER2-enriched group showed increased expression of FGFR4, HER1/EGFR, and HER2 genes as well as other genes present within the HER2 amplicon. In contrast, HER2-positive tumors, which clustered with the luminal subtype, showed amplification of other luminal genes, such as GATA3, BCL2, and ESR1. Furthermore, TP53 mutations were more frequent in the Her-2–enriched group, whereas GATA-3 mutation was identified more frequently in the luminal group.[97]

Increased frequency of PIK3CA gene mutations were noted in up to 39% of this group.

No specific DNA methylation patterns were identified associated with this group.

Protein expression correlated with the subtypes identified, including high correlation with Her-2 protein expression, which has been established as a clinical target.

The Cancer Genome Atlas and basal-like carcinoma High frequency of TP53 mutations were identified in up to 80% of basal-like carcinoma and these consisted of mainly nonsense and frameshift mutations. RB1 and BRCA1 mutations are also commonly present in basal-like carcinomas. PIK3CA gene mutations, commonly present in breast cancer overall, was also present in basal-like carcinoma, with a frequency of 9%; however, the impact of these mutations via downstream pathway events was more significant in basal-like breast carcinoma compared with luminal carcinomas. Similar gene mutations have been reported in other studies.[99,102]

Similar molecular abnormalities were identified between basal-like carcinoma and ovarian serous carcinoma, including mutations inTP53, BRCA1, RB1, cyclin D1, cMYC genes.[97] Also there were similar copy number alterations between basal-like breast carcinoma and ovarian serous carcinoma, such as common gains of 1q, 3q, 8q, and 12p, and loss of 4q, 5q, and 8p. These common genetic abnormalities detected in basal-like and ovarian serous carcinoma imply that these may be driver mutations for these very aggressive tumors.

Cell-free nucleic acid analysis

Although solid tissue–based analysis has been the mainstay of breast cancer diagnosis, analysis of cell-free samples via interrogation of circulating miRNA and cell-free DNA (cfDNA) in fluids including serum, plasma, urine, spinal fluid has proved beneficial for diagnosis and prognosis of breast carcinoma.[103] To this end, miRNA, including miR-1, miR-92a, miR-133a, and miR-133b, has been found to be increased, whereas let-7b, miR-381, miR-10b, miR-125a-5p, miR-335, miR-205, and miR-145, among others, have been found to be downregulated in patients with breast cancer.[104] cfDNA has also been reported to be useful for detecting PIK3CA gene mutation in breast cancer,[105] especially for metastatic disease. However, although a recent meta-analysis concluded that cfDNA is a promising test in screening and diagnosis of breast cancer, the caveat that using population-based standardization of test methods before clinical use would be required has been noted.[106] Further studies will help elucidate the ideal application of circulating nucleic acids in breast cancer.

SUMMARY

The most significant contribution of molecular subtyping of breast carcinomas has been the identification of estrogen-positive and estrogen-negative tumor subtypes. These two entities are distinct, with differing prognoses and requiring different therapy. Also, molecular and genetic analyses can provide prognostic information; however, thorough histopathologic evaluation with evaluation of the predictive biomarkers (ER, PR, and Her-2/neu) is able to provide similar information. Knowledge of genetic alterations in these tumors will help clinicians identify novel therapeutic targets, which might have significant impact on prognosis. Understanding the progression pathways involved in the transition of in situ carcinoma to invasive carcinoma might lead to efficient risk stratification in these patients.

The Cancer Genome Analysis Network has collected genomic and epigenomic data across multiple interrogative platforms and tumor types to provide comprehensive information regarding carcinogenesis and pathway interactions. Prime examples are the similarities elucidated between triple-negative breast carcinoma and ovarian serous carcinoma. Such information improves understanding of the disease process and also provides more accurate information toward identifying targetable mutations for treatment.

REFERENCES

1. Siegel R, Naishadham D, Jemal A. Cancer statistics, 2013. CA Cancer J Clin 2013;63:11–30.
2. Tavassoli FA, Devilee P, editors. World Health Organization classification of tumor. Pathology and genetics of tumors of the breast and female genital organs. Lyon (France): IARC Press; 2003.
3. O'Brien KM, Cole SR, Tse CK, et al. Intrinsic breast tumor subtypes, race, and long-term survival in the Carolina Breast Cancer Study. Clin Cancer Res 2010; 16:6100–10.

4. Patani N, Martin LA, Dowsett M. Biomarkers for the clinical management of breast cancer: international perspective. Int J Cancer 2013;133:1–13.
5. Hammond ME. ASCO-CAP guidelines for breast predictive factor testing: an update. Appl Immunohistochem Mol Morphol 2011;19:499–500.
6. Perou CM, Sorlie T, Eisen MB, et al. Molecular portraits of human breast tumours. Nature 2000;406:747–52.
7. Sorlie T, Perou CM, Tibshirani R, et al. Gene expression patterns of breast carcinomas distinguish tumor subclasses with clinical implications. Proc Natl Acad Sci U S A 2001;98:10869–74.
8. Sotiriou C, Neo SY, McShane LM, et al. Breast cancer classification and prognosis based on gene expression profiles from a population-based study. Proc Natl Acad Sci U S A 2003;100:10393–8.
9. Prat A, Cheang MC, Martin M, et al. Prognostic significance of progesterone receptor-positive tumor cells within immunohistochemically defined luminal A breast cancer. J Clin Oncol 2013;31:203–9.
10. Park S, Koo JS, Kim MS, et al. Characteristics and outcomes according to molecular subtypes of breast cancer as classified by a panel of four biomarkers using immunohistochemistry. Breast 2012;21:50–7.
11. Voduc KD, Cheang MC, Tyldesley S, et al. Breast cancer subtypes and the risk of local and regional relapse. J Clin Oncol 2010;28:1684–91.
12. Goldhirsch A, Wood WC, Coates AS, et al, Panel Members. Strategies for subtypes–dealing with the diversity of breast cancer: highlights of the St. Gallen International Expert Consensus on the primary therapy of early breast cancer 2011. Ann Oncol 2011;22:1736–47.
13. Kim HS, Park I, Cho HJ, et al. Analysis of the potent prognostic factors in luminal-type breast cancer. J Breast Cancer 2012;15:401–6.
14. Cheang MC, Chia SK, Voduc D, et al. Ki67 index, HER2 status, and prognosis of patients with luminal B breast cancer. J Natl Cancer Inst 2009;101:736–50.
15. Wirapati P, Sotiriou C, Kunkel S, et al. Meta-analysis of gene expression profiles in breast cancer: toward a unified understanding of breast cancer subtyping and prognosis signatures. Breast Cancer Res 2008;10:R65.
16. Guiu S, Michiels S, Andre F, et al. Molecular subclasses of breast cancer: how do we define them? The IMPAKT 2012 working group statement. Ann Oncol 2012;23:2997–3006.
17. Ono M, Tsuda H, Yunokawa M, et al. Prognostic impact of Ki-67 labeling indices with 3 different cutoff values, histological grade, and nuclear grade in hormone-receptor-positive, HER2-negative, node-negative invasive breast cancers. Breast Cancer 2015;22(2):141–52.
18. Hu Z, Fan C, Oh DS, et al. The molecular portraits of breast tumors are conserved across microarray platforms. BMC Genomics 2006;7:96.
19. Natrajan R, Weigelt B, Mackay A, et al. An integrative genomic and transcriptomic analysis reveals molecular pathways and networks regulated by copy number aberrations in basal-like, HER2 and luminal cancers. Breast Cancer Res Treat 2010;121:575–89.
20. Wiechmann L, Sampson M, Stempel M, et al. Presenting features of breast cancer differ by molecular subtype. Ann Surg Oncol 2009;16:2705–10.
21. Dowsett M, Procter M, McCaskill-Stevens W, et al. Disease-free survival according to degree of HER2 amplification for patients treated with adjuvant chemotherapy with or without 1 year of trastuzumab: the HERA trial. J Clin Oncol 2009;27:2962–9.

22. Smith I, Procter M, Gelber RD, et al, HERA study team. 2-year follow-up of trastuzumab after adjuvant chemotherapy in HER2-positive breast cancer: a randomised controlled trial. Lancet 2007;369:29–36.

23. Gennari A, Sormani MP, Pronzato P, et al. HER2 status and efficacy of adjuvant anthracyclines in early breast cancer: a pooled analysis of randomized trials. J Natl Cancer Inst 2008;100:14–20.

24. Hayes DF, Thor AD, Dressler LG, et al, Cancer and Leukemia Group B (CALGB) Investigators. HER2 and response to paclitaxel in node-positive breast cancer. N Engl J Med 2007;357:1496–506.

25. Pritchard KI, Messersmith H, Elavathil L, et al. HER-2 and topoisomerase II as predictors of response to chemotherapy. J Clin Oncol 2008;26:736–44.

26. Goldstein NS, Decker D, Severson D, et al. Molecular classification system identifies invasive breast carcinoma patients who are most likely and those who are least likely to achieve a complete pathologic response after neoadjuvant chemotherapy. Cancer 2007;110:1687–96.

27. Nguyen PL, Taghian AG, Katz MS, et al. Breast cancer subtype approximated by estrogen receptor, progesterone receptor, and HER-2 is associated with local and distant recurrence after breast-conserving therapy. J Clin Oncol 2008;26: 2373–8.

28. Kennecke H, Yerushalmi R, Woods R, et al. Metastatic behavior of breast cancer subtypes. J Clin Oncol 2010;28:3271–7.

29. Smid M, Wang Y, Zhang Y, et al. Subtypes of breast cancer show preferential site of relapse. Cancer Res 2008;68:3108–14.

30. Livasy CA, Karaca G, Nanda R, et al. Phenotypic evaluation of the basal-like subtype of invasive breast carcinoma. Mod Pathol 2006;19:264–71.

31. Bosch A, Eroles P, Zaragoza R, et al. Triple-negative breast cancer: molecular features, pathogenesis, treatment and current lines of research. Cancer Treat Rev 2010;36:206–15.

32. Carey LA, Perou CM, Livasy CA, et al. Race, breast cancer subtypes, and survival in the Carolina Breast Cancer Study. JAMA 2006;295:2492–502.

33. Prat A, Parker JS, Karginova O, et al. Phenotypic and molecular characterization of the claudin-low intrinsic subtype of breast cancer. Breast Cancer Res 2010; 12:R68.

34. Farmer P, Bonnefoi H, Becette V, et al. Identification of molecular apocrine breast tumours by microarray analysis. Oncogene 2005;24:4660–71.

35. Bhargava R, Striebel J, Beriwal S, et al. Prevalence, morphologic features and proliferation indices of breast carcinoma molecular classes using immunohistochemical surrogate markers. Int J Clin Exp Pathol 2009;2:444–55.

36. Moinfar F, Okcu M, Tsybrovskyy O, et al. Androgen receptors frequently are expressed in breast carcinomas: potential relevance to new therapeutic strategies. Cancer 2003;98:703–11.

37. Mellinghoff IK, Vivanco I, Kwon A, et al. HER2/neu kinase-dependent modulation of androgen receptor function through effects on DNA binding and stability. Cancer Cell 2004;6:517–27.

38. Bromberg JF, Horvath CM, Wen Z, et al. Transcriptionally active Stat1 is required for the antiproliferative effects of both interferon alpha and interferon gamma. Proc Natl Acad Sci U S A 1996;93:7673–8.

39. Rakha EA, Lee AH, Evans AJ, et al. Tubular carcinoma of the breast: further evidence to support its excellent prognosis. J Clin Oncol 2010;28:99–104.

40. Colleoni M, Rotmensz N, Maisonneuve P, et al. Outcome of special types of luminal breast cancer. Ann Oncol 2012;23:1428–36.

41. Montagna E, Maisonneuve P, Rotmensz N, et al. Heterogeneity of triple-negative breast cancer: histologic subtyping to inform the outcome. Clin Breast Cancer 2013;13:31–9.
42. Weigelt B, Horlings HM, Kreike B, et al. Refinement of breast cancer classification by molecular characterization of histological special types. J Pathol 2008; 216:141–50.
43. Iorfida M, Maiorano E, Orvieto E, et al. Invasive lobular breast cancer: subtypes and outcome. Breast Cancer Res Treat 2012;133:713–23.
44. Castellana B, Escuin D, Perez-Olabarria M, et al. Genetic up-regulation and overexpression of PLEKHA7 differentiates invasive lobular carcinomas from invasive ductal carcinomas. Hum Pathol 2012;43:1902–9.
45. Gruel N, Lucchesi C, Raynal V, et al. Lobular invasive carcinoma of the breast is a molecular entity distinct from luminal invasive ductal carcinoma. Eur J Cancer 2010;46:2399–407.
46. Eusebi V, Magalhaes F, Azzopardi AG. Pleomorphic lobular carcinoma of the breast: an aggressive tumor showing apocrine differentiation. Hum Pathol 1992;23:655–62.
47. Middleton LP, Palacios DM, Bryant BR, et al. Pleomorphic lobular carcinoma: morphology, immunocytochemistry and molecular analysis. Am J Surg Pathol 2000;24:1650–6.
48. Monhollen L, Morrison C, Ademuyiwa FO, et al. Pleomorphic lobular carcinoma: a distinctive clinical and molecular breast cancer type. Histopathology 2012;61: 365–77.
49. Buchanan CL, Flynn LW, Murray MP, et al. Is pleomorphic lobular carcinoma really a distinct clinical entity? J Surg Oncol 2008;98:314–7.
50. Venable JG, Schwartz AM, Silverberg SG. Infiltrating cribriform carcinoma of the breast: a distinctive clinicopathologic entity. Hum Pathol 1990;21:333–8.
51. Riener MO, Nikolopoulos E, Herr A, et al. Microarray comparative genomic hybridization analysis of tubular breast carcinoma shows recurrent loss of the CDH13 locus on 16q. Hum Pathol 2008;39:1621–9.
52. Capella C, Eusebi V, Mann B, et al. Endocrine differentiation in mucoid carcinoma of the breast. Histopathology 1980;4:613–30.
53. Weigelt B, Geyer FC, Horlings HM, et al. Mucinous and neuroendocrine breast carcinomas are transcriptionally distinct from invasive ductal carcinomas of no special type. Mod Pathol 2009;22:1401–14.
54. Lacroix-Triki M, Suarez PH, MacKay A, et al. Mucinous carcinoma of the breast is genomically distinct from invasive ductal carcinomas of no special type. J Pathol 2010;222:282–98.
55. Duprez R, Wilkerson PM, Lacroix-Triki M, et al. Immunophenotypic and genomic characterization of papillary carcinomas of the breast. J Pathol 2012;226: 427–41.
56. Liu ZY, Liu N, Wang YH, et al. Clinicopathologic characteristics and molecular subtypes of invasive papillary carcinoma of the breast: a large case study. J Cancer Res Clin Oncol 2013;139:77–84.
57. Chen L, Fan Y, Lang RG, et al. Breast carcinoma with micropapillary features: clinicopathologic study and long-term follow-up of 100 cases. Int J Surg Pathol 2008;16:155–63.
58. Marchio C, Iravani M, Natrajan R, et al. Genomic and immunophenotypical characterization of pure micropapillary carcinomas of the breast. J Pathol 2008;215: 398–410.

59. Yamaguchi R, Tanaka M, Kondo K, et al. Characteristic morphology of invasive micropapillary carcinoma of the breast: an immunohistochemical analysis. Jpn J Clin Oncol 2010;40:781–7.

60. Thor AD, Eng C, Devries S, et al. Invasive micropapillary carcinoma of the breast is associated with chromosome 8 abnormalities detected by comparative genomic hybridization. Hum Pathol 2002;33:628–31.

61. Dellapasqua S, Maisonneuve P, Viale G, et al. Immunohistochemically defined subtypes and outcome of apocrine breast cancer. Clin Breast Cancer 2013; 13:95–102.

62. Tsutsumi Y. Apocrine carcinoma as triple-negative breast cancer: novel definition of apocrine-type carcinoma as estrogen/progesterone receptor-negative and androgen receptor-positive invasive ductal carcinoma. Jpn J Clin Oncol 2012;42:375–86.

63. Hennessy BT, Gonzalez-Angulo AM, Stemke-Hale K, et al. Characterization of a naturally occurring breast cancer subset enriched in epithelial-to-mesenchymal transition and stem cell characteristics. Cancer Res 2009;69:4116–24.

64. Weigelt B, Kreike B, Reis-Filho JS. Metaplastic breast carcinomas are basal-like breast cancers: a genomic profiling analysis. Breast Cancer Res Treat 2009; 117:273–80.

65. Geyer FC, Weigelt B, Natrajan R, et al. Molecular analysis reveals a genetic basis for the phenotypic diversity of metaplastic breast carcinomas. J Pathol 2010; 220:562–73.

66. Martinez SR, Beal SH, Canter RJ, et al. Medullary carcinoma of the breast: a population-based perspective. Med Oncol 2011;28:738–44.

67. Li CI. Risk of mortality by histologic type of breast cancer in the United States. Horm Cancer 2010;1:156–65.

68. Vu-Nishino H, Tavassoli FA, Ahrens WA, et al. Clinicopathologic features and long-term outcome of patients with medullary breast carcinoma managed with breast-conserving therapy (BCT). Int J Radiat Oncol Biol Phys 2005;62:1040–7.

69. Reinfuss M, Stelmach A, Mitus J, et al. Typical medullary carcinoma of the breast: a clinical and pathological analysis of 52 cases. J Surg Oncol 1995; 60:89–94.

70. Ridolfi RL, Rosen PP, Port A, et al. Medullary carcinoma of the breast: a clinico-pathologic study with 10 year follow-up. Cancer 1977;40:1365–85.

71. Bertucci F, Finetti P, Cervera N, et al. Gene expression profiling shows medullary breast cancer is a subgroup of basal breast cancers. Cancer Res 2006;66: 4636–44.

72. Vincent-Salomon A, Gruel N, Lucchesi C, et al. Identification of typical medullary breast carcinoma as a genomic sub-group of basal-like carcinomas, a heterogeneous new molecular entity. Breast Cancer Res 2007;9:R24.

73. McDivitt RW, Stewart FW. Breast carcinoma in children. JAMA 1966;195:388–90.

74. Oberman HA. Secretory carcinoma of the breast in adults. Am J Surg Pathol 1980;4:465–70.

75. Lae M, Freneaux P, Sastre-Garau X, et al. Secretory breast carcinomas with ETV6-NTRK3 fusion gene belong to the basal-like carcinoma spectrum. Mod Pathol 2009;22:291–8.

76. Lambros MB, Tan DS, Jones RL, et al. Genomic profile of a secretory breast cancer with an ETV6-NTRK3 duplication. J Clin Pathol 2009;62:604–12.

77. Vasudev P, Onuma K. Secretory breast carcinoma: unique, triple-negative carcinoma with a favorable prognosis and characteristic molecular expression. Arch Pathol Lab Med 2011;135:1606–10.

78. Brill LB 2nd, Kanner WA, Fehr A, et al. Analysis of MYB expression and MYB-NFIB gene fusions in adenoid cystic carcinoma and other salivary neoplasms. Mod Pathol 2011;24:1169–76.
79. Wetterskog D, Lopez-Garcia MA, Lambros MB, et al. Adenoid cystic carcinomas constitute a genomically distinct subgroup of triple-negative and basal-like breast cancers. J Pathol 2012;226:84–96.
80. Persson M, Andren Y, Mark J, et al. Recurrent fusion of MYB and NFIB transcription factor genes in carcinomas of the breast and head and neck. Proc Natl Acad Sci U S A 2009;106:18740–4.
81. Collins LC, Tamimi RM, Baer HJ, et al. Outcome of patients with ductal carcinoma in situ untreated after diagnostic biopsy: results from the Nurses' Health Study. Cancer 2005;103:1778–84.
82. Tsikitis VL, Chung MA. Biology of ductal carcinoma in situ classification based on biologic potential. Am J Clin Oncol 2006;29:305–10.
83. Chaudhuri B, Crist KA, Mucci S, et al. Distribution of estrogen receptor in ductal carcinoma in situ of the breast. Surgery 1993;113:134–7.
84. Barnes R, Masood S. Potential value of hormone receptor assay in carcinoma in situ of breast. Am J Clin Pathol 1990;94:533–7.
85. Karayiannakis AJ, Bastounis EA, Chatzigianni EB, et al. Immunohistochemical detection of oestrogen receptors in ductal carcinoma in situ of the breast. Eur J Surg Oncol 1996;22:578–82.
86. Provenzano E, Hopper JL, Giles GG, et al. Biological markers that predict clinical recurrence in ductal carcinoma in situ of the breast. Eur J Cancer 2003;39: 622–30.
87. Poller DN, Roberts EC, Bell JA, et al. p53 protein expression in mammary ductal carcinoma in situ: relationship to immunohistochemical expression of estrogen receptor and c-erbB-2 protein. Hum Pathol 1993;24:463–8.
88. Allred DC, Wu Y, Mao S, et al. Ductal carcinoma in situ and the emergence of diversity during breast cancer evolution. Clin Cancer Res 2008;14:370–8.
89. Wiechmann L, Kuerer HM. The molecular journey from ductal carcinoma in situ to invasive breast cancer. Cancer 2008;112:2130–42.
90. Gupta SK, Douglas-Jones AG, Fenn N, et al. The clinical behavior of breast carcinoma is probably determined at the preinvasive stage (ductal carcinoma in situ). Cancer 1997;80:1740–5.
91. Wallis MG, Clements K, Kearins O, et al. The effect of DCIS grade on rate, type and time to recurrence after 15 years of follow-up of screen-detected DCIS. Br J Cancer 2012;106:1611–7.
92. Reis-Filho JS, Lakhani SR. The diagnosis and management of pre-invasive breast disease: genetic alterations in pre-invasive lesions. Breast Cancer Res 2003;5:313–9.
93. King TA, Sakr RA, Muhsen S, et al. Is there a low-grade precursor pathway in breast cancer? Ann Surg Oncol 2012;19:1115–21.
94. Allinen M, Beroukhim R, Cai L, et al. Molecular characterization of the tumor microenvironment in breast cancer. Cancer cell 2004;6:17–32.
95. Ma XJ, Salunga R, Tuggle JT, et al. Gene expression profiles of human breast cancer progression. Proc Natl Acad Sci U S A 2003;100:5974–9.
96. Knudsen ES, Ertel A, Davicioni E, et al. Progression of ductal carcinoma in situ to invasive breast cancer is associated with gene expression programs of EMT and myoepithelia. Breast Cancer Res Treat 2012;133:1009–24.
97. The Cancer Genome Atlas Network. Comprehensive molecular portraits of human breast tumors. Nature 2012;490:61–70.

98. Ciriello G, Sinha R, Hoadley KA, et al. The molecular diversity of Luminal A breast carcinoma. Breast Cancer Res Treat 2013;14(3):409–20.

99. Heliosa H, Milioli HH, Tischenko I, et al. Basal-like breast cancer: molecular profiles, clinical features and survival outcomes. BMC Med Genomics 2017;10:19.

100. Jonsson G, Staaf J, Vallon-Christerrson J, et al. Genomic subtypes of breast cancer identified by array-comparative genomic hybridization display distinctive molecular and clinical characteristics. Breast Cancer Res 2010;12(3):R42.

101. Holm K, Hegardt C, Staaf J, et al. Molecular subtypes are associated with characteristic DNA methylation patterns. Breast Cancer Res 2010;12(3):R36.

102. Weisman PS, Ng CK, Brogi E, et al. Genetic alterations of triple negative breast cancer by targeted next-generation sequencing and correlation with tumor morphology. Mod Pathol 2016;29(5):476–88.

103. Traver S, Assou S, Scalici E, et al. Cell-free nucleic acids as non-invasive biomarkers of gynecological cancers, ovarian, endometrial and obstetric disorders and fetal aneuploidy. Hum Reprod Update 2014;20:905–23.

104. Liu J, Mao Q, Liu Y, et al. Analysis of miR-205 and miR-155 expression in the blood of breast cancer patients. Chin J Cancer Res 2013;25:46–54.

105. Zhou Y, Wang C, Zhu H, et al. Diagnostic accuracy of PIK3CA mutation detection by circulating free DNA in breast cancer: a meta-analysis of diagnostic test accuracy. PLoS One 2016;11:e0158143.

106. Wang H, Liu Z, Xie J, et al. Quantitation of cell-free DNA in blood is a potential screening and diagnostic maker of breast cancer: a meta-analysis. Oncotarget 2017;8:102336–45.

Gynecologic Cancers
Molecular Updates 2018

Eman Abdulfatah, MD[a], Quratulain Ahmed, MD[b], Baraa Alosh, MD[a],
Sudeshna Bandyopadhyay, MD[a],*, Martin H. Bluth, MD, PhD[c,d],
Rouba Ali-Fehmi, MD[a]

KEYWORDS

- Molecular pathogenesis • Ovarian carcinoma • Uterine carcinoma
- Endometrial carcinoma • Cell free nucleic acid

KEY POINTS

- Understanding the molecular basis of of uterine and ovarian carcinoma to explain prognosis in these tumors.
- Updates from The Cancer Genome Atlas (TCGA) in classifying endometrial carcinoma.
- New frontiers in early detection and monitoring of gynecologic disease.

MOLECULAR PATHOGENESIS OF EPITHELIAL OVARIAN CANCER

Globally, ovarian cancer is the sixth most common cancer in women and ranks seventh among the most lethal cancers. The estimated number of new cases yearly is about 204,000, and there are 125,000 deaths annually.[1] In the United States, there are 22,240 new cases and 14,030 deaths from ovarian cancer annually.[2]

The new molecular studies led to a division of ovarian cancer into 2 types based on clinical, pathologic, and genetic features. A dualistic model of ovarian carcinogenesis has been proposed. Type I tumors include low-grade endometrioid, low-grade serous, clear cell, mucinous, and Brenner tumors. The behavior of these tumors is not aggressive and they are usually confined to the ovaries (International Federation of Gynecology and Obstetrics [FIGO] stage I). The indolent progression of type I tumors reflects their relative genetic stability and they have multiple types of somatic mutations such as KRAS, phosphatase and tensin homolog (PTEN), BRAF, CTNNB, PIK3CA, PPP2R1A, ARID1A, and rarely TP53.[3,4] Type II tumors include high-grade serous

---

This article has been updated from a version previously published in *Clinics in Laboratory Medicine*, Volume 33, Issue 4, December 2013.

[a] Department of Pathology, Detroit Medical Center Harper University Hospital, Wayne State University, 3990 John R Detroit, MI 48201, USA; [b] Michigan Diagnostic pathologists, Providence Hospital, 16001 W Nine Mile Road, Southfield, MI 48075, USA; [c] Department of Pathology, Wayne State University, School of Medicine, 540 East Canfield Street, Detroit, MI 48201, USA; [d] Pathology Laboratories, Michigan Surgical Hospital, 21230 Dequindre Road, Warren, MI 48091, USA
* Corresponding author.
E-mail address: SBandyop@dmc.org

Clin Lab Med 38 (2018) 421–438
https://doi.org/10.1016/j.cll.2018.02.007
0272-2712/18/© 2018 Elsevier Inc. All rights reserved.

carcinoma (HGSC), high-grade endometrioid, malignant mixed Müllerian tumor, and undifferentiated carcinoma. The behavior of these tumors is more aggressive in comparison with type I tumors and they invade rapidly (FIGO stages II–IV). The genetic characteristics are highly unstable and TP53 mutations are present in more than 95% of cases.[5] The mutations that exist in type I are rarely found in type II; P53 mutations are mostly restricted to type II.[6]

Type I Tumors

Low-grade serous carcinoma

Low-grade serous carcinoma (LGSC) represents a minority of ovarian serous carcinomas.[7] The morphologic and genetic evidence support the notion that cystadenomas/adenofibromas are precursors of LGSC. In this model, serous cystadenoma progresses to an atypical proliferative serous tumor, noninvasive micropapillary serous carcinoma, and finally to invasive LGSC.[8]

It is widely accepted that HGSC and LGSC are different type of tumors and have distinctive characteristics. LGSCs have a strong association with serous borderline tumors and express KRAS and BRAF mutations and do not express TP53 mutations, which have a strong expression in HGSCs.[9] Epidemiology studies have showed the differences in survival, age, annual incidence, and other parameters between LGSC and HGSC.[7] These data support the distinct identity of LGSC in comparison with HGSC.

Clear cell carcinoma

The presentation of clear cell carcinoma of the ovary (**Fig. 1**D) is characterized by a large adnexal mass, FIGO stage I, and highly malignant behavior. Some studies

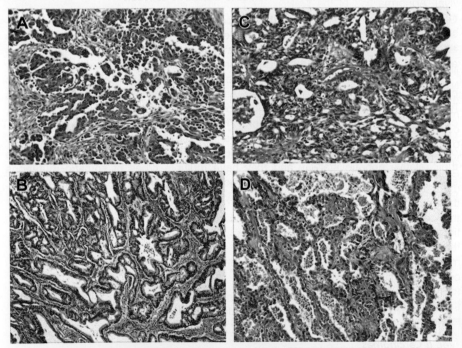

Fig. 1. (A) Ovarian serous carcinoma. (B) Ovarian mucinous carcinoma. (C) Ovarian endometrioid carcinoma. (D) Ovarian clear cell carcinoma (stain: hematoxylin and eosin; original magnification ×20). (From Ahmed Q, Alosh B, Bandyopadhyay S, et al. Gynecologic cancers: molecular updates. Clin Lab Med 2013;33(4):912; with permission.)

suggest clear cell fibroadenoma can be a clonal precursor of clear cell carcinoma. This evidence for this association was provided by the identical loss of heterozygosity pattern in both clear cell fibroadenoma and clear cell carcinoma.[10] In addition, there is a well-known association between clear cell carcinoma and endometriosis.[11] Retrograde menstruation has been suggested as a mechanism of endometriotic implants; however, the origin of endometriosis has not been firmly established. Based on many genetic and molecular studies, the most common genetic abnormality is an inactivating mutation of ARID1A in 50% of tumors,[4] an activating mutation of PIK3CA in 50% of cases,[12] deletion of PTEN and a tumor suppressor gene involved in the PI3K/PTEN signaling pathway in 20%.[13] In addition to these results, single nucleotide polymorphism array analysis has established a deletion of the CDKN2A/2B locus and amplification of the ZNF2017 locus, which identify the important role of these pathways in the development of clear cell carcinoma of the ovary.[13]

Low-grade endometrioid carcinoma

The origin of low-grade endometrioid carcinoma resembles the origin of clear cell carcinoma. Both develop from endometriotic cysts and are associated with implants of endometriosis outside the ovaries.[11] Intrinsic genetic abnormalities were observed in eutopic endometrium found in patients with endometriosis.[14] The genetics and molecular pathogenesis of low-grade endometrioid carcinoma are similar to the pathogenesis of clear cell carcinoma. The mutations that affect the PI3KCA/PTEN signaling pathway are common in low-grade endometrioid carcinoma.[15] Deregulation of the Wnt/β-catenin signaling pathway was observed in 40% of endometrioid ovarian carcinomas. This pathway plays an important role in proliferation, motility, and survival. Abnormalities of the Wnt/β-catenin signaling pathway may rely on activation of mutation of CTNNB1, a gene that encodes β-catenin.[16] The mutation of CTNNB1 has been associated with well-known features of low-grade endometrioid carcinoma such as squamous differentiation, low grade, and a relatively good prognosis.[17–19]

Mucinous carcinoma

Mucinous carcinomas are not well-understood because they are rare (3% of epithelial ovarian cancers). Mucinous carcinomas (**Fig. 1**B) have a strong association with KRAS mutations (75%). KRAS mutations have been shown in mucinous carcinomas and adjacent mucinous cystadenomas, and in borderline tumors, supporting tumor progression in ovarian mucinous neoplasms.[20,21] Many studies have shown that most gastrointestinal-type tumors that involve the ovary are secondary.[22] The origin of mucinous tumors and Brenner tumors is challenging, because unlike serous, endometrioid, and clear cell tumors, they do not display a Müllerian phenotype. Some researchers have suggested that mucinous tumors have a relationship to the endocervix; the mucinous epithelium that characterizes them more closely resembles gastrointestinal mucosa. The association of Brenner tumors and mucinous tumors has been well-recognized. A study reported that, after extensive sectioning, mucinous cystadenomas contained foci of Brenner tumor in 18% of cases.[23] Frequently, mucinous tumors were associated with Walthard cell nests, which are composed of benign transitional-type epithelium and are found frequently in paraovarian and paratubal locations. This similarity raises the possibility that mucinous tumors and Brenner tumors have the same origin.[24] Ovarian mature cystic teratomas have been suggested as an origin of gastrointestinal-type mucinous tumors.[25]

Type II Carcinomas

Serous carcinoma

Serous carcinoma represents about 70% of ovarian malignancies.[26] The epithelium of serous carcinomas is similar to fallopian tube epithelium, especially HGSCs (**Fig. 1**A).

These similarities suggest the fallopian origin of ovarian HGSC.[27] In the past, the fallopian tubes were not examined thoroughly because of a logical assumption that the precursors of ovarian carcinomas are in the ovaries and not in the fallopian tubes. However, in the last few years, this idea has changed dramatically and now many researchers believe that serous tubal intraepithelial carcinoma (STIC) may be the precursor of HGSC, especially if this lesion is in the fimbria.[8,20] Some studies show that STIC was found in 50% to 60% of patients who have negative BRCA mutations (ie, sporadic ovarian cancer).[28–32] A gene profiling study showed that the profile of gene expression in HGSC is more related to fallopian tube epithelium than the epithelium of the ovarian surface.[33] The identical TP53 mutations in STIC and HGSC support the theory that STIC is a precursor of HGSC.[33–35] Further studies have confirmed that both HGSA and STIC share expression of p53, p16, Rsf-1, FAS, and cyclin E1.[35] HGSCs express PAX8, a Müllerian marker, but do not express calretinin, a mesothelial marker that is seen in ovarian epithelium.[36] During ovulation, the fimbria of the fallopian tube come close to the ovary, which may explain the implantation of fallopian epithelium onto the surface of the ovary and cortical inclusion cyst formation. The free radical environment of ovulation itself and other factors such as inflammation may play a role in ovarian carcinogenesis.[36] This is consistent with epidemiologic studies that showed the risk of ovarian cancers decreases with anovulation (oral contraceptive, multiparty).[37,38]

High-grade endometrioid carcinomas

Although low-grade endometrioid carcinomas are easily recognized, it is difficult to distinguish between high-grade endometrioid carcinoma (**Fig. 1**C) and HGSC. This similarity raises the question whether high-grade endometrioid carcinoma is a variant of HGSC. These difficulties reflect the genetics and molecular similarities between high-grade endometrioid carcinomas and HGSC. Low-grade endometrioid carcinomas have mutations that deregulate the canonical Wnt/β-catenin and PI3K/PTEN signaling pathways and lack TP53 mutations, whereas high-grade endometrioid carcinomas lack Wnt/b catenin or PI3K/PTEN signaling pathway defects and frequently have TP53 mutations.[17] A few high-grade endometrioid carcinomas exhibit mutations found in low-grade endometrioid carcinomas in addition to TP53 mutations, which suggest that some low-grade endometrioid carcinomas may progress to high-grade carcinomas. Similar findings have been seen in serous tumors, so the general consensus is that low-grade and high-grade carcinomas develop independently, but rarely does a low-grade tumor progress to a high-grade tumor. The high frequency of TP53 mutation that occurs in both high-grade endometrioid carcinoma and HGSC suggests that they both develop in a similar fashion and explains why high-grade endometrioid carcinoma is closely related to HGSC.

Clinical Implications of the Dualistic Model of Ovarian Carcinogenesis

Molecular and genetics studies have led to a better understanding of the pathogenesis of epithelial ovarian carcinomas. The old concepts regarding the origin of epithelial ovarian carcinoma as ovarian have been changed, and these new concepts will have many clinical implications and will help in improving early detection and management of ovarian neoplasms.

Some researchers argue that type I tumors do not need urgent biomarker screening tests because they are slow growing, present as a large mass when diagnosed, and are still confined to the ovaries. They are easy to detect by pelvic ultrasonography or pelvic examination, and responsible for about 10% of deaths from ovarian cancer.[25] In contrast, type II tumors constitute 75% of ovarian cancers, account for approximately 90% of deaths from ovarian cancer,[25] and are rarely confined to the ovaries at diagnosis. These features of type II tumors emphasize the importance of developing a screening or biomarker test that detects very small tumors even if outside the ovary. For type I tumors confined to the ovary, oophorectomy alone may be sufficient treatment in some cases. Chemotherapy is effective if these tumors spread outside the ovary. An understating of the pathogenesis and deregulation of signaling pathways may lead to new medications. For instance, mutations in KRAS or BRAF may cause activation of the MAPK signaling pathway, so it is logical to assume that MAPK kinase inhibitors could benefit survival.

In contrast, treatment of type II tumor should start early. Early treatment depends on the development of a new screen or biomarkers that detect the tumor at an early stage. With the advances of molecular testing, several genomic and molecular alterations have emerged in ovarian high-grade serous carcinomas, including the somatic and germline defects in genes of the homologous recombination pathway (BRCA1, BRCA2, and others),[39] which have been implicated in cancer predisposition and have been associated with high-sensitivity to platinum-based chemotherapies and targeted therapies (such as PARP inhibitors).[40,41]

UTERINE CARCINOMAS: MOLECULAR FEATURES AND PATHOGENESIS

Endometrial carcinoma is the most common gynecologic malignancy in the United States with 61,389 new cases and 10,920 deaths estimated in 2017.[42] The dualistic model established on morphologic basis more than 20 years ago divides endometrial carcinoma into 2 broad subtypes, defined as types I and II. Type I carcinoma is related to hyperestrogenism by association with endometrial hyperplasia, which usually develops in perimenopausal women with frequent expression of estrogen and progesterone receptors, whereas type II carcinoma is unrelated to estrogen, associated with atrophic endometrium, frequent lack of estrogen and progesterone receptors, and older age.[43] Recently, 4 prognostically significant molecular subtypes of endometrial carcinoma were recognized by The Cancer Genome Atlas group based on a combination of somatic nucleotide substitutions, microsatellite instability (MSI) and somatic copy number alterations, namely: ultramutated (POLE), MSI, copy number low, and copy number high subtypes.[44]

By histology, endometrioid and mucinous carcinomas are considered type I, and serous and clear cell carcinomas are type II. Among these, the most frequent tumor type is endometrioid adenocarcinoma (**Fig. 2B**) and they can show many histologic variants including a villoglandular pattern, secretory changes, and squamous differentiation.[43] It has also been shown that molecular alterations involved in the development of type I carcinomas are different from type II carcinoma.

Type I Uterine Carcinoma

Four main molecular genetic alterations have been described in type I uterine carcinoma: MSI, which occurs in 25% to 30% of cases; PTEN mutations in 37% to 61%; kRAS mutations in 10% to 30%; and CTNNB1 mutations with nuclear protein accumulation in 25% to 38% of cases. Although MI, PTEN, or kRAS mutations may coexist in many cases, these molecular abnormalities are not usually associated with β-catenin alterations. Type II tumors exhibit alterations of p53, loss of heterozygosity on several chromosomes, as well as other molecular alterations (STK15, p16, E-cadherin, and C-erb B2).

Microsatellite instability

Microsatellite DNA sequences are short tandem repeats distributed throughout the genome. The most common dinucleotide sequence in eukaryotes is the (CA)n repeat,

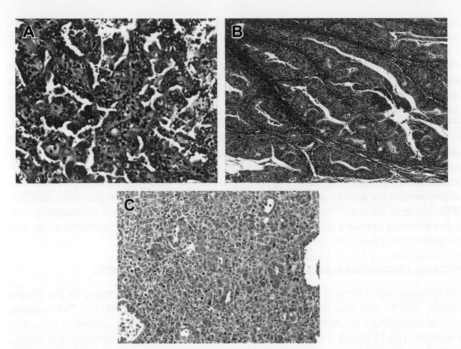

Fig. 2. (*A*) Uterine serous carcinoma. (*B*) Endometrioid carcinoma. (*C*) Carcinosarcoma (stain: hematoxylin and eosin; original magnification ×20). (*From* Ahmed Q, Alosh B, Bassndyopadhyay S, et al. Gynecologic cancers: molecular updates. Clin Lab Med 2013;33(4):915; with permission.)

and there are 50,000 to 100,000 (CA)n repeats in the entire human genome. The genes responsible for MI encode proteins involved in DNA mismatch repair (hMSH-2, hMLH-1, hPMS1, or hPMS2). Mutations of these genes alter the ability of the cells to repair errors produced during DNA replication. Therefore, cells with mutated mismatch repair genes replicate DNA mistakes more frequently than normal cells.[45]

MSI was initially found in cancers from patients with the hereditary nonpolyposis colon cancer (HNPCC) syndrome; it was also found in some sporadic tumors. EC is the second most common neoplasm encountered in patients with HNPCC. MSI has been detected in 75% of cases of EC associated with HNPCC but also in 25% to 30% of cases of sporadic EC.[45] Histopathologic features suggestive of HNPCC-related carcinoma are well-characterized in the colon, but not in the uterus. However, when examining an EC in a patient less than 50 years of age or with a personal or family history of colon carcinoma, it is important to consider the possibility of an HNPCC-related endometrial carcinoma. In these cases, testing for defective DNA mismatch repair may be performed by immunohistochemistry (MSH1, MLH2, MLH6, and PMS2 antibodies are commercially available). Loss of MSH2 expression essentially always indicates the Lynch syndrome and MSH6 is related to MSH2. HNPCC-related EC is predominantly associated with MSH2 mutations and MLH6 mutations in particular. PMS2 loss is often associated with loss of MLH1 and is only independently meaningful if MLH1 is intact. In addition, polymerase chain reaction assays can be used to detect high levels of microsatellite alterations (MSI), a condition that is, definitive for defective DNA mismatch repair. This testing is performed on paraffin-embedded tissue and compares the results of tumor DNA with those of nonneoplastic tissues from the same patient.

Although data are controversial regarding the prognostic significance of MI, it is usually associated with a high histologic grade. Patients who have HNPCC and EC have an inherited germline mutation in MLH-1, MSH-2, MSH-6, or PMS-2 (first hit), but EC develops only after the instauration of a deletion or mutation in the contralateral MLH-1,MSH-2, MSH-6, or PMS-2 allele (second hit) in endometrial cells.[46-48] Once the 2 hits occur, the deficient mismatch repair role of the gene (MLH-1, MSH-2, MSH-6, or PMS-2) causes the acquisition of MSI, and the development of the tumor. In sporadic EC, MLH-1 inactivation by promoter hypermethylation is the main cause of mismatch repair deficiency, which usually occurs at the precursor (atypical hyperplasia) lesion. Thus, MLH-1 hypermethylation is an early event in the pathogenesis of type I carcinoma, which precedes the development of MSI. The prognostic significance of MI is under debate, but there is some convincing evidence suggesting an association with favorable outcome.[45-48]

Phosphatase and tensin homolog

The tumor suppressor gene termed PTEN, located at chromosome10q23, encodes a protein (PTEN) with tyrosine kinase function and behaves as a tumor suppressor gene. PTEN has been reported to be altered in up to 83% of endometrioid carcinomas and 55% of precancerous lesions. PTEN inactivation is caused by mutations that lead to a loss of expression and, to a lesser extent, by a loss of heterozygosity. Thus, loss or altered PTEN expression results in aberrant cell growth and apoptotic escape. Loss of PTEN is, furthermore, probably an early event in endometrial tumorigenesis, as shown by its presence in precancerous lesions, and is likely initiated in response to known hormonal risk factors. Its expression is highest in an estrogen-rich environment; in contrast, progesterone promotes involution of PTEN-mutated endometrial cells.

Loss of heterozygosity at the PTEN region occurs in 40% of cases of EC. Somatic PTEN mutations are also common and found predominantly in endometrioid endometrial carcinoma, occurring in 37% to 61% of cases. PTEN mutations have been identified in endometrial hyperplasias with and without atypia (19% and 21%, respectively).[49]

Furthermore, PTEN mutations have been detected in hyperplasias coexisting with MI-positive EC, which suggests that PTEN mutations are early events in the development of EC. Data are controversial regarding the prognostic significance of PTEN mutations in EC, but there are some results that suggest an association with favorable prognostic factors.[50] This testing is performed on paraffin-embedded tissue, using immunohistochemistry.

The RAS-RAF-MEK-ERK signaling pathway

The RAS-RAF-MEK-ERK signaling pathway plays an important role in tumorigenesis. The frequency of kRAS mutations in EC ranges between 10% and 30%. In some series, KRAS mutations have been reported to be more frequent in EC showing MI. During tumorigenesis, activated RAS is usually associated with enhanced proliferation, transformation, and cell survival. BRAF, another member of the RAS-RAF-MEK-ERK pathways, is infrequently mutated in EC. RAS effectors like RASSF1A are supposed to have an inhibitory growth signal, which needs to be inactivated during tumorigenesis. RASSF1A inactivation by promoter hypermethylation may contribute significantly to increased activity of the RAS-RAF-MEK-ERK signaling pathway.[47]

PIK3CA

Mutations in PIK3CA, which codes for the p110a catalytic subunit of PI3K, have been described in various tumors and may contribute to the alteration of the PI3K/AKT signaling pathway in EC. PI3K is a heterodimer enzyme consisting of a catalytic subunit and a regulatory subunit.

The PIK3CA gene, located on chromosome3q26.32, codes for the p110a catalytic subunit of PI3K. A high frequency of mutations in the PIK3CA gene has been reported recently in EC. Mutations are located predominantly in the helical (exon 9) and kinase (exon 20) domains, but they can also occur in exons 1 to 7. PIK3CA mutations occur in 24% to 39% of cases, and coexist frequently with PTEN mutations. Oda and colleagues[51] described mutations in the PIK3CA gene in ECs for the first time. In this series, PIK3CA mutations occurred in 36% of cases, and coexisted frequently with PTEN mutations. Subsequent studies have shown that PIK3CA mutations, particularly in exon 20, are frequent in EC, and are associated with adverse prognostic factors such as high histologic grade, myometrial invasion, and vascular invasion.

β-Catenin gene (CTNNB1)

The β-catenin gene (CTNNB1) maps to 3p21. β-Catenin seems to be important in the functional activities of both APC and E-cadherin. β-Catenin is a component of the E-cadherin–catenin unit, which is important for cell differentiation and maintenance of the normal tissue architecture. β-Catenin is also important in signal transduction.[52] Mutations in exon 3 of CTNNB1 result in stabilization of the β-catenin protein, cytoplasmic and nuclear accumulation, and participation in signal transduction and transcriptional activation through the formation of complexes with DNA binding proteins.[47,53] They seem to be independent of the presence of MI, and the mutational status of PTEN and kRAS. These mutations are believed to be homogeneously distributed in different areas of the tumors, which suggest that they do play a role in the early steps of endometrial tumorigenesis. Alterations in β-catenin have been described in endometrial hyperplasias that contain squamous metaplasia (morules). Data are controversial regarding the prognostic significance of β-catenin mutations in EC, but they probably occur in tumors with a good prognosis.[54,55]

In routine practice, pathologists are faced with tumors showing mixed, morphologic, and molecular characteristics. Serous and clear cell carcinomas have been classified within the same category of type II carcinomas, based on high nuclear grade and aggressive behavior. However, recent studies have shown that these carcinomas are actually distinct tumor types.[44] They exhibit different clinical, immunohistochemical, and molecular features. Another controversial setting is cases between high-grade (predominantly solid) type I and type II ECs. Distinction between these 2 types of tumors is difficult; conversely, high-grade type I EC occasionally exhibits molecular alterations typical of type II EC such as TP53 mutations. Because of the controversial prognostic usefulness and therapeutic modalities, MSI testing and PTEN are routinely offered using paraffin-embedded tissue; however, the role of other molecular tests in daily practice has yet to be elucidated.

Treatment Modalities

Recent advances in the understanding of the molecular and genetic basis of EC have led to the development of targeted therapies that inhibit cellular signaling pathways involved in cell growth and proliferation. Several of these targeted agents are currently being investigated in EC. Inactivating mutations of PTEN, a tumor suppressor gene, are found in 40% to 60% of endometrial cancers. PTEN-deficient cells are sensitive to mammalian target of rapamycin (mTOR) inhibitors in vitro because loss of PTEN leads to constitutive activation of Akt, which in turn upregulates mTOR activity. Hence, there was interest in testing mTOR inhibitors in the treatment of EC. These inhibitors are expected to be effective in cancers like EC with PTEN mutations, PIKECA mutations, and receptor tyrosine kinase-dependent activation. Combinations of mTOR inhibitors with hormonal therapy, chemotherapy, or other targeted therapies such as epidermal growth factor receptor (EGFR) inhibitors and antiangiogenic agents have been promising in the preclinical setting, and numerous trials to develop and test such combinations are under way.

Type II Uterine Carcinoma

Type II uterine carcinomas arise in postmenopausal women, are associated with atrophy, and by definition are graded as high grade. These tumors are reported to have a poor prognosis.
  These include:

1. Serous carcinoma,
2. Clear cell carcinoma, and
3. Carcinosarcoma.

Uterine serous carcinoma

Uterine serous carcinomas accounting for approximately 15% of cases, approximately 50% of deaths owing to uterine carcinomas are caused by this subtype.[56] This highlights the aggressive nature of this disease compared with the more indolent endometrioid carcinoma and its variants. Significant differences in survival have been reported between stage-matched serous carcinoma and FIGO grade 3 endometrioid carcinoma; serous carcinomas have a lower survival.[56] In most cases, the tumor presents at a late stage with extrauterine involvement possibly the underlying cause of the poor prognosis of these tumors.[57–59] The rate of recurrence even in seemingly limited disease is high ranging from 31% to 80%.[60–62] More recent data have shown that low-stage disease, confined to the endometrium and polyp, was associated with a poor outcome.[63] Even the presence of a small amount of serious histology (<10%) in an EC is reported to have a poorer prognosis compared with pure grade 3 endometrioid carcinoma.[64]

  Histologically, the morphology of this tumor, as described by Hendrickson and colleagues,[65] is similar to ovarian serous carcinoma. Cytologically, high-grade nuclei with gland formation/clefting and papillary configuration with floating tufts of neoplastic cells make up the morphology of this tumor (**Fig. 2A**). It is well-documented that uterine serous carcinomas are more common in older women[66] and have been described in an atrophic background.[67] Increasing evidence shows that endometrial intraepithelial carcinoma is the precursor of uterine serous carcinoma. This lesion is described as malignant cells lining the surface of the endometrium or glands without invasion.

TP53

The most common mutation seen in uterine serous carcinoma is mutations in the p53 gene. This is a tumor suppressor gene present on chromosome 17p and its activities include cell cycle control and apoptosis. Loss of the normal activity prevents apoptosis and promotes tumor progression.[68] Mutations in this gene result in an abnormal protein that, although dysfunctional, is more stable and can be stained by immunohistochemistry.[69] Other mutations prevent transcription of any protein and thus show no staining by immunohistochemistry.[68] These alterations have been reported in about 90% of cases of serous carcinoma.[68] It has been postulated that the hypoxic environment of atrophic endometrium promotes selection of cells, which are able to overcome apoptosis, thereby selecting for cells that already contain p53 mutations. In addition, these mutations have also been documented in endometrial intraepithelial carcinoma and concordant mutations occurring in the endometrial intraepithelial carcinoma component and concurrent serous carcinoma have also been identified, implying that these mutations occur early in the pathogenesis of serous carcinomas.[68]

Her-2/neu

The success of trastuzumab in breast cancer treatment has led to interest in assessing this gene and its function in EC. Her-2/neu receptor is a membrane-bound tyrosine kinase receptor with an extracellular ligand-binding domain, a transmembrane component, and an intracellular component related to tyrosine kinase enzyme. Her-2/neu gene amplification results in overexpression of the receptors with homodimerization and ultimately in activation of the tyrosine kinase enzyme and related pathways, resulting in increased cell proliferation.[70]

Variable levels of Her-2/neu protein expression and gene amplification have been reported in uterine serous carcinomas,[71] with a lack of concordance between the two. This most likely is due to the small number of cases in each study. Higher levels of Her-2/neu expression have been reported in African Americans with this disease alluding to race-related biological differences affecting this tumor type.[71] A relatively poor prognosis has been attributed to tumors bearing overexpression and amplification of Her-2/neu, including recurrence and overall survival.[72,73] Although it has prognostic significance, treatment with trastuzumab does not seem to confer any benefit to these patients.

Epidermal growth factor receptor

EGFR is a transmembrane tyrosine kinase receptor (belonging to the same family as Her-2), similarly composed of an extracellular ligand-binding domain, intracellular tyrosine kinase activity, and a portion spanning the cell membrane. Ligands associated with EGFR are epidermal growth factor and transforming growth factor-α. Mutant variants of EGFR, although they do not bind a ligand, have activated tyrosine kinase, resulting in increased cell progression and inhibition of apoptosis. Although the studies are limited in the literature, EGFR overexpression has been reported in a significant subset of serous carcinomas, although EGFR mutations were not documented in these cases.[74,75] However, downstream PIK3CA mutations were identified in a small proportion of these cases.[75] The purpose of identifying these mutations in addition to understanding the pathogenesis of these tumors provides a foundation for new therapeutic molecules.

Other alterations seen more frequently in serous carcinomas are p16 inactivation and decreased E-cadherin expression.[76] Mutation analyses have identified a high frequency of mutations involving TP53 as expected, PPP2R1A, and PI3KCA.[77]

Clear Cell Carcinoma

These tumors have a distinctive histologic appearance composed of cuboidal cells with clear or eosinophilic cytoplasm, hyalinized cores, extracellular globules, and hyperchromatic nuclei. The cells exhibit hob nailing and are arranged in glandular and papillary configurations (see **Fig. 2**B). They are often present in association with serous carcinoma as mixed tumors. They are associated with a poor prognosis.

Meaningful studies on this tumor type have been limited because of its rarity. Although some degree of p53 alterations are seen in clear cell carcinoma, they seem to be much less compared with serous carcinoma. Also, PTEN mutations are rare and reported KRAS mutations are rare.[78] EGFR is reported to be overexpressed.[79]

Carcinosarcoma (Malignant Mixed Müllerian Tumor)

These tumors comprise 2% to 5% of all ECs. Although more commonly reported in the postmenopausal age group, they have been reported in younger women who might have undergone pelvic radiation for unrelated causes.[80] Stage for stage, this subtype has a poorer prognosis than other subtypes.[81]

Morphologically, these tumors are composed of carcinomatous and sarcomatous components, which are intimately admixed with each other (**Fig. 2C**). Studies have concluded that the 2 components are clonal. Recent studies have shown immunohistochemical expression of p53, MSH2, and MSH6 corresponding to epithelial and mesenchymal components, confirming the monoclonal origin of uterine carcinosarcomas. Therefore, the proposal that these tumors represent metaplasia of the carcinomatous component into sarcomatous components is being increasingly accepted.[80,82] Chromosomal alterations were identified using comparative genomic hybridization analysis. Gains were seen more commonly than losses (85% vs 30%). The epithelial component is either endometrioid or serous, whereas the sarcomatous component is composed of homologous or heterologous elements. Mutational analyses have subtyped carcinosarcomas into 2 categories: the serous type with TP53 and PPP2R1A mutations and the endometrioid type with mutations involving PTEN and ARID1A.[77] As expected, p53 expression is associated with a nonendometrioid epithelial tumor component and expression patterns of MMR proteins, PTEN, and hormone receptors are seen in endometrioid component carcinomas.[83]

MOLECULAR CLASSIFICATION OF ENDOMETRIAL CARCINOMAS

The stratification of patients with endometrial carcinoma into several risk groups is currently based on postoperative pathologic information, including histologic type, tumor grade, stage, and lymphovascular and myometrial invasion. However, high-grade endometrial cancers cannot be reliably classified by histomorphologic criteria with moderate to poor interobserver agreement for histotype and tumor grade.[84] In addition, 8% to 10% of early stage endometrial carcinoma develops recurrence and distant metastasis, hence the need for more reliable systems to categorize and classify endometrial carcinomas to inform clinical management.

Using a combination of whole genome sequencing, exome sequencing, MSI assays, and copy number analysis, The Cancer Genome Atlas group classified endometrial cancers into 4 prognostically significant molecular subtypes: POLE ultramutated, MSI hypermutated, copy number low, and copy number high.

The molecular classification of endometrial carcinoma has shown great promise, proving to be reproducible, demonstrating associations with clinical outcomes, and providing valuable prognostic and predictive information.

POLE Ultramutated Subtype

POLE encodes the major catalytic subunits of the DNA polymerase epsilon enzyme complex, which is involved in nuclear DNA replication and repair.[85] The proofreading exonuclease domain functions to ensure low mutation rates in replicating cells.[86] POLE exonuclease domain mutations (EDM) involving 2 hotspot regions (V411L and P286R) are identified in 5% to 8% of sporadic endometrial cancers. These mutations reduce the proofreading activity during DNA replication and thereby contribute to a very high mutation burden, among the highest found in human cancers and hence exhibit an "ultramutated" phenotype.[87] POLE EDM characterize a subtype of endometrial carcinoma with endometrioid histology, younger age at diagnosis and higher tumor grade (FIGO grade 3). These tumors also predominately exhibit normal DNA mismatch repair (microsatellite stable) and harbor several somatic mutations involving the PTEN (94%), PIK3R1 (65%), PIK3CA (71%), and KRAS (53%) genes.[88]

Clinically, patients in the POLE ultramutated group have favorable outcomes even within the high-grade tumors.[89] This could be partly explained by the high neoantigen load and immune-rich microenvironment in tumors with POLE EDM. Testing for POLE EDM may help to identify a subset of endometrial carcinoma with high-grade histology but a relatively indolent clinical course.

Microsatellite Instability (Hypermutated) Subtype

MSI, determined by a panel of 4 mononucleotide repeat loci (BAT25, BAT26, BAT40, and transforming growth factor receptor type II) and 3 dinucleotide repeat loci (CA repeats in D2S123, D5S346, and D17S250), characterized this group of endometrial carcinomas. Most of the tumors had MLH1 promoter methylation. In addition, frequent KRAS gene mutations were also identified.

Epigenetic/methylation events in mismatch repair have different implications on tumor characteristics and clinical outcomes than germline defects. Immune environment, intrinsic biologic behavior, and toleration of adjuvant therapy/response to cell injury may vary significantly in these individuals. Microsatellite unstable tumors are most commonly of endometrioid histology, with increased tendency to involve the lower uterine segment, increased tumor infiltrating lymphocytes and peritumoral lymphocytic infiltrate (Crohn-like) and are associated with increased risk of dedifferentiation.

Applying the molecular classification to endometrial carcinoma enables early identification of women who may have an inherited genetic syndrome (Lynch syndrome) who would benefit from additional screening or interventions for other Lynch-associated cancers or in whom specific therapies for their endometrial carcinomas may be more effective.

Copy Number Low Subtype

Copy number was determined using Affymetrix SNP 6.0 microarrays. All tumors that did not belong to the POLE ultramutated group were microsatellite stable and had infrequent somatic copy number alterations were termed copy number low. Moreover, tumors within this group had a frequency of CTNNB1 mutations. Increased progesterone receptor expression was also noted in this group, suggesting responsiveness to hormonal therapy.

Copy Number High Group

The copy number high cluster, which included most of the serous carcinomas and 25% of FIGO grade 3 endometrioid carcinomas, exhibited high somatic copy number alterations and the greatest transcriptional activity exemplified by increased cell cycle deregulation (CCNE1, PIK3CA, MYC, and CDKN2A) and TP53 mutation. The copy number high group also had decreased levels of phospho-AKT, consistent with downregulation of the AKT pathway.

CELL-FREE NUCLEIC ACID ANALYSIS

Although solid tissue based analysis has been the mainstay of gynecologic diagnosis of disease analysis of cell free samples via interrogation of circulating microRNA and cell-free DNA in fluids including serum, plasma, urine, and spinal fluid has proven beneficial for diagnosis and prognosis of gynecologic diseases.[90] To this end, microRNA including miR-205 and miR-92 have been found to be increased, whereas miR-145 and let-7f have been found to be decreased in ovarian cancer.[91–93] Furthermore, miR-21, miR-27b, miR-103, and miR-155 have been found to be increased and miR-132 and miR-320 have been found to be decreased in polycystic ovary disease,[94,95] the expression of which was related to obesity in certain respects. Cell-free DNA has also been reported to be useful in the early detection and monitoring of gynecologic diseases including ovarian cancer[96] and endometrial cancer.[97,98] Further studies will help to elucidate the ideal application of circulating nucleic acid utilization in gynecologic disorders.

SUMMARY

An integrated clinicopathologic and molecular classification of gynecologic malignancies has the potential to refine the clinical risk prediction of patients with cancer and to provide more tailored treatment recommendations.

ACKNOWLEDGMENTS

We would like to thank Ms. Heya Batah for proofreading and editing the manuscript.

REFERENCES

1. Boyle P, Levin B. World cancer report 2008. Lyon (France): World Health Organization; 2008.
2. Siegel R, Naishadham D, Jemal A. Cancer statistics, 2013. CA Cancer J Clin 2013;63(1):11–30.
3. Shih Ie M, Kurman RJ. Ovarian tumorigenesis: a proposed model based on morphological and molecular genetic analysis. Am J Pathol 2004;164(5):1511–8.
4. Jones S, Wang TL, Shih Ie M, et al. Frequent mutations of chromatin remodeling gene ARID1A in ovarian clear cell carcinoma. Science 2010;330(6001):228–31.
5. Ahmed AA, Etemadmoghadam D, Temple J, et al. Driver mutations in TP53 are ubiquitous in high grade serous carcinoma of the ovary. J Pathol 2010;221(1):49–56.
6. Karamurzin Y, Leitao MM Jr, Soslow RA. Clinicopathologic analysis of low-stage sporadic ovarian carcinomas: a reappraisal. Am J Surg Pathol 2013;37(3):356–67.
7. Plaxe SC. Epidemiology of low-grade serous ovarian cancer. Am J Obstet Gynecol 2008;198(4):459.e1-8 [discussion: 459.e8–9].
8. Vang R, Shih Ie M, Kurman RJ. Fallopian tube precursors of ovarian low- and high-grade serous neoplasms. Histopathology 2013;62(1):44–58.
9. Prat J. New insights into ovarian cancer pathology. Ann Oncol 2012;23(Suppl 10): x111–7.
10. Yamamoto S, Tsuda H, Takano M, et al. Clear-cell adenofibroma can be a clonal precursor for clear-cell adenocarcinoma of the ovary: a possible alternative ovarian clear-cell carcinogenic pathway. J Pathol 2008;216(1):103–10.
11. Veras E, Mao TL, Ayhan A, et al. Cystic and adenofibromatous clear cell carcinomas of the ovary: distinctive tumors that differ in their pathogenesis and behavior: a clinicopathologic analysis of 122 cases. Am J Surg Pathol 2009;33(6):844–53.
12. Campbell IG, Russell SE, Choong DY, et al. Mutation of the PIK3CA gene in ovarian and breast cancer. Cancer Res 2004;64(21):7678–81.
13. Sato N, Tsunoda H, Nishida M, et al. Loss of heterozygosity on 10q23.3 and mutation of the tumor suppressor gene PTEN in benign endometrial cyst of

the ovary: possible sequence progression from benign endometrial cyst to endometrioid carcinoma and clear cell carcinoma of the ovary. Cancer Res 2000; 60(24):7052–6.

14. Bulun SE. Endometriosis. N Engl J Med 2009;360(3):268–79.

15. Obata K, Morland SJ, Watson RH, et al. Frequent PTEN/MMAC mutations in endometrioid but not serous or mucinous epithelial ovarian tumors. Cancer Res 1998;58(10):2095–7.

16. Cho KR, Shih Ie M. Ovarian cancer. Annu Rev Pathol 2009;4:287–313.

17. Wu R, Hendrix-Lucas N, Kuick R, et al. Mouse model of human ovarian endometrioid adenocarcinoma based on somatic defects in the Wnt/beta-catenin and PI3K/Pten signaling pathways. Cancer Cell 2007;11(4):321–33.

18. Gamallo C, Palacios J, Moreno G, et al. Beta-catenin expression pattern in stage I and II ovarian carcinomas: relationship with beta-catenin gene mutations, clinicopathological features, and clinical outcome. Am J Pathol 1999;155(2):527–36.

19. Saegusa M, Okayasu I. Frequent nuclear beta-catenin accumulation and associated mutations in endometrioid-type endometrial and ovarian carcinomas with squamous differentiation. J Pathol 2001;194(1):59–67.

20. Kurman RJ, Shih Ie M. Molecular pathogenesis and extraovarian origin of epithelial ovarian cancer–shifting the paradigm. Hum Pathol 2011;42(7):918–31.

21. Gemignani ML, Schlaerth AC, Bogomolniy F, et al. Role of KRAS and BRAF gene mutations in mucinous ovarian carcinoma. Gynecol Oncol 2003;90(2):378–81.

22. Riopel MA, Ronnett BM, Kurman RJ. Evaluation of diagnostic criteria and behavior of ovarian intestinal-type mucinous tumors: atypical proliferative (borderline) tumors and intraepithelial, microinvasive, invasive, and metastatic carcinomas. Am J Surg Pathol 1999;23(6):617–35.

23. Seidman JD, Khedmati F. Exploring the histogenesis of ovarian mucinous and transitional cell (Brenner) neoplasms and their relationship with Walthard cell nests: a study of 120 tumors. Arch Pathol Lab Med 2008;132(11):1753–60.

24. Seidman JD, Yemelyanova A, Zaino RJ, et al. The fallopian tube-peritoneal junction: a potential site of carcinogenesis. Int J Gynecol Pathol 2011;30(1):4–11.

25. Vang R, Gown AM, Zhao C, et al. Ovarian mucinous tumors associated with mature cystic teratomas: morphologic and immunohistochemical analysis identifies a subset of potential teratomatous origin that shares features of lower gastrointestinal tract mucinous tumors more commonly encountered as secondary tumors in the ovary. Am J Surg Pathol 2007;31(6):854–69.

26. McCluggage WG. Morphological subtypes of ovarian carcinoma: a review with emphasis on new developments and pathogenesis. Pathology 2011;43(5): 420–32.

27. Erickson BK, Conner MG, Landen CN Jr. The role of the fallopian tube in the origin of ovarian cancer. Am J Obstet Gynecol 2013;209(5):409–14.

28. Callahan MJ, Crum CP, Medeiros F, et al. Primary fallopian tube malignancies in BRCA-positive women undergoing surgery for ovarian cancer risk reduction. J Clin Oncol 2007;25(25):3985–90.

29. Shaw PA, Rouzbahman M, Pizer ES, et al. Candidate serous cancer precursors in fallopian tube epithelium of BRCA1/2 mutation carriers. Mod Pathol 2009;22(9):1133–8.

30. Finch A, Shaw P, Rosen B, et al. Clinical and pathologic findings of prophylactic salpingo-oophorectomies in 159 BRCA1 and BRCA2 carriers. Gynecol Oncol 2006;100(1):58–64.

31. Medeiros F, Muto MG, Lee Y, et al. The tubal fimbria is a preferred site for early adenocarcinoma in women with familial ovarian cancer syndrome. Am J Surg Pathol 2006;30(2):230–6.

32. Przybycin CG, Kurman RJ, Ronnett BM, et al. Are all pelvic (nonuterine) serous carcinomas of tubal origin? Am J Surg Pathol 2010;34(10):1407–16.

33. Marquez RT, Baggerly KA, Patterson AP, et al. Patterns of gene expression in different histotypes of epithelial ovarian cancer correlate with those in normal fallopian tube, endometrium, and colon. Clin Cancer Res 2005;11(17):6116–26.

34. Lee Y, Miron A, Drapkin R, et al. A candidate precursor to serous carcinoma that originates in the distal fallopian tube. J Pathol 2007;211(1):26–35.

35. Sehdev AS, Kurman RJ, Kuhn E, et al. Serous tubal intraepithelial carcinoma up-regulates markers associated with high-grade serous carcinomas including Rsf-1 (HBXAP), cyclin E and fatty acid synthase. Mod Pathol 2010;23(6):844–55.

36. Kurman RJ, Shih Ie M. The origin and pathogenesis of epithelial ovarian cancer: a proposed unifying theory. Am J Surg Pathol 2010;34(3):433–43.

37. Beral V, Bull D, Green J, et al, Million Women Study Collaborators. Ovarian cancer and hormone replacement therapy in the Million Women Study. Lancet 2007; 369(9574):1703–10.

38. Lurie G, Thompson P, McDuffie KE, et al. Association of estrogen and progestin potency of oral contraceptives with ovarian carcinoma risk. Obstet Gynecol 2007; 109(3):597–607.

39. Frey MK, Pothuri B. Homologous recombination deficiency (HRD) testing in ovarian cancer clinical practice: a review of the literature. Gynecol Oncol Res Pract 2017;4:4.

40. Audeh MW, Carmichael J, Penson RT, et al. Oral poly(ADP-ribose) polymerase inhibitor olaparib in patients with BRCA1 or BRCA2 mutations and recurrent ovarian cancer: a proof-of-concept trial. Lancet 2010;376(9737):245–51.

41. Tutt A, Robson M, Garber JE, et al. Oral poly(ADP-ribose) polymerase inhibitor olaparib in patients with BRCA1 or BRCA2 mutations and advanced breast cancer: a proof-of-concept trial. Lancet 2010;376(9737):235–44.

42. Siegel RL, Miller KD, Jemal A. Cancer statistics, 2017. CA Cancer J Clin 2017; 67(1):7–30.

43. Llobet D, Pallares J, Yeramian A, et al. Molecular pathology of endometrial carcinoma; practical aspects from the diagnostic and therapeutical view points. J Clin Pathol 2009;62:777–85.

44. Talhouk A, McConechy MK, Leung S, et al. A clinically applicable molecular-based classification for endometrial cancers. Br J Cancer 2015;113(2):299–310.

45. Caduff RF, Johnston CM, Svoboda-Newman SM, et al. Clinical and pathological significance of microsatellite instability in sporadic endometrial carcinoma. Am J Pathol 1996;148:1671–8.

46. Duggan BD, Felix JC, Muderspach LI, et al. Microsatellite instability in sporadic endometrial carcinoma. J Natl Cancer Inst 1994;86:1216–21.

47. Matias-Guiu X, Prat J. Molecular pathology of endometrial carcinoma. Histopathology 2013;62(1):111–23.

48. Kobayashi K, Sagae S, Kudo R, et al. Microsatellite instability in endometrial carcinomas: frequent replication errors in tumors of early onset and/or of poorly differentiated type. Genes Chromosomes Cancer 1995;14:128–32.

49. Risinger JI, Berchuck A, Kohler MF, et al. Genetic instability of microsatellites in endometrial carcinoma. Cancer Res 1993;53:5100–3.

50. Matias-Guiu X, Catasus L, Bussaglia E, et al. Molecular pathology of endometrial hyperplasia and carcinoma. Hum Pathol 2001;32:569–77.

51. Oda K, Stokoe D, Taketani Y, et al. High frequency of coexistent mutations of PIK3CA and PTEN genes in endometrial carcinoma. Cancer Res 2005;65: 10669–73.

52. Catasus L, Matias-Guiu X, Machin P, et al. Frameshift mutations at coding mononucleotide repeat microsatellites in endometrial carcinomas with microsatellite instability. Cancer 2000;88:2290–7.
53. Catasus L, Gallardo A, Cuatrecasas M, et al. PIK3CA mutations in the kinase domain (exon 20) of uterine endometrial adenocarcinomas are associated with adverse prognostic parameters. Mod Pathol 2008;21:131–9.
54. Catasus L, D'Angelo E, Pons C, et al. Expression profiling of 22 genes involved in the PI3K–AKT pathway identifies two subgroups of high-grade endometrial carcinomas with different molecular alterations. Mod Pathol 2010;23:694–702.
55. Rudd ML, Price JC, Fogoros S, et al. A unique spectrum of somatic PIK3CA (p110alpha) mutations within primary endometrial carcinomas. Clin Cancer Res 2011;17:1331–40.
56. Slomovitz BM, Burke TW, Eifel PJ, et al. Uterine papillary serous carcinoma (UPSC): a single institution review of 129 cases. Gynecol Oncol 2003;91:463–9.
57. Trope C, Kristensen GB, Abeler VM. Clear-cell and papillary serous cancer: treatment options. Best Pract Res Clin Obstet Gynaecol 2001;15:433–46.
58. Matthews RP, Hutchinson-Colas J, Maiman M, et al. Papillary serous and clear cell type lead to poor prognosis of endometrial carcinoma in black women. Gynecol Oncol 1997;65:206–12.
59. Soslow RA, Bissonnette JP, Wilton A, et al. Clinicopathologic analysis of 187 high-grade endometrial carcinomas of different histologic subtypes: similar outcomes belie distinctive biologic differences. Am J Surg Pathol 2007;31:979–87.
60. Wu W, Slomovitz BM, Celestino J, et al. Coordinate expression of Cdc25B and ER-alpha is frequent in low-grade endometrioid endometrial carcinoma but uncommon in high-grade endometrioid and nonendometrioid carcinomas. Cancer Res 2003;63:6195–9.
61. Naumann RW. Uterine papillary serous carcinoma: state of the state. Curr Oncol Rep 2008;10:505–11.
62. Bristow RE, Asrari F, Trimble EL, et al. Extended surgical staging for uterine papillary serous carcinoma: survival outcome of locoregional (Stage I-III) disease. Gynecol Oncol 2001;81:279–86.
63. Semaan A, Mert I, Munkarah AR, et al. Clinical and pathologic characteristics of serous carcinoma confined to the endometrium: a multi-institutional study. Int J Gynecol Pathol 2013;32:181–7.
64. Boruta DM 2nd, Gehrig PA, Groben PA, et al. Uterine serous and grade 3 endometrioid carcinomas: is there a survival difference? Cancer 2004;101:2214–21.
65. Hendrickson M, Ross J, Eifel P, et al. Uterine papillary serous carcinoma: a highly malignant form of endometrial adenocarcinoma. Am J Surg Pathol 1982;6:93–108.
66. Lachance JA, Everett EN, Greer B, et al. The effect of age on clinical/pathologic features, surgical morbidity, and outcome in patients with endometrial cancer. Gynecol Oncol 2006;101:470–5.
67. Ambros RA, Sherman ME, Zahn CM, et al. Endometrial intraepithelial carcinoma: a distinctive lesion specifically associated with tumors displaying serous differentiation. Hum Pathol 1995;26:1260–7.
68. Tashiro H, Isacson C, Levine R, et al. p53 gene mutations are common in uterine serous carcinoma and occur early in their pathogenesis. Am J Pathol 1997;150:177–85.
69. Reihsaus E, Kohler M, Kraiss S, et al. Regulation of the level of the oncoprotein p53 in non-transformed and transformed cells. Oncogene 1990;5:137–45.

70. Perez-Soler R. HER1/EGFR targeting: refining the strategy. Oncologist 2004;9: 58–67.

71. Santin AD, Bellone S, Van Stedum S, et al. Amplification of c-erbB2 oncogene: a major prognostic indicator in uterine serous papillary carcinoma. Cancer 2005; 104:1391–7.

72. Slomovitz BM, Broaddus RR, Burke TW, et al. Her-2/neu overexpression and amplification in uterine papillary serous carcinoma. J Clin Oncol 2004;22: 3126–32.

73. Lukes AS, Kohler MF, Pieper CF, et al. Multivariable analysis of DNA ploidy, p53, and HER-2/neu as prognostic factors in endometrial cancer. Cancer 1994;73: 2380–5.

74. Konecny GE, Venkatesan N, Yang G, et al. Activity of lapatinib a novel HER2 and EGFR dual kinase inhibitor in human endometrial cancer cells. Br J Cancer 2008; 98:1076–84.

75. Hayes MP, Douglas W, Ellenson LH. Molecular alterations of EGFR and PIK3CA in uterine serous carcinoma. Gynecol Oncol 2009;113:370–3.

76. Holcomb K, Delatorre R, Pedemonte B, et al. E-cadherin expression in endometrioid, papillary serous, and clear cell carcinoma of the endometrium. Obstet Gynecol 2002;100:1290–5.

77. McConechy MK, Ding J, Cheang MC, et al. Use of mutation profiles to refine the classification of endometrial carcinomas. J Pathol 2012;228:20–30.

78. Lax SF. Molecular genetic pathways in various types of endometrial carcinoma: from a phenotypical to a molecular-based classification. Virchows Arch 2004; 444:213–23.

79. Khalifa MA, Mannel RS, Haraway SD, et al. Expression of EGFR, HER-2/neu, P53, and PCNA in endometrioid, serous papillary, and clear cell endometrial adenocarcinomas. Gynecol Oncol 1994;53:84–92.

80. Yamada SD, Burger RA, Brewster WR, et al. Pathologic variables and adjuvant therapy as predictors of recurrence and survival for patients with surgically evaluated carcinosarcoma of the uterus. Cancer 2000;88:2782–6.

81. Amant F. The rationale for comprehensive surgical staging in endometrial carcinosarcoma. Gynecol Oncol 2005;99:521–2 [author reply: 522–3].

82. McCluggage WG. Uterine carcinosarcomas (malignant mixed Mullerian tumors) are metaplastic carcinomas. Int J Gynecol Cancer 2002;12:687–90.

83. de Jong RA, Nijman HW, Wijbrandi TF, et al. Molecular markers and clinical behavior of uterine carcinosarcomas: focus on the epithelial tumor component. Mod Pathol 2011;24:1368–79.

84. Han G, Sidhu D, Duggan MA, et al. Reproducibility of histological cell type in high-grade endometrial carcinoma. Mod Pathol 2013;26(12):1594–604.

85. Pursell ZF, Isoz I, Lundström EB, et al. Yeast DNA polymerase epsilon participates in leading-strand DNA replication. Science 2007;317(5834):127–30.

86. Briggs S, Tomlinson I. Germline and somatic polymerase epsilon and delta mutations define a new class of hypermutated colorectal and endometrial cancers. J Pathol 2013;230(2):148–53.

87. Rayner E, van Gool IC, Palles C, et al. A panoply of errors: polymerase proofreading domain mutations in cancer. Nat Rev Cancer 2016;16(2):71–81.

88. Billingsley CC, Cohn DE, Mutch DG, et al. Polymerase varepsilon (POLE) mutations in endometrial cancer: clinical outcomes and implications for Lynch syndrome testing. Cancer 2015;121(3):386–94.

89. Cancer Genome Atlas Research, Network, Kandoth C, Schultz N, Cherniack AD, et al. Integrated genomic characterization of endometrial carcinoma. Nature 2013;497(7447):67–73.
90. Traver S, Assou S, Scalici E, et al. Cell-free nucleic acids as non-invasive biomarkers of gynecological cancers, ovarian, endometrial and obstetric disorders and fetal aneuploidy. Hum Reprod Update 2014;20:905–23.
91. Zheng H, Zhang L, Zhao Y, et al. Plasma miRNAs as diagnostic and prognostic biomarkers for ovarian cancer. PLoS One 2013;8:e77853.
92. Guo F, Tian J, Lin Y, et al. Serum microRNA-92 expression in patients with ovarian epithelial carcinoma. J Int Med Res 2013;41:1456–61.
93. Wu H, Xiao Z, Wang K, et al. MiR-145 is downregulated in human ovarian cancer and modulates cell growth and invasion by targeting p70S6K1 and MUC1. Biochem Biophys Res Commun 2013;441:693–700.
94. Murri M, Insenser M, Fernández-Durán E, et al. Effects of polycystic ovary syndrome (PCOS), sex hormones, and obesity on circulating miRNA-21, miRNA-27b, miRNA-103, and miRNA-155 expression. J Clin Endocrinol Metab 2013;98:E1835–44.
95. Sang Q1, Yao Z, Wang H, et al. Identification of microRNAs in human follicular fluid: characterization of microRNAs that govern steroidogenesis in vitro and are associated with polycystic ovary syndrome in vivo. J Clin Endocrinol Metab 2013;98:3068–79.
96. No JH, Kim K, Park KH, et al. Cell-free DNA level as a prognostic biomarker for epithelial ovarian cancer. Anticancer Res 2012;32:3467–71.
97. Tanaka H, Tsuda H, Nishimura S, et al. Role of circulating free alu DNA in endometrial cancer. Int J Gynecol Cancer 2012;22:82–6.
98. Dobrzycka B, Terlikowski SJ, Mazurek A, et al. Circulating free DNA, p53 antibody and mutations of KRAS gene in endometrial cancer. Int J Cancer 2010;127:612–21.

Moving?

Make sure your subscription moves with you!

To notify us of your new address, find your **Clinics Account Number** (located on your mailing label above your name), and contact customer service at:

Email: journalscustomerservice-usa@elsevier.com

800-654-2452 (subscribers in the U.S. & Canada)
314-447-8871 (subscribers outside of the U.S. & Canada)

Fax number: 314-447-8029

Elsevier Health Sciences Division
Subscription Customer Service
3251 Riverport Lane
Maryland Heights, MO 63043

*To ensure uninterrupted delivery of your subscription, please notify us at least 4 weeks in advance of move.

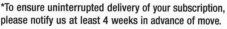